Midwifery and Public Health: future directions, new opportunities

For Churchill Livingstone:

Senior Commissioning Editor: Mary Seager
Development Editor: Rebecca Nelemans
Project Manager: Caroline Horton
Designer: Judith Wright

Midwifery and Public Health: future directions, new opportunities

Edited by

Pádraig Ó Lúanaigh MSc(Psych) BSc(Hons) RGN RM RHV DipHE(Mid) AdvDipEd PGDE

Dean, Faculty of Health and Science, Western Institute of Technology, New Plymouth, New Zealand

Cindy Carlson BA MPH PGCertEdTHE MFPH(Hon)

Health Specialist, DFID Health Resource Centre, London, United Kingdom

Foreword by

Dame Karlene Davis

General Secretary, Royal College of Midwives, United Kingdom,
Director, WHO Collaborating Centre for Midwifery,
Vice President, International Confederation of Midwives

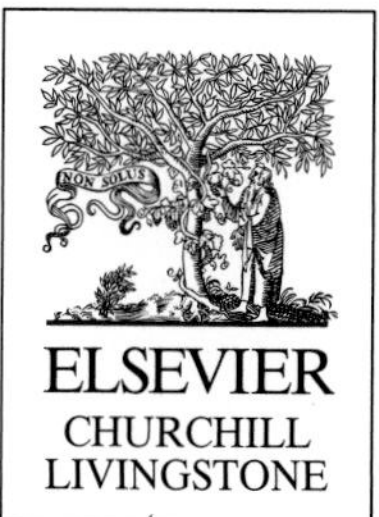

ELSEVIER
CHURCHILL LIVINGSTONE

EDINBURGH LONDON NEW YORK OXFORD PHILADELPHIA ST LOUIS SYDNEY TORONTO 2005

ELSEVIER
CHURCHILL
LIVINGSTONE

ISBN 0 443 10235 X

British Library Cataloguing in Publication Data
A catalogue record for this book is available from the British Library

Library of Congress Cataloging in Publication Data
A catalog record for this book is available from the Library of Congress

Knowledge and best practice in this field are constantly changing. As new research and experience broaden our knowledge, changes in practice, treatment and drug therapy may become necessary or appropriate. Readers are advised to check the most current information provided (i) on procedures featured or (ii) by the manufacturer of each product to be administered, to verify the recommended dose or formula, the method and duration of administration, and contraindications. It is the responsibility of the practitioner, relying on their own experience and knowledge of the patient, to make diagnoses, to determine dosages and the best treatment for each individual patient, and to take all appropriate safety precautions. To the fullest extent of the law, neither the publisher nor the editors and contributors assume any liability for any injury and/or damage.

The Publisher

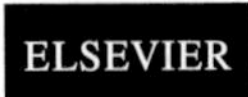

Printed in China

Contents

Contributors

Debra Bick RM, FPCert, BA(Hons), MMedSc, PhD
Professor of Midwifery and Women's Health, Faculty of Health and Human Sciences, Thames Valley University, UK.
Debra has responsibility for co-ordinating and developing research across the midwifery subject group at Thames Valley. Prior to taking up her current post, she was a Senior Research and Development Fellow at the Royal College of Nursing Institute, and had responsibility for the development of national guidelines to inform nursing practice. As a Research Fellow in the Department of Public Health and Epidemiology, University of Birmingham, Debra worked on several large studies examining the impact on women's health of interventions during and after pregnancy. Her doctoral thesis presented data on midwife implementation of a new model of midwifery-led care and impact on women's physical and psychological well-being at four months post partum compared with current care in a cluster randomised controlled trial. Her current research interests include postnatal health and well-being, organisation of maternity services and knowledge utilisation and transfer.

Carole Butterfield RGN, RM, DPSM, BSc(Hons)
Midwifery Mainstream Coordinator, The Pennine Acute Hospitals NHS Trust, Greater Manchester, UK.
Carole qualified as a midwife in 1985 and has had a varied career, including having working clinically in a refugee camp in Thailand for 2 years, and developed a teaching programme for lay midwives. For many years she was a community midwife in North Manchester and was involved in a Trailblazer Sure Start programme. Her current role involves working with colleagues to mainstream the principles of Sure Start and develop a public health approach within midwifery for The Pennine Acute Hospitals NHS Trust. Carole is also a part-time lecturer/practitioner at the University of Manchester.

Cindy Carlson BA, MPH, PGCertEdTHE, MFPH(Hon)
Health Specialist, DFID Health Resource Centre, London, UK.
Cindy works as a public health specialist for the UK Department for International Development's Health Resource Centre, based at the Institute for Health Sector Development in London. She has 23 years of public health experience, focusing primarily on maternal/child health and sexual health programmes. Prior to joining the resource centre Cindy worked with the Public Health Resource Unit in Oxford as Director of Learning and Development, while also undertaking specific public health-related projects. She also designed, developed and led the MSc in Public Health at Oxford Brookes University for a number of years. Cindy's main areas of work now are in researching and developing public health topics to help inform DFID policy and practice, as well as supporting a range of other international development-related work done within the resource centre.

Claire Chambers MSc, PGDip(Prof)Ed, HV(Dip), CPT, RGN
Principal Lecturer in Health Visiting, School of Health and Social Care, Oxford Brookes University, Oxford, UK.
Claire leads the Public Health Nursing/Health Visiting Programme at Oxford Brookes University. She has a particular interest in diversity issues and encouraging students to increase their knowledge and develop their practice by understanding how individuals, groups and communities can be disadvantaged in life. Health professionals can then be proactive in empowering individuals and communities to make positive life changes when possible and to enable them to receive appropriate and accessible care in professional practice.

Jacqueline Dunkley-Bent MSc ADM, PGCEA, RM, RGN, MRIPH
Counsellor in Rape and Sexual Assault; Consultant Midwife Public Health, Guy's and St Thomas' NHS Trust, St Thomas' Hospital, London, UK.
Jacqueline has been a Consultant Midwife since September 2001. She teaches at Kings College, London University, and runs a specialist consultant midwives community clinic. Referrals to the clinic include women who have had a traumatic childbirth experience, survivors of rape and sexual assault, women who have experienced domestic violence, women who have a fear of childbirth and women who request caesarean section. A major part of her work is focused toward collaboration with the primary care sector, community organisations and social service colleagues to improve areas of inequality in health and health care provision. She previously worked as senior lecturer in midwifery for ten years.

Maralyn Foureur RM, RGON, BA, Grad Dip Clin Epidem, PhD, FACMI
Clinical Professor, Midwifery and Women's Health, Graduate School of Nursing and Midwifery, Victoria University of Wellington, New Zealand.
Maralyn has a joint appointment with Victoria University and Capital and Coast District Health Board in Wellington. She is also Director of the Collaborating Centre for Midwifery and Nursing Education, Practice and Research, a joint venture between the university and the district health board. The Centre facilitates programmes of education and research to improve practice and health care outcomes. Her main interests are in the organisation of maternity services, evidence-based practice, the birth environment and the physiology of birth and breastfeeding. Her PhD was a randomised controlled trial of continuity of midwifery care.

Jill Gullidge BSc(Hons), RM, RN
Community Midwife, Peterborough Maternity Hospital, UK.
Jill has a variety of clinical experience, having worked as a Registered Nurse and Registered Midwife. She studied fertility treatment and previously was employed as a Fertility Nurse Specialist. She then undertook her midwifery training and graduated from Oxford Brookes University with a First Class honours degree. Jill now works as a Community Midwife, employed through Peterborough and Stamford Hospitals NHS Trust. She is responsible for the care of a large caseload of women within the city centre.

Caroline Homer RM, RN, MN, PhD
Midwifery Consultant: Practice Development, Division of Women's and Children's Health, St George Hospital, Kogarah, Australia.
Caroline's current role incorporates research, teaching, leadership and clinical practice in the public hospital setting in New South Wales, Australia. Her practice and research interests include the development and evaluation of new models of midwifery care, the translation of research into clinical practice and, more recently, the experience and outcomes of women with hypertension in pregnancy. She is also involved in teaching through the University of Technology Sydney and the University of New South Wales. She works as a consultant for Health Departments in NSW and in Samoa and works in partnership with two other midwives providing care for a small caseload of women through the St George Hospital's Birth Centre.

Tina Miller BA(Hons), MSc, PhD
Senior Lecturer, School of Social Sciences and Law, Oxford Brookes University, Oxford, UK.
Tina's research and teaching interests include mothering and caring responsibilities, health and illness experiences, narrative and qualitative research methods. Her recent publications include an edited collection *Ethics in Qualitative Research* (with Melanie Mauthner, Maxine Birch and Julie Jessop; Sage, 2002), Shifting Perceptions of Expert Knowledge: Transition to Motherhood (*Human Fertility*, 2003) and Losing the Plot: Narrative construction and Longitudinal Childbirth Research (*Qualitative Health Research*, 2000). Most recently she has completed a sole authored book, *Making Sense of Motherhood: A Narrative Approach* (Cambridge University Press, 2005). Tina is also a member of the Women's Workshop on Qualitative Household/Family Research.

Pádraig Ó Lúanaigh MSc(Psych), BSc(Hons), RGN, RM, RHV, DipHE(Mid), AdvDipED, PGDE
Dean, Faculty of Health and Science, Western Institute of Technology, New Plymouth, New Zealand.
Pádraig has a broad clinical background, having practised as a registered nurse, midwife and health visitor. He has previously worked with midwifery students as a lecturer and as head of a midwifery department. Having practised in a variety of areas in the UK, he is now living and working in New Zealand. Pádraig is currently completing a Doctorate in Education exploring the measurement and assessment of clinical competence.

Stephen Peckham BSc(Hons), MA(Econ), Hon FFPHM
Head of Department of Sociology, School of Social Sciences and Law, Oxford Brookes University, Oxford, UK.
Stephen is Reader in Health Policy and a Head of Department. He has been involved in health and social policy research and teaching for 12 years and previously worked in the voluntary and local government sectors. He is course director for the MA in Social Policy and teaches undergraduate and postgraduate modules in social policy, health policy and policy process and evaluation. His main research interests are in health policy analysis, inter-agency collaboration, primary care, public health and public involvement. He is currently working on two research projects: one is examining the links between community organisations and primary care on public health issues and the other concerns carers and primary care. Stephen is particularly interested in promoting a broader model of health and examining multi-disciplinary and lay approaches to addressing health issues.

Eileen Stringer RGN, RM, DPSM, BSc(Hons)
Consultant Midwife, Public Health, Pennine Acute Hospitals Trust, Greater Manchester, UK.
Eileen has been a midwife for 20 years, working within and managing many different areas of the midwifery service. Throughout her career she has developed an interest and expertise in addressing public health issues, culminating in her current post, which she has held since February 2003. The post entails working clinically and with local communities and PCTs to address health inequalities and influence maternity strategy in order to strengthen the role of the midwife in public health. Eileen is also currently completing a Master's degree in Evidence for Population Health.

Suzanne Tyler BA(Hons), MA, PhD
Senior Research Fellow, Health Services Management Centre, University of Birmingham, UK.
Suzanne is a health policy analyst with 15 years' experience of working in national health organisations. She has worked most recently with managers, as Deputy Chief Executive of the Institute of Healthcare Management (IHM) and previously with clinicians, as Head of Policy at the Royal College of Midwives (RCM) and with users as Research Officer at the Association of CHCs. She is Vice Chair of the Management Committee of Maternity Alliance, a voluntary organisation concerned with issues around poverty in pregnancy, and is a member of IHM.

Foreword

For me, public health is a framework that refuses to isolate individual health within a purely medical perspective; instead it is placed within the context of an individual's family and community, and within a society's physical, environmental, psychological and political well-being. And it is clear to me that this framework lies at the heart of midwifery care, so I am delighted to introduce this very timely book exploring both trends in public health policy, but more importantly its application by midwives to improving the health and happiness of women and babies. It is of course a truism to state that midwives are the best placed to encourage a healthy start to life; as a midwife I am also very clear that the well-being of mothers is key to the well-being of babies and of entire families. This book is in part a celebration of midwives' work in reaching out to provide this best start to some of society's most vulnerable and needy women. All readers of this book will recognise the traditional role of the midwife in educating women about nutrition, promoting breastfeeding, exercise and smoking cessation, as well as screening and preventative measures, which encapsulate their contribution to public health. As our understanding of the links between the wider world and health increase, so does the midwife's ambit. Take for example the care of diabetic women, who continue to experience poorer perinatal outcomes in terms of mortality and morbidity. Throughout the industrialised world the incidence of diabetes is increasing, linked to rising rates of obesity – a public health issue in itself. For midwives this means more women with diabetes are likely to be presenting for maternity care. Whilst responsibility for a woman with a pre-existing medical complication lies firmly with doctors, recent work shows clearly that midwives can make an important contribution to improving the health of these women and their babies, through support in making lifestyle changes, adopting a healthy diet, stopping smoking and drinking, and support in maintaining blood sugar levels (Hutcherson 2004). The care of diabetic women nicely illustrates the paradox of a public health approach to midwifery – on the one hand treating every woman as an individual, responding to her personal circumstances, needs and preferences, not making assumptions based on pre-existing medical or indeed social factors; and yet at the same time having in mind an understanding of how the environment, origins, background and lifestyle of that woman may impact on her health and well-being. It also illustrates how a public health approach is fundamental to all elements of midwifery practice – developing trusting relationships, offering flexible care, informing the wider community about self care, involvement in health education and raising awareness in the general population about the need for lifestyle changes prior to pregnancy. In the United Kingdom politicians and planners have acknowledged the key role that midwives can play in public health. For example, the Department of Health in England outlined the implications of the NHS Plan for maternity services as:

> ... this means knowing where pregnant women are and how they want and need their care delivered and

> configured. It means understanding the local patterns of disadvantage and exclusion; and designing services that reach out to ensure those most in need have prompt access to the support they need.
>
> (House of Commons Health Committee 2003)

Health modernisation in Wales, Scotland and Northern Ireland similarly focuses on targeting those most in need. It seems to me that this is an aspiration that midwives throughout the world share and I am sure that midwives beyond the UK will find much to reflect on and consider within this book.

I urge all midwives not only to appreciate and value their existing public health expertise, but to develop this role further by:

- Articulating a midwifery philosophy in the context of public health policy in order to win greater resources and commitment
- Contributing midwifery expertise and information to demographic profiling, local needs assessment and health strategy
- Developing alliances with other health professionals, with local government, with voluntary and community organisations
- Identifying groups who have particular needs, or who are missing out on maternity care and working with them to develop services that are appropriate, acceptable and accessible to them
- Building the maternity service's dialogue with, and involvement of, its users and local communities.

The lessons from this book are that achieving this requires interdependence – rather than the independence midwives have traditionally cherished. More can be achieved through community action, participation and partnership than through the application of our clinical skills in isolation. Despite the domination of medicine in health care around the world, most improvements in maternal and child health are the result of improvements in women's economic and social status. The examples and case studies included in this book should encourage many midwives to tap into local resources in their communities and to work in collaboration with statutory and non-statutory services. I hope it will help you think about the additional needs the women you care for might have, and help you think about how to reach out to the women who do not access services.

Dame Karlene Davis

References

House of Commons Health Committee 2003 Eighth report of Session 2002–2003: Inequalities in access to maternity services. The Stationery Office, London

Hutcherson A 2004 Does midwifery involvement in care have an effect on perinatal outcome for insulin dependent diabetic women? MIDIRS Midwifery Digest 13(4):469–476

Preface

Public health has always been a core part of midwifery practice, though perhaps not always recognised as such. Every time a midwife counsels a woman on how best to protect her unborn child, with advice on nutrition and smoking, and every time midwives stand up and argue for changes in health care practices that will improve the health of women and children, midwives are practising public health. Public health is an integral part of midwives' work, whether they are based in hospitals or in the community. This book brings together various perspectives on why this should be so, from the wider policies that support public health midwifery to specific programmes that demonstrate good public health practice amongst midwives.

If public health has always been so important for midwives, why this book now? Public health in Britain has taken on increasing importance in the last decade, especially with changes in government in 1997. In 2004 the British government consulted on and produced a new public health White Paper to further hone the debate begun in its 1999 White Paper 'Saving Lives'. While some of the arguments arise out of economic concerns about the ever-rising cost of health care in an ageing population whose main health problems are, at least at first glance, linked to behavioural determinants of health, there remain highly justified concerns about increasing inequalities in health and the social impact this has on communities and individuals. Public health practice has never been so needed since the nineteenth century, when working-class conditions inspired Victorian health and social reformers to work towards improving living conditions for the least fortunate in their societies. Midwives, who serve all communities and who often see and support women and families who are at the sharp end of social inequalities, have become involved in a range of programmes to improve the life chances of women and their babies. Even as we planned and prepared this text we could not have anticipated the amazingly clear driver to come from the UK government for midwives to play a much greater role in promoting public health. In July 2003 the Chief Nurse for England launched the *Delivering the Best* website, and the National Service Framework for children, young people and maternity services published in September 2004 contains a defined role for midwifery in terms of promoting public and community health.

As editors we were fortunate to have been able to work with a range of excellent contributors from the UK, Australia and New Zealand who found time in their busy lives to write for us. It was equally gratifying to be able to involve practising midwives and those who are leading innovation and a public health focus to their work. The other contributors, while not midwives, all have extensive experience of working with midwifery students, midwives in practice or maternity services. This textbook represents a global and interdisciplinary collaborative approach which we believe is a key strength of this work.

The book is divided into three sections which take the reader from a broad concept to a more focused practice perspective. However, each section and chapter is structured to be read in isolation, which allows the reader to be selective in the aspects of public health on which to focus.

The first section, *Building blocks for practice*, provides an overview of the general policy context of public health as well as giving an in-depth view of the 'art' and 'science' of public health as it is and could be practised.

Chapter 1 explores public health both from a historical context and its particular evolution in the UK, as well as from the policy context arising out of these historical peculiarities. Public health law aims to protect the health of whole populations, and so policy making is crucial to how the public's health can be maintained and improved.

Chapter 2 situates midwifery practice within a public health perspective. The concept of disadvantage is explored and examined in the context of providing services to refugees and asylum seekers, and of people with emotional disturbance. The chapter skillfully draws on examples from practice to illustrate issues around the adequacy of health service provision and inequalities in health and care provision. The examples given provide a credible argument for midwives to increase their knowledge and application of public health concepts to their practice.

Chapter 3 discusses the common types of data collected and used to inform public health midwifery. It also examines what is meant by public health practice for midwives in more detail by considering how midwifery practice fits within the Ten Key Standard Areas of Public Health, as they are currently understood in the UK context. These are compared to other countries' own definitions of public health practice and found to map well across the international public health scene.

The second section, *Developing ideas and opportunities*, looks at the social contexts of practising public health midwifery, from understanding health inequalities or how community development techniques can be used in public health to providing services that are sensitive to the diversity of individuals, to having a sociological perspective of women's experience of childbirth.

In Chapter 4 we explore and attempt to clarify the term 'inequalities', while highlighting that the concept of 'health inequalities' itself is somewhat contested and needs unpicking to bring greater clarity to the ongoing debates on inequalities. International and UK examples help inform the discussion of what social elements make up the inequalities picture, as well as opportunities that provide levers for change.

Chapter 5 examines the differing forms of diversity within society and how a poor understanding of ethnic, social class or religious differences can lead to mistrust between midwife, mothers and families. Midwives are frequently faced with a highly diverse clientele, many of whom are socially isolated or excluded for a variety of reasons. This chapter provides concrete examples of the types of social situation midwives might find themselves in and suggests interventions and approaches that may be useful.

The concepts of need and community needs assessment and profiling are explored in Chapter 6. Central to recent health policy is a drive to involve communities and professionals in the identification of health needs. This chapter provides an overview of the possible approaches that can be taken in carrying out a community profile.

Chapter 7 focuses on a key, but sometimes neglected, aspect of public health: how other disciplines such as sociology or anthropology can help inform public health practice. Through an examination of women's own statements about different aspects of pregnancy and childbirth through a lens of sociological theory, different insights into how women react to this key time in their lives are gained, giving food for thought to those developing ways to improve services for mothers-to-be.

The third section, *The practice reality*, focuses on specific areas of public health midwifery practice, providing examples and case studies that can help inform ideas for local initiatives.

In Chapter 8 we provide an account of a midwifery-led research project conducted in Australia. The project had a strong focus on providing continuity of care for women through a new model of midwifery care provision, and the chapter highlights the identified benefits achieved through this approach.

In Chapter 9 teenage pregnancy is identified as a key priority area. This chapter provides an in-depth discussion around teenage pregnancy with a specific focus on the midwives' role around sex education for young people.

Drawing on the strong practice focus of this section, Chapter 10 provides insight and examination of a Sure Start programme from a midwifery perspective.

Chapter 11 further explores the possibilities of implementing a public health focus within clinical practice with a clear emphasis on providing midwifery postnatal care which is flexible and tailored to needs of women, their babies and their families.

The final section of the book, *Moving forward*, considers the future of public health in midwifery practice.

Chapter 12 provides a clear call to midwives to 'keep birth normal' and through a commitment to this approach will allow midwives to make their greatest contribution to the public health agenda.

We do not expect that all the answers will be found in this book; however, we are confident that readers will gain an appreciation and understanding of public health as it relates to midwifery and more importantly will see opportunities to improve and develop their practice.

Pádraig Ó Lúanaigh — New Plymouth

Cindy Carlson — Oxford

2005

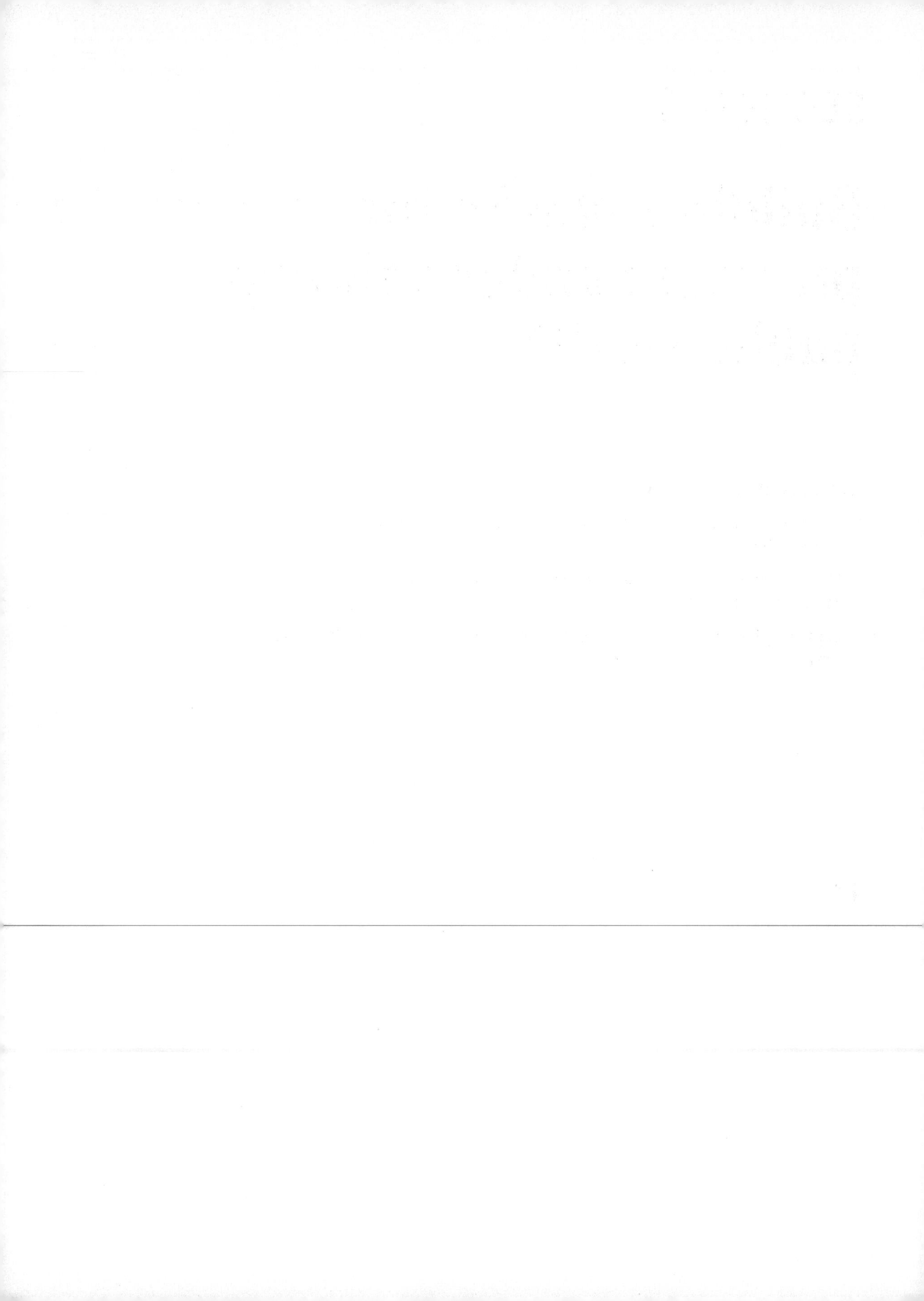

SECTION 1

Building blocks for practice: understanding public health

SECTION CONTENTS

Chapter 1

The 'New' Public Health: political rhetoric or real opportunities?

Suzanne Tyler

CHAPTER CONTENTS

SUMMARY

It is now widely recognised that whilst health at the beginning of life is the foundation for health throughout life, too many babies start life with a less than optimal chance of enjoying health and happiness. Tackling the unacceptable variations in health that exist across social class, income, educational status and ethnic origin is at the heart of both the public agenda and the agenda of maternity services.

This chapter demonstrates the close historical links that exist between developments in public health and in midwifery care, as well as the significance of today's public health policy initiatives for the organisation and delivery of maternity care. It argues that midwives today should demonstrate a commitment to improving maternal and perinatal outcomes through effective health promotion and education, targeted support for women with particular needs and cross-sectoral partnership working to reduce health and social inequalities.

INTRODUCTION

Public health is about more than just the health of the public. Today, it is an expression used to encapsulate the aims and methods of all of those whose concern it is to protect and promote the health of all citizens in the interests of both each individual and society as a whole. It includes health promotion activities, disease prevention programmes and the treatment of illness as well as care of those who are disabled or disadvantaged.

This definition makes it immediately clear why public health is the concern and province of every midwife. After all, the well-being of mothers is the key to the well-being of babies and of entire families in both the long and short term, and midwifery care is all about assisting each woman to achieve a happy and healthy pregnancy and birth.

What is more, a public health perspective in midwifery is one that explicitly acknowledges the impact that an individual woman's social, economic and psychological life, as well as personal behaviour, has on their health. Infant mortality is in fact one of the most sensitive indices we possess of social welfare and of sanitary administration (Louden 1992).

For midwives this means effective care must focus on the wider context within which each woman's pregnancy occurs if we are to maintain and improve outcomes for mothers and babies.

The Royal College of Midwives (2000) has adopted the following definition of public health, which is a useful aid to reflecting on how the maternity services you work in are organised and your approach to practice:

> A way of looking at health that brings together all the factors which shape and influence the health of individuals and communities:
>
> - A perspective which encompasses the roots and causes of health and ill health, as well as its treatment, and
> - Which sees health within its overall social and political context, rather than as an isolated medical event, and
> - Which looks for solutions in wider social action, individual empowerment and community development, as well as clinical interventions.

In this chapter we explore the changing nature of public health, principally in the United Kingdom, and its growing political importance and ask whether this is all just rhetoric or if the public health agenda presents midwives with real opportunities to make a real difference to the lives of women and babies.

WHY INEQUALITIES MATTER

Inequalities in maternity care operate at two levels. Firstly, there is now a wealth of evidence to suggest that pregnant women from vulnerable and deprived communities, socially excluded and black and minority ethnic women experience significantly worse outcomes in terms of their own and their babies' health and well-being (Rowe et al 2003). Secondly, research suggests that these women are disproportionately amongst those least likely to access and enjoy the highest quality maternity services available, particularly the important psycho-social aspects of care, and are therefore less likely to exert choice and control in their care.

This reflects the well-documented inverse care law in health, which states: '*the availability of good medical care tends to vary inversely with the need of the population served*' (Hart 1971).

Table 1.1 summarises what we know about the key determinants of health outcome for pregnant women.

Whilst these two dimensions of inequality are not necessarily causally related, they are linked and midwives will have witnessed their impact on each other. Indeed, this is a complex relationship; some women will present with multiple 'risk' factors, such as the black teenager or the woman living on means-tested benefits who is in an abusive relationship. At the same time it cannot be presumed that all women falling within an 'at risk' group are equally vulnerable. Not all women in social class V will have a low birth-weight baby, not all women whose first language is not English will experience difficulty communicating with their caregivers. The significance of this for the public health role of midwives is the importance of understanding and recognising the impact of inequalities on groups within society at a macro level, whilst at the same time designing and delivering services at a micro level to treat each woman as an individual with care packages tailored to her specific and personal needs and desires.

One of the long-standing criticisms of the UK National Health Service is that it has been, since its inception in 1948, a 'sickness' service concerned with treating morbidity, rather than a 'wellness' service concerned to promote health. In policy terms this means that public health, preventative programmes and health promotion have traditionally been accorded a lower priority than curative hospital services and resource allocation has been drastically steered towards treatment rather than prevention. In the next section we chart the rise of a public health approach within UK health care in response to increasing public expectations for intervention before people become ill enough to become patients.

HISTORICAL CONTEXT

Over the last 150 years, since the first public health measures were taken in the UK, we have seen along with other developed countries dramatic changes in demographic structures, in the patterns of health and disease and in the capacity of interventions to make a difference.

Table 1.1 Relationship between external factors and health and well-being of women and babies

Key determinants of health outcome	Impact on health and well-being of mother and baby
Social class (women in social classes IV and V are more likely to experience)	• Low birth weight (associated with increased risk of death in first year and increased risk of disability and special educational need) • Preterm birth • Still birth and infant mortality • Maternal death • Smoking • Lower rates of successful breastfeeding
Deprivation[1]	• Still birth and infant mortality • Congenital abnormalities • Smoking • Lower rates of successful breastfeeding
Teenage parenting	• Postnatal depression • Smoking • Domestic violence • Inadequate diet • Establishing successful breastfeeding
Ethnic origin[2]	• Low birth weight (associated with increased risk of death in first year and increased risk of disability and special educational need) • Maternal death • Establishing successful breastfeeding (inverse relationship)
First language not English	• Higher caesarean section rate?
Smoking	• Low birth weight • Fetal and neonatal death • Sudden infant death syndrome • Childhood development
Inadequate diet	• Low birth weight • Coronary heart disease • Diabetes
Drug and alcohol misuse	• Miscarriage • Developmental abnormalities • Fetal alcohol syndrome • Sudden infant death syndrome
Domestic violence (associated with younger couples, separation, financial pressures, drug/alcohol abuse, Asian populations, refugees)	• Premature death • Low birth weight • Fetal injury • Placental abruption
Lack of social support	• Postnatal depression
Homelessness	• Low birth weight • Miscarriage • Still birth • Infant mortality • Childhood accidents
Asylum seekers	• Rape • Poor maternal health • Depression • Poor nutrition
Disability	• Accessing services • Communication

[1] Measured by receipt of welfare benefits, unemployment, younger parents, low educational attainment, poor and overcrowded housing
[2] Existing data relates only to women born outside the UK

Table 1.2 A history of public health development in England

1847	Appointment of first Medical Officers for Health
1848	First Public Health Act concentrates on sanitation and clean water
1860	Florence Nightingale's *Nursing Notes* highlight significance of hygiene
1868	Poor Law Amendment Act introduces separate infirmaries
1902	Midwives Act introduces standards and registration of midwives
1906	Introduction of free school meals and school health services
1907	Notification of Births Act – formalises health visiting
1918	Maternity and Child Welfare Act clarifies provision of antenatal and postnatal care
1919	Creation of the Ministry of Health
1948	Introduction of the NHS
1977	World Health Organization: *Health for All by the Year 2000*
1980	Inequalities in Health (*Black Report*) points to health divide in UK, but is blocked by Government
1997	Independent Inquiry into Health Inequalities commissioned by incoming Labour Government
1998	*Our Healthier Nation* (Green Paper) issued for consultation
1998	Independent Inquiry (Acheson Report) published
1999	*Saving Lives: Our Healthier Nation* published in response to Acheson
1999	*Reducing Health Inequalities: An Action Plan* published
2000	NHS Plan including national health inequalities targets
2000	Inequalities and Public Health Task Force established
2001	National health inequalities targets announced
2001	*From vision to reality* – consultation on plan for delivery
2002	*Tackling health inequalities* – Update
2003	Wanless II: Review of NHS funding linked to improving health

Table 1.2 charts the development of public health legislation and innovation in the UK. Ashton (1997) illustrates this progress by comparing the changing patterns of health in northwest England over the 50 years since the NHS was founded. In 1948 there were around 40,000 births annually in the region; by 1994 this had fallen to around 30,000. Whereas in 1948 childbearing commonly began in the teens and early 20s with large families commonplace, by the end of the 1990s family size had halved and childbearing was deferred until the late twenties. In 1948, 50 out of every 1000 children died before their first birthday; by 1998 this had fallen to fewer than 7, of which most were attributable to genetic causes.

THE ORIGINS OF PUBLIC HEALTH

The earliest public health approaches date from the nineteenth century and coincide with the rapid growth of industrial towns, often accompanied by overcrowded living space, poor sanitation and nutrition and the spread of communicable diseases. It was civil servant Edwin Chadwick who in the UK was one of the first to make the connection between the environment that people lived in and their health status: his select committee into the causes of mortality and morbidity in the 1830s set the tone for decades of investment and action to improve sanitation, provide clean water supplies, build drainage systems and enable the safe removal of sewage. The impact was extraordinary; in 1842 Chadwick estimated that the life expectancy of a working class child born in any of the provincial cities was between 12 and 15 years. In 1900 infant mortality stood at

156 per 1000 live births, and this had been reduced to 36 per thousand by 1946 and today, as described above, it stands at under 7 per thousand.

Throughout the twentieth century public health expanded beyond public sanitation and epidemiology to include health education programmes to encourage individuals to adopt healthier lifestyles.

The impact of improvements in public health have had a direct correlation with improvements in maternal and infant health. Tew demonstrates how declining mortality was brought about by the improving fitness of child-bearing women, through improvements in diet and living conditions at the end of the nineteenth century:

> Maternal and perinatal mortality are critically dependent on standards of maternal nutrition both during the gestation period and no less importantly, during the mother's life since her own conception. The process is cumulative over generations. (Tew 1995)

PUBLIC HEALTH TO 1997: FROM WHO TO BOBBLE HATS

In 1977 the World Health Organization adopted an explicitly public health approach in its Health For All by the Year 2000 campaign (HFA 2000). This policy reflected the agreement of the world community that '*the main social target of governments and of the WHO should be the attainment by all the people of the world by the year 2000 of a level of health that will permit them to lead a socially and economically productive life…*' HFA 2000 marks the beginning of more than 20 years of an approach to protecting and promoting the health of the population, emphasising more than just health services. This was further codified in WHO principles that remain a pertinent checklist for every midwife in every encounter with a client (see Box 1.1).

Whilst throughout the 1980s much of the western industrialised world was translating the Health For All targets into tangible policies, the UK's Conservative Government resisted all analysis that indicated that action by the state could overcome or alleviate the impact of inequalities in health. Its health policies focused instead largely on the need to produce changes in individual behaviour, concentrating on lifestyles and involving mass health education and public information campaigns. Not only did the Government refuse to develop a national Health For All strategy,

Box 1.1
WHO Ottawa Charter for Health Promotion: How do midwives respond?

- Health promotion actively involves the population in the setting of everyday life rather than focusing on people who are at risk for specific conditions and in contact with medical services.
- Health promotion is directed at action on the causes of ill health.
- Health promotion uses many different approaches, which combine to improve health. These include education and information, community development and organisation, health advocacy and legislation.
- Health promotion depends particularly on public participation.
- Health professionals – especially those in primary care – have an important part to play in nurturing health promotion and enabling it to take place.

but it also rejected the recommendations of its own Chief Scientist who had been charged with exploring the broader factors influencing health. The Black Report (named after the Chairman of a Health Department working group) was a shocking indication of the gap in health status between the wealthiest and poorest citizens and the socio-economic factors that lay behind this.

No discussion of public health can be value free, and it is clear that a political ideology that is based around free markets, and the inevitable (and desirable?) inequalities that result from it, will not sit easily with a public health agenda focused on eliminating the social and economic inequalities that determine much ill health. The approach of the UK Government throughout the 1980s and early 1990s is best illustrated by its health minister Edwina Currie whose advice to old people who were threatened with hypothermia because they could not afford heating was to wear woolly hats and stay in bed; whilst Secretary of State Virginia Bottomley recommended (Jay 1997) that the solution to high rates of heart disease was to eat fewer biscuits and run up and down stairs!

In midwifery the consequences of the prevailing political climate were evident in the Government's response to a House of Commons Select Committee Report into maternity services (the Winterton Report). The Winterton Report not only explored the provision of health services for pregnant women and new babies and issues around quality, outcomes and women's experience, it also focused on the social context within which maternity care is provided. It provided compelling evidence of the inequalities that exist both in outcomes and in access for disadvantaged and excluded women. It made recommendations about the social security and benefits systems relating to pregnant women, as well as looking at the social support available for vulnerable women in their transition to motherhood. However, the Government's response published in 1994, the Cumberledge Report, which remains the essential blueprint for maternity services, ignored all of these elements. *Changing Childbirth* focused exclusively on individual women's experiences and its mantra of 'choice, continuity and control' arguably did little for women from the most vulnerable and excluded groups.

Indeed the emphasis on individual preferences and choice may have distorted the broader perspective of equity and equality: 'what is best for one, may not be best for all' (Klein 1994). The 'trickle-down' rationale, which assumes that gains made by middle-class women for home births, homeopathy and water birth will in time alter the structure and provision of care for all, has been demonstrated to be false. In fact, policies such as *Changing Childbirth* may lead indirectly to a sharpening of the inverse care law and the widening of health inequalities, with women who are most in need of the emotional, psychological and practical support of good midwifery care, least likely to access it.

THE NEW PUBLIC HEALTH

The new public health, launched by WHO in 1977 and ignored by the UK Government until 1997, puts much greater emphasis on the socio-economic environment and in particular the impact of poverty and health inequalities. More specifically the new public health has recognised that it is not poverty itself that is crucial to health outcomes but inequalities, what is sometimes called relative poverty, the prevalence and distribution of social position, job insecurity, unemployment, social mobility, education, social networks, family disruption and stress (Kaufmann 2002). The new public health recognises that the causes of ill health are complex. Midwives will know that of course, smoking, obesity, drug misuse and reckless sexual behaviour relate to poor health status. However, what epidemiology shows us is that it is not the differences between individuals that are significant, but the differences between groups – defined by income levels, social deprivation, employment status, educational attainment and ethnicity. So we see that unhealthy lifestyles are not randomly distributed throughout society; rather they are found concentrated at the lower end of the socio-economic spectrum amongst these vulnerable groups (Evans 2002).

The election in 1997 of a Labour Government in the UK heralded a shift towards a left-leaning administration that stated its commitment to improving standards of care, especially amongst the poorest sections of society. In May 1997 the then Minister for Health, Tessa Jowell, invited former Chief Medical Officer Donald Acheson 'to review and summarise inequalities in health in England and to identify priority areas for policies to reduce them'. The Acheson Report (Independent Inquiry into Inequalities) was published a year later and provided a socio-economic explanation of health inequalities, highlighting the significance of variations in income, education, employment and environment, as well as lifestyle. The influence of the new public health was visible in the Government's recognition that the NHS alone could not ensure good health. Rather initiatives since 1997 have called for a compact between government, communities and individuals with each recognising its responsibilities. The Acheson Report was just one of a raft of initiatives launched by the government to approach inequalities and social exclusion through programmes of neighbourhood renewal to build capacity and cohesion within local communities (Coote 2000). In the next section we explore in more detail the policy initiatives enacted since 1997 to develop a public health approach in the UK.

THE POLICY ARENA

ACHESON REPORT

The Independent Inquiry into Inequalities in Health chaired by Sir Donald Acheson (1998) found that inequalities in health range across geographical areas, social class, gender and ethnicity.

The report recommended that the needs of pregnant women, young families and infants should be a high priority for efforts to reduce inequalities in health, to ensure a healthier nation (see Box 1.2).

It emphasised the need to tackle maternal poverty through policies that support women in choosing either to return to work or remain at home, and its wide-ranging recommendations covered tax and benefits, education, employment, housing, the environment and transport. The Government's response was a major initiative to eradicate child poverty

Box 1.2
Key areas of the Acheson Report relating to mothers and pre-school children (Brocklehurst & Costello 2003)

- Introduction of free milk to first born and to children in large families
- Reviews of antenatal and child health provision and accessibility in order to increase uptake in the early months of pregnancy
- Savings made from the reduction in the school population to be redirected into the provision of new services for the under 5s
- School health to be integrated into generic community medical services, and health screening and surveillance in areas of special need to be intensified
- Abolition of child poverty as a priority
- Action to be taken to reduce accidents to children.

by 2020 and lift 1 million children out of poverty by 2004. It has implemented a series of interrelated multi-dimensional policies including reform of the tax and benefit system, the New Deal for Lone Parents, Sure Start and Health Action Zones, as well as national teenage pregnancy, domestic violence and smoking cessation strategies.

The Sure Start programme targets the 20% most deprived neighbourhoods throughout England to combine nursery education, family support, employment advice, childcare and health services on one site. Although each Sure Start programme has been developed to meet local needs and priorities, they all share the aim of achieving better outcomes for children, parents and communities by increasing the availability of childcare for all children; improving health, education and emotional development for young children; and supporting parents in their role and in developing their employment aspirations.

Around the country many maternity services and primary care trusts (PCTs) are working with their local Sure Start programmes to raise the quality of maternity services for vulnerable women by helping services develop in disadvantaged areas, while providing financial help to enable parents to afford quality childcare. Sure Start is discussed in greater detail in Chapter 10.

The limitations of the Acheson Report lie in its ambition. The report's 74 separate recommendations are not prioritised, nor does it give pointers to how they might best be implemented. The recommendations range from the very general to the very specific, which makes them difficult for individual practitioners to relate to – just where should efforts be placed to make a difference (Exworthy et al 2003)?

Despite these criticisms the Acheson Report has been instrumental in fostering a new and widespread recognition of health inequalities and the wider determinants of health. In a review of policy initiatives across Government since Acheson, researchers at University College London (Exworthy et al 2003) concluded its legacy was:

- It acted as a prompt for new policies
- It engendered a climate of opinion favouring policies to tackle health inequalities

- It introduced a health inequalities dimension to mainstream policies
- It acts as a reference book.

SAVING LIVES: OUR HEALTHIER NATION, THE STRATEGY IN ENGLAND

The White Paper *Saving Lives: Our Healthier Nation*, published in 1999, is an action plan to tackle poor health and sets out how the Government planned to implement the Acheson recommendations. It has two key aims: to increase length of life and number of years free from illness; and to improve the health of the worst off in society at a faster rate than for other groups and narrow the health gap. It sets out the Government's strategy for England, the goals and targets and how they will be reached. Deliberately the Government choose to select only four priority areas, on the basis that if everything is a priority nothing is a priority. The strategy therefore is concentrated on the four biggest causes of premature death and long term ill health:

- Cancer
- Coronary heart disease
- Accidents
- Mental health.

Maternity care and obstetric outcomes are not therefore central to the strategy – because compared to these other areas, outcomes in pregnancy and childbirth are good, with low levels of morbidity or mortality. However, this does not mean that *Saving Lives* has no relevance for midwives: indeed it explicitly recognises the important public health role that midwives play. Table 1.3 illustrates how *Saving Lives* gives midwifery the

Table 1.3 Midwifery contribution to Government health priorities

Priority area	Target	Midwifery contribution
Cancer	By 2010 reduce deaths by cancer by one fifth	Maternity care provides opportunities to identify risk factors and provide advice on health-promoting behaviours. Breastfeeding is known to decrease the risk of both breast and ovarian cancer in pre-menopausal women (Heining & Dewey 1997)
Coronary heart disease and stroke	By 2010 reduce deaths from coronary heart disease and stroke by two fifths	Good maternity care is significant in promoting and sustaining breastfeeding; breastfed infants are likely to be at reduced risk of CHD throughout life (Wilson et al 1998)
Accidents	By 2010 reduce deaths by accidents by one fifth and serious injury by two fifths	Many accidents happen in the home, often involving infants and young children. Parenting education and domiciliary visits provide opportunities to discuss these risks and how to avoid them
Mental health	By 2010 reduce deaths by suicide by one fifth	10–15% of new mothers experience depression, and around one in 500 experience puerperal psychosis. It is not known how many women experience post-traumatic stress disorder following childbirth because it often fails to be accurately diagnosed or is put down to depression. Appropriate professional support has been shown to lead to more rapid remission of symptoms, fewer problems in the mother–child relationship and fewer child behavioural problems

opportunity to extend its traditional boundaries and demonstrate how its contribution to making a difference to the health and well-being of families actually impacts on the Government's key health targets.

Saving Lives sets out ten core functions that describe and guide the practice of all public health in England. Again there is a clear and unique midwifery contribution to each of these, should midwives be prepared to make it.

Health surveillance, monitoring and analysis

Analysing data on health and on the population provides valuable information on current and future health trends. It enables the public health system to plan for change, for example the ageing of the population, or variations in the pattern of disease or lifestyle risk factors.

- Midwifery perspective:

Where midwives really know their local communities and the health and other issues they face, they have been able to target care to those who need it most. By using the available local data on demographics, health outcomes, etc., midwives can re-orientate their services to make sure priority is given to women with the highest needs.

Investigation of disease outbreaks, epidemics and risks to health

Protecting the health of the population is a key part of public health. This includes investigating disease outbreaks and epidemics and dealing with emergencies and disasters including terrorist attacks, chemical leaks and nuclear accidents.

- Midwifery perspective:

The bedrock of effective midwifery is the promotion of healthy lifestyles, providing information, advice and support on smoking, nutrition, exercise and infant feeding. These essentially personal messages are reinforced by midwives' monitoring of women's overall well-being during and after pregnancy, picking up on domestic violence or postnatal depression or worries about money, housing or childcare.

Establishing, designing and managing health promotion and disease prevention programmes

Promoting good health and preventing disease are important aspects of public health. Public health information campaigns using the media can achieve high awareness.

- Midwifery perspective:

Midwives meet women at a period of their lives when they are particularly open to health promotion, and midwifery care provides many opportunities for health education through antenatal visits, parentcraft classes and postnatal support.

Enabling and empowering communities

Key to health improvement and the reduction in health inequalities is community empowerment. To enable a community to develop its own health and well-being requires support.

- Midwifery perspective:

Midwives can help build women's self-confidence by acting as their advocates, seeing each woman as an active partner in her own care and encouraging women and their communities to influence sensitive, responsive and flexible maternity services. Rather than maintaining traditional hierarchical power relations, midwifery creates the opportunity for non-authoritarian relationships and shared responsibility with their clients. This approach seeks to promote trust and communication between woman and service, and may encourage women to both access appropriate support and adopt healthier lifestyles (Mottl-Santiago 2002).

Creating and sustaining cross-government and intersectoral partnerships to improve health and reduce inequalities

Tackling health inequalities and improving health requires active commitment by departments across Government and by groups at all levels, national, regional and local. Joint working, partnerships, networking, shared funding and resources are crucial to ensuring the public health agenda can be taken forward.

- Midwifery perspective:

The success of the Sure Start initiative demonstrates how midwives can achieve far more, working collaboratively with colleagues, than they do in isolation. Working in a multi-disciplinary and multi-sectoral team means midwives can facilitate women's interaction with the 'right' people at the 'right' time.

Looking at one of midwives' top health promotion priorities, breastfeeding support services can certainly be purchased and provided within a health care system, but if the population's overall health status is to be raised, then lifestyle changes and the opportunity for healthy choices must be extended within a multi-sectoral environment.

Ensuring compliance with regulations and laws to protect and promote health

There are a wide range of laws and regulations that protect and promote health and a number of different agencies and bodies involved in enforcement and providing guidance and advice on compliance.

- Midwifery perspective:

Although not regulated, screening has the potential to save lives or improve the quality of life through early diagnosis of serious conditions. Midwives have a crucial role in maintaining high compliance with antenatal screening and testing that allows women to make informed choices about a range of infections and congenital conditions that could affect them or their babies.

Developing and maintaining a well-educated and trained multi-disciplinary public health workforce

Public health involves a wide range of disciplines. It is important that those involved in taking forward public health improvements are professionally competent, skilled and well trained.

- Midwifery perspective:

With their history of caring for vulnerable women, midwives have an expertise that has contributed to the wider understanding of the health needs of diverse groups. But to maintain this it is every midwife's responsibility to keep up to date: 'In refocusing on health rather than simply health care, there is a need for midwives to be self determining and self sufficient, confident in their knowledge base to address issues of social justice and service development' (Hillier & Caan 2002). Midwives and other primary care workers must work together to standardise care, to maintain knowledge and to strengthen professional development.

Ensuring the effective performance of NHS services to meet goals in improving health, preventing disease and reducing inequalities

The Department of Health is responsible in England for ensuring effective guidance is issued to NHS services for them to implement practice measures for improving health, preventing disease and reducing health inequalities. It is also responsible for setting national targets and performance indicators, which provide goals and benchmarks to be met and a measure of progress.

- Midwifery perspective:

The midwifery impact is being demonstrated where they are taking lead responsibility for service improvement for vulnerable and excluded women such as teenagers, asylum seekers and drug users, etc. In a recent survey UK Heads of Midwifery recognised the need to re-organise maternity services and redistribute resources to facilitate a public health approach that would enable midwives to effectively deliver a public health-oriented service, emphasising:

- Screening and support
- Parent preparation
- Integrated working, and
- Involvement with specific groups (Henderson 2002).

Research development evaluation and innovation

Research is crucial to developing evidence-based public health policies, initiatives and interventions. It therefore has to be developed and evaluated and new methods and ideas used to gain knowledge and understanding and to develop creative ideas from the outcomes of research.

- Midwifery perspective:

Midwives need to recognise public health as a core function, not as a bolt-on series of additional tasks. Whilst we have a strong evidence base for the causes of poor maternal and infant health, we are still lacking a sound basis for demonstrating which midwifery interventions are most successful.

Quality assuring the public health function

The exercise of public health functions supports the commissioning process in PCTs and in service delivery in acute and mental health trusts. It provides evidence of effectiveness of interventions and supports capacity planning through service modelling and planning. Evaluation of services, setting standards and auditing against these standards is a public health skill to support continuous improvement in service provision.

- Midwifery perspective:

Midwives are experienced in networking across health care, social services and local voluntary organisations and can utilise their skills and contacts to build alliances and multi-sectoral initiatives. They can demonstrate their effectiveness in monitoring the health of pregnant women and their unborn children.

THE NHS PLAN

Whilst the NHS Plan is primarily concerned with the organisation and delivery of health services in England, the 10-year plan for modernisation of the NHS does include a chapter dedicated to improving public health and reducing inequalities. The NHS Plan reflects the themes from both Acheson and *Saving Lives* to focus on:

- Setting a national inequalities target
- Reducing inequalities in access to NHS services
- Prioritising children to ensure a healthy start in life
- Reducing smoking
- Improving diet and nutrition
- Tackling drugs and alcohol
- Forging new partnerships to tackle inequality.

The first national target for reducing inequalities was set for infant mortality, and there are now four targets that relate directly to the care that midwives provide which are a key part of the performance framework for primary care and acute trusts (see Box 1.3).

Achieving sustainable long-term benefits of reducing health inequalities requires the integration of a comprehensive range of policies into mainstream policy and planning. In maternity care this has implications for modernisation which must involve appropriate systems and processes to support existing and new policies, such as the comprehensive smoking cessation service.

MAKING A DIFFERENCE

This national strategy for nursing, midwifery and health visiting launched in 1999 called for an enhanced midwifery role in maximising women's health and in contributing to public health targets. It recognises that the context of care is changing and that midwives face new challenges; it also recognises that midwives are often constrained by structures that limit development and innovation. However, it places midwives as central to improving the nation's health through extending their role to include wider responsibilities for women's health.

In particular it calls on midwives to work with school nurses and health visitors to ensure young people are well informed about healthy lifestyles including contraception, sexual health, relationships and responsibilities associated with pregnancy and childbirth. It suggests midwives can play

Box 1.3
National Health inequalities targets

- Starting with children under 1 year, by 2010, to reduce by at least 10% the gap in mortality between manual groups and the population as a whole
- By achieving agreed local conception reduction targets to reduce the national under-18 conception rates by 15% by 2004 and 50% by 2010, while reducing the gap in rates between the worst fifth of electoral wards and the average by one quarter
- To achieve a 10% reduction in the number of mothers who smoke during pregnancy in the 500 Sure Start areas by 2004
- To reduce the number of children living on low income by at least one quarter by 2004, as a contribution towards the broader target of halving child poverty by 2010 and eradicating it by 2020.

a bigger role in health promotion by assisting women to make informed choices about diet, exercise, smoking and obesity. It challenges midwives to make services more responsive to vulnerable women by providing antenatal classes and parentcraft sessions in the evenings and weekends and in places that are welcoming and conveniently located.

It goes on to highlight the contribution midwives can make to educating women about breast and cervical screening, so preparing women for a healthy life after childbirth. Furthermore it sees scope for midwives to extend the contact they have with women to improve and refer women suffering postnatal depression, through, for example, active debriefing sessions.

It calls on NHS organisations to explore opportunities to make the best use of the knowledge and skills of the entire midwifery team and in particular to create midwife consultant posts enabling expert experienced midwives to remain in practice and provide strong leadership.

DELIVERING THE BEST

In June 2003 the English Chief Nursing Officer launched a new midwifery website entitled 'Delivering the Best' which explored five big challenges of modernisation for midwives, including improving public health. This sets out how midwives can emphasise their role to ensure pregnancy is not viewed in isolation from the other important factors that influence health and outcome (see Box 1.4). It explores a number of national health improvement targets that relate specifically to pregnancy and childbirth, including reducing the number of women smoking during pregnancy, increasing the number of women breastfeeding and reducing the number of teenage conceptions, and suggests that by adopting a public health approach individual midwives can become more effective in:

- Sharing information to give women control over their lives and health
- Considering the whole picture of a woman's life

Box 1.4
Adopting a Public Health approach – a checklist for individual midwives (DH 2003)

- Think about the backgrounds of your clients, the realities of their daily lives and what their priorities are likely to be
- Recognise the link between social inequality, poverty and ill health, using your daily experiences and national and local data and information
- Challenge judgemental attitudes and relinquish professional power
- Make links with local statutory and voluntary organisations to provide information, support and advice to vulnerable women
- Find out how your PCT approaches Health Needs Assessment and get involved to feed in your local knowledge
- Look for the opportunities to collaborate with local community development initiatives
- Be creative and work differently when expressing health messages
- Search for and share examples of good practice with other midwives.

- Discovering simple methods to assist women
- Working more effectively with vulnerable clients who have complex needs
- Fostering women's belief in normality and helping to build their self-esteem.

Using examples from around the country of midwifery units that are adopting a public health approach, the website offers individual midwives a simple checklist for delivering a better start in life.

MATERNITY NATIONAL SERVICE FRAMEWORK

Implementation of the government's strategy for health in England is being driven through a series of National Service Frameworks that set blueprints for the organisation and delivery of services. NSFs are intended to ensure the uniform application of best practice, solidly founded on research evidence. To date NSFs have been produced for the four priority areas: CHD, mental health, and cancer. In September 2004 the government issued the Children's NSF, which includes a separate and distinct maternity section. Work on the maternity NSF has been divided between antenatal, intrapartum and postnatal care with additional work on both user involvement and the reduction of inequalities.

The Children's NSF provides the blueprint for maternity service modernisation by breaking down professional boundaries and promoting partnerships between agencies. Its central principle is a holistic approach to caring for children and pregnant women that places them at the centre of care. The emphasis within the NSF on reducing health inequalities and improving health outcomes will be a significant driver for improving services for vulnerable and socially excluded families.

TOWARDS A HEALTHY SCOTLAND – THE SCOTTISH STRATEGY

The Government's vision for improving the health of all Scotland was published in 1999, and the main thrust is to reduce inequalities. Scotland is near the top of the international league for CHD, cancer and stroke, ensuring that these diseases have a much higher political and public profile. The Scottish strategy explicitly recognises that good health comes about through improving physical, mental and social well-being, fitness and quality of life. The planks of the Scottish approach are:

- A co-ordinated attack on health inequalities
- A programme of activities aimed at improving and sustaining the health of children and young people
- Major initiatives to prevent CHD and cancer
- Like the English strategy, teenage pregnancy is a priority area in Scotland where the target is to reduce the pregnancy rate of 13–15-year-olds by 20% by 2010.

THE WELSH APPROACH TO PUBLIC HEALTH

The Welsh Assembly created in 1998 has adopted both a devolved and an integrated approach to public health, in its stated aim to promote health and develop health services, not illness services. *Wellbeing in Wales* (2000) sets out how the Assembly Government intends to work to improve health and reduce inequalities through an integrated approach to policies and programmes. This is now being implemented through a framework of local health, social care and well-being strategies. At the same time resource allocation is being targeted at specific communities linked to action to help people improve their health.

The radical approach being taken in Wales includes an explicit recognition of the multi-dimensional nature of social and economic policies and the impact that various areas of Government policy have on each other. This is illustrated by the approach to joined-up policy making.

Policy Area	Policy Area	Policy Area	Policy Area	Policy Area	Policy Area	Policy Area
Economic development	Agriculture & rural affairs	Training & education	Health & social services	Transport & environment	Culture, arts & sport	Communities housing
Challenges and solutions Poverty – ill health – social exclusion – equal opportunities – sustainable development						

Health policy in Wales is now structured around these cross-cutting themes, but it is to be actioned through local strategies spanning the whole spectrum from preventative action and regulation to improve health and reduce the risk of ill health through to care services provided by local government, the NHS, voluntary and private organisations. In addition the Assembly has a national strategy for children and young people founded in the UN Convention on the Rights of the Child.

PUBLIC HEALTH IN NORTHERN IRELAND

In Northern Ireland, Initiative for Health has been launched and involves all Government departments. The four health and social services boards are working to establish Investing for Health partnerships in their area at board level to develop long-term local cross-sectoral health improvement plans. These plans will address the identified needs of their local populations by action to improve health and well-being and reduce health inequalities (NHS Confederation 2003).

MIDWIFERY'S RESPONSE TO THE NEW PUBLIC HEALTH

Whilst it is enormously helpful in planning and designing services to recognise and understand the socio-economic, cultural, behavioural and other determinants of health access and outcomes, such determinants should be viewed with caution when approaching the care of individual women. It is enormously unhelpful for practitioners to make simplistic assumptions based on a woman's social or cultural background or to use these as a short cut to determining what she really needs or wants.

The central factor in delivering services to address or alleviate health inequalities must be the recognition that this is not a homogeneous group for whom there is a simple formula for 'how to get it right'. In maternity care this means that getting it right in terms of reducing health inequalities rests on the same principles as mainstream maternity care. That is, personalised, flexible and responsive services that are tailored to each individual woman's needs, not those of professionals or the service. This is not to say that providing appropriate, flexible and responsive maternity services for vulnerable women is easy; indeed there is considerable research evidence to demonstrate current service failings: from failure to communicate in language that is understood, through to providing inappropriate foods, misunderstanding cultural customs and failing to screen for genetic conditions, our services are all too often insensitive and inappropriate.

Equal access means ensuring that everyone has equal and full access to the health care that is available. It doesn't mean offering the same service to everyone and assuming that each person will therefore receive the same service. Rather it means providing flexible responsive services in which differing needs are identified and accommodated so that each person benefits equally. Midwives should treat all women with respect and parity to other clients, regardless of their own feelings about the woman and her family, their lifestyle or the life choices they make.

Having established the factors that give rise to inequalities in health outcome and experience and the interventions that are likely to alleviate these inequalities, the next step is to consider what health services in collaboration with local agencies and communities can do to provide appropriate and effective services. There is a moral and ethical obligation on health services and all practitioners to minimise inequalities, whilst human rights legislation and sex, race and disability discrimination legislation provide a legal responsibility for health providers not to discriminate against women. Minimising the effects of inequalities must be a central element of maternity care, and ensuring that vulnerable women receive appropriate care to overcome their problems must be central to every practitioner's approach. Achieving this is rooted in planning, commissioning, designing and delivering services underpinned by correct identification of disadvantaged clients, making their care individual, and recognition of the parallel services available to them.

Identifying women who are likely to experience inequalities of access or outcome

Before maternity stakeholders (commissioners and providers) can deliver comprehensive care and support to vulnerable women, they need to develop a local strategy derived from regular local needs assessment and mapping, together with identification and networking with relevant local statutory and voluntary agencies. Developing a strategic approach to reducing health inequalities will enable maternity services to identify who leads on care, what other help is required and what support is required in each individual case. Further discussion on health needs assessment is covered in Chapter 4.

Local strategies need to be kept up to date and functional by harnessing local intelligence networks and by promoting common development and learning opportunities from staff across agencies.

Planning, commissioning and delivering care that is individual and personal for each woman

Ensuring that vulnerable women receive appropriate care that starts to overcome inequalities in outcome and access must be a central part of every practitioner's practice. Care needs to be individual, flexible and personal for each woman, with consideration of her circumstances. Carers should not jump to conclusions and make assumptions about a woman's appearance, ability to communicate her past history, culture or religion. Chapter 7 explores issues around diversity in health care. Personal opinions and judgements should be kept out of professional practice, as should subjective comments.

Family and social circumstances often change during pregnancy. It cannot be assumed that a woman's needs will be constant throughout pregnancy, labour, childbirth and the postnatal period and these should be continually reassessed in collaboration with the woman.

Recognising that care of a pregnant woman and her family is not exclusive to the NHS

Effective care of vulnerable pregnant women and their families relies on collaboration between local statutory and voluntary agencies, who may play an essential role in service provision and deliver key support structures and mechanisms. Whilst staff in maternity units will not know of every local agency in detail, they should be able to signpost vulnerable women to other professionals, voluntary groups and agencies that have relevant specialist expertise.

CONCLUSIONS: POLITICAL RHETORIC OR REAL OPPORTUNITIES?

Midwives would have every right to be sceptical about any Government suggestions that midwifery care alone can ameliorate the impact of health, social, economic and geographical inequalities on the health outcomes for mothers and their babies. They also have the right to look askance at the priority public health is given in terms of Government funding and its relative investment compared to, say, waiting lists. For all the talk of the health of local populations the focus of policymakers seems to remain firmly based on hospital services, acute care, beds, waiting times and bricks and mortar issues.

However, it is undoubtedly true that since 1997 the focus of politicians, health service policymakers and managers has been on the broader context within which individual professionals deliver care.

By establishing four dedicated cross-cutting departmental units – Sure Start, Teenage Pregnancy Unit, Neighbourhood Renewal and the Social Exclusion Unit – the Government has put in the political will to achieving joined-up solutions to public health issues. The early evaluations of Sure Start, the teenage pregnancy strategy and the anti-smoking campaigns show that these are having an effect. In its programme for addressing health inequalities published in July 2003 the Department of Health emphasised the need to support families, mothers and children to ensure the best possible start in life and break the inter-generational cycle of health.

Table 1.4 Refocusing midwifery to a public health perspective

If you already do this . . .	You could also . . .
Focus on the individual	Focus on the community
Deliver woman-centred care	Focus on inequalities
Engage with women through Maternity Services Liaison Committees	Engage with women through health improvement programmes
Provide midwifery-led care	Provide primary care-led partnerships
Undertake postnatal examinations	Develop postnatal support
Give smoking cessation advice	Give substance misuse advice
Provide parental education	Provide parenting education
Give advice on diet	Understand the consequences of food poverty
Undertake antenatal screening	Undertake well woman screening
Include partners	Understand relationship issues
Deliver good care for all	Prioritise efforts to targeted outreach

The problem is as always sustaining political commitment, will and resourcing. Promoting health equality requires real investment and to date less than 1% of total NHS spending has been specifically earmarked for public health. It is also still to be seen whether the NHS performance management framework which emphasises waiting times and waiting lists will be robust enough to keep attention focused on public health – with star ratings largely determining managers' careers it is not surprising that these are the issues that attract most attention.

Midwives will know that politicians, governments and political fancies come and go; this year's priority may not be next year's. However, this should not be a reason to dismiss adopting a public health approach in midwifery care. The changes in demography, epidemiology and possibilities and expectations alluded to in this chapter are transforming the task facing public health. Dame Karlene Davis, General Secretary of the Royal College of Midwives, outlined how midwives could refocus their existing activities (Davis 2002, see Table 1.4) by taking some of their core skills and using them outside the box of the traditional obstetric parameters. This involves working from a health perspective and working alongside people in a way designed to be health enhancing rather than health damaging.

Midwifery at its best sees each woman holistically, taking into account her social, psychological and emotional as well as physical needs. Where midwives practise most effectively they recognise that a woman's confidence and her sense of control, her relationships with those around her and her domestic situation are as important as – perhaps more significant than – any clinical interventions she may receive during pregnancy. Maternity care offers a unique window of opportunity through which midwives working within a public health model can effect real change in women's lives; after all, users of maternity services are not by definition sick, but experiencing a normal physiological life event. Therefore obstacles that beset emergency services to intervening in environment or influencing behaviour do not apply. Furthermore, users of maternity services potentially have time to become informed during their pregnancy about the range of health and social services on offer and to participate in discussions about the appropriateness of these.

Much has been written about the impact of the medicalisation of childbirth on the profession of midwifery. The realities of working as a midwife within the restrictions of the powerful medical model have restricted the freedom of many to develop the vision of what a public health approach to maternity care might look like. For example the emphasis on obstetrics and labour deflects attention and resources away from women's needs in the postnatal period, leading to significant rates of undetected morbidities, postnatal depression and failure to sustain breastfeeding. This book is one attempt to redress that balance by demonstrating how midwives can reclaim their public health role and by showing how, when midwives do have the freedom to practise autonomously, there is evidence of improvement in women's lives.

References

Ashton J 1997 Health for All: The New Millennium. In: Scally G (ed.) Progress in Public Health. Royal Society of Medicine Press, London

Brocklehurst R, Costello J 2003 Health inequalities: The Black Report and beyond. In: Costello J, Haggart M (eds) Public Health and Society. Palgrave Macmillan, Basingstoke

Coote A 2000 New Labour's public health policy: theory good, practice middling to poor. Health Care UK, Winter 2000

Davis K 2002 The Midwife in the United Kingdom and Public Health, paper delivered at International Confederation of Midwives Triennial Congress, Vienna. ICM, London

Department of Health 2003 Delivering the Best. Online. Available: http://www.publications.doh.gov.uk/cno/midwives.pdf

Evans R 2002 Interpreting and Addressing Inequalities in Health: from Black to Acheson. Office of Health Economics, London

Exworthy M, Stuart M, Blane D, Marmot M 2003 Tackling Health Inequalities since the Acheson Inquiry. Polity Press, London

Hart J T 1971 The inverse care law. Lancet 1971(i):405–412

Heining M J, Dewey K G 1997 Health effects of breastfeeding for mothers: a critical review. Nutrition Research Reviews 10:35–56

Henderson C 2002 The public health role of the midwife. British Journal of Midwifery 10(5):268–269

Hillier D, Caan W 2002 Researching the public health role of the midwife. British Journal of Midwifery 10(9):545–546

Jay (Baroness) 1997 Speech in House of Lords Debate on Poverty and Ill Health. Hansard 12/2/97 Column 247

Kaufmann T 2002 Midwifery and public health. MIDIRS Midwifery Digest 12, Supplement 1:S23–S24

Klein R 1994 The politics of participation. In: Maxwell R, Weaver N (eds) Public Participation in Health – Towards a clearer view. King's Fund, London

Louden I 1992 Death in Childbirth. Clarendon Press, Oxford

Mottl-Santiago J 2002 Women's public health policy in the 21st century. Journal of Midwifery and Women's Health 47(4)

NHS Confederation 2003 Prevention is Better than Cure. NHS Confederation, London

Rowe R, Jayaweera H, Henderson J, Garcia J, Macfarlane A 2003 Inequalities in Mother and Baby Health in England. National Perinatal Epidemiology Unit, Oxford

Royal College of Midwives 2000 Midwives and the New NHS Paper 4: Public Health. RCM, London

Tew M 1995 Safer Childbirth? A Critical History of Maternity Care, 2nd edn. Chapman & Hall, London

Wilson A C, Stewart Forsyth J, Greene S A et al 1998 Relation of infant diet to childhood health: seven year follow up of cohort of children in Dundee infant feeding study. British Medical Journal 316:21–25

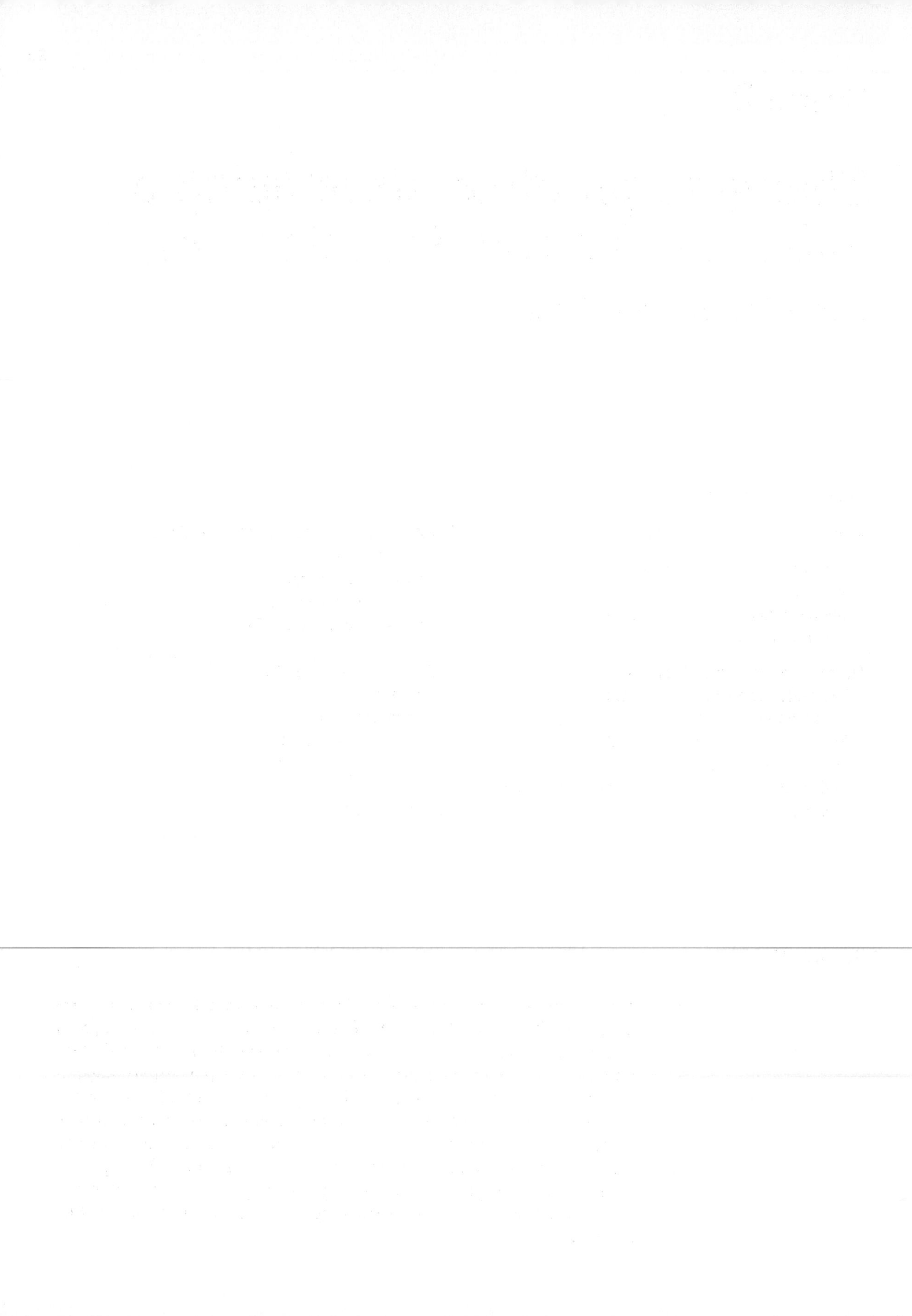

Chapter 2

Changing practice: developing a public health role for midwives

Jacqueline Dunkley-Bent

CHAPTER CONTENTS

SUMMARY

This chapter aims to explore the midwife's role within the context of public health. The scope of the midwife's role within this area of practice is broad and the impact on health outcome has significant potential. Two defined areas of practice are explored in this chapter, providing the reader with examples of public health in practice. The health disadvantage of asylum seekers and refugees and emotional disturbances across the childbirth continuum are two topical areas of midwifery practice worthy of further discussion and are presented in the following text. Baseline knowledge of the physiology of pregnancy will enable the reader to have a deeper understanding of the issues discussed in this chapter.

RECOGNISING THE MIDWIFE'S PUBLIC HEALTH ROLE

The midwife is described as a public health practitioner who enhances long-term health (RCM 2000). Heller et al (2003) define public health as the use of theory, experience and evidence derived through the population sciences to improve the health of the population in a way that best meets the implicit and explicit needs of the community. The use of evidence to inform practice and the responsibility to collect evidence that will improve the health of the population is integral to this definition. Midwives have an important role to play in public health but the public health role is focused toward the individual rather than a population approach. Data collection is vitally important if process, impact and outcome evaluation are to be taken seriously by key stakeholders.

Education about the scope and purpose of the midwife's role is not always apparent and understood. In order to establish a database of public health practitioners, researchers developed a tool to identify the public health workforce, including those people whose work contributes to the wider public health function. Public health practitioners identified included health visitors, school nurses and dentists, but despite the contribution that midwifery care makes to public health, midwives were not recognised as public health practitioners (Sim et al 2002). To raise awareness about the scope and purpose of the midwife's role and its contribution toward public health it is important that midwifery services collaborate with primary care trusts and public health practitioners. It is also important that focused liaison with primary care colleagues, social services and voluntary organisations is developed when informing the midwifery contribution to public health.

THE BENEFITS OF ANTENATAL CARE – AN OVERVIEW

The antenatal period provides the midwife with a window of opportunity for contributing to the reduction in maternal and neonatal morbidity and mortality rates. Early and comprehensive antenatal care is the cornerstone of improving maternal and perinatal health outcomes. Women who book early for antenatal care create an opportunity for health education and screening. Delayed or no antenatal care increases the risk of undetected complications of pregnancy that can result in severe maternal and fetal morbidity and sometimes death (Centers for Disease Control and Prevention 2000). Women who receive little or no antenatal care are three times more likely to have a low birth-weight infant when compared with women who receive early antenatal care (US Department of Health 1990). Evidence suggests that a baby's birth weight is influenced most strongly during the preconception stage and first trimester of pregnancy. Individual interventions aimed at influencing the woman's behaviour during the preconception period are problematic, as 50% of pregnancies are unplanned. The efficiency of preconception care is therefore reduced. Despite this the benefits of preconception care are well documented (Cefalo et al 1995, Hellerstedt et al 1998), but this area of practice is sparse and fragmented. Some aspects of care are concentrated within primary care provision and targeted toward potentially modifiable factors including diet and nutrition, weight, exercise, smoking, drinking, substance misuse, type of work and domestic violence. Women who would most benefit from preconception care are those least likely to access, or be able to access, the service. A whole-population approach to preconception care has been adopted, including fortification of food with folic acid to help reduce the incidence of neural tube defect. This approach to health promotion is focused to one area of health gain and leaves little room for education and understanding.

Midwifery services have a responsibility to ensure that all services are appropriate, effective, flexible, accessible, and focused to meet the needs of local communities and do not embrace the inverse care law, whereby the greatest need for health care is associated with the poorest provision (Hart 2000).

Reflection on practice

> Think about the health problems of asylum seekers you have supported. Reflect on the health problems presented and the ability of the service you provide to meet these needs.

REFUGEES AND ASYLUM SEEKERS

A refugee is a person who has fled the country of origin or is unable to return because he/she fears persecution due to race, religion, nationality, political opinion or membership of a social group. The term refugee is used to describe displaced people all over the world. In the legal context in the UK, a person is a refugee when their asylum claim has been accepted by the Home Office.

There is no breakdown of gender available for asylum seekers supported by the London boroughs, but figures from July 2001 show that the total number of women dispersed by the National Asylum Support Service (NASS) since April 2000 was 2,510 out of a total of 28,000 asylum seekers dispersed at that time. NASS is a department of the Home Office that was set up in 2000. When under the NASS system, an asylum seeker applies for support in an induction centre. If NASS accepts the claim for support the asylum seeker is allocated an accommodation centre where they may remain for up to 6 months, during which time their application is considered. The United Kingdom's Immigration and Asylum Act of 1999 set out a legislative framework for the location of asylum seekers outside of London and the Home Counties. The main aim of the dispersal arrangements was to relieve pressure on public services in London and the South East to provide support to asylum seekers in dispersal areas.

It has been recognised that asylum seekers have difficulties in adapting to a different environment and language. Cultural differences limit access to health services.

THE HEALTH OF PREGNANT REFUGEES AND ASYLUM SEEKERS

The health of pregnant asylum seekers is frequently compromised by lack of antenatal care, stressful, tortuous journeys from countries of origin, turmoil caused by war and oppression, and poor nutrition. Their health disadvantage increases the risk of perinatal mortality and morbidity

(DH 2001) and renders them ill-prepared for childbirth and parenting, particularly if antenatal care has been sparse. Screening and health promotion programmes tend to have a low uptake of asylum seekers. Pregnant women seeking asylum have experienced inequality in health care and health care provision. Their limited knowledge of the health care system has reduced their access to primary and acute care services and as such has reduced the level of maternity care received (McLeish 2002). The perinatal mortality and morbidity rates of this client group are higher in comparison to British nationals (DH 2001). The risk of maternal death in England and Wales is known to be higher in women born abroad compared with the indigenous population, and is higher in ethnic minority women (Ibison et al 1996, RCOG 2001). The risk of operative delivery in ethnic minority women is higher than in women born in England and Wales, and this may predispose to the higher maternal mortality and morbidity rates (Braveman et al 1995, Ibison 2005). It is not uncommon for women seeking asylum to be pregnant as a result of rape, increasing their chances of contracting HIV. The Black Women's Rape Action Project estimates that at least half of all women asylum seekers are pregnant as a result of rape (Cowen 2001). More than 10,000 asylum seekers have so far been dispersed throughout the UK, many of whom are from regions with HIV and Aids epidemics (Heath et al 2003).

A recent study revealed the antenatal booking patterns of asylum seekers. Out of a sample size of 61 women, two thirds were seen in antenatal care for the first time at 22 weeks or over, and 38% of these at 30 weeks or over (Kennedy & Murphy-Lawless 2001). Twenty percent of women who were reported to the 1997–1999 Confidential Enquiries into Maternal Deaths report (DH 2001) booked for maternity care after 24 weeks' gestation and had missed over four routine antenatal visits. Pregnant women who are seeking asylum enter pregnancy physically and mentally compromised, and without antenatal care they continue on a downward spiral of health disadvantage as the pregnancy advances. They are more likely to give birth to low birth-weight babies who are at an increased risk of illness or death during the first year of life. It is suggested that women from poorer social backgrounds are 1.5 times more likely to produce a low birth-weight baby or suffer perinatal death than those from other social classes (Donaldson & Donaldson 2000). They are 20 times more likely to die than those in the higher social classes. Women from minority ethnic groups, particularly those who speak little or no English, are two times more likely to die than women in the white group (DH 2001). Barker (1997) suggests that people who are born weighing less than 2.5 kg are at an increased risk of developing coronary heart disease, non-insulin dependent diabetes and stroke as adults. During pregnancy, language barriers reduce the woman's ability to make informed decisions about her care (Kirkham 2002) in an environment that is frequently viewed as alien and hostile (McLeish 2002).

MIDWIVES AND ASYLUM SEEKERS

Midwives should offer maternity care that is flexible, accessible and culturally sensitive, thereby maximising the uptake of maternity care services. When providing care the midwife should be aware of the practical problems asylum seekers and refugees face, as well as the physical and emotional effects they may have experienced in their country of origin. Although they are not a homogeneous group of people there are some experiences that may be common to all. Midwives should be mindful that counselling approaches as understood in the western culture may be seen as alien concepts to many asylum seekers and refugees. Talking about past trauma may not be a culturally acceptable way of dealing with unhappy memories, particularly when talking to a stranger.

A qualitative study that explored the experiences of pregnant asylum seekers quoted one woman's experiences of counselling.

> It was making me angry to talk about it, because you tell someone … you go, you cry every day and someone says 'Oh you cry as much as you like'. I was feeling like, he's laughing at me, like you enjoy watching me cry. I used to run away so they changed me to another and another and another. If you talk and tell someone, it won't change, it's me. Because I try to live with this myself. I try to pretend … but still my life is not changing. It's like it will never change. Where is the hope?
>
> (McLeish 2002)

Disclosure of a pregnancy if the woman is unmarried is difficult for some cultural groups, even if the woman is pregnant as a result of rape. It is not uncommon for some women to believe that the pregnancy negatively influences their asylum claim. It is important that midwives work closely with refugee councils to ensure that disclosure of pregnancy is encouraged as early as possible to ensure early antenatal care. Frequently interpreting services are used across the childbirth continuum. Midwives and other health care professionals rely heavily on accurate translation of information both from the woman to the midwife and from the midwife to the woman. It is important when working with the interpreter to ask for the nuance and body language to be interpreted as well as the spoken word, or parts of the conversation may be omitted. Despite tight resource allocation, resources should be flexible enough to allow for choice of gender when seeking professional interpreter services, as women frequently experience torture, rape and sexual assault during travel from their country of origin. Many women request female interpreter services because of religious and/or culture needs. Regardless of the reason for requesting a female interpreter, the disclosure of important, sensitive information may be withheld if the interpreter is male (see Box 2.1).

When supporting women whose pregnancies are considered to be high risk, midwives have a responsibility to exercise their autonomy and interrupt the dispersal process, reducing the risks associated with travel and high-risk pregnancy. Presenting a legitimate case to NASS is acceptable and can delay the dispersal process until the woman is deemed fit to travel.

The benefits should not be underestimated of encouraging the development of community groups and social support networks in an environment where women often feel depressed, lonely and isolated. Midwives are in a unique position to help refugees and asylum seekers forge community links through antenatal and postnatal education forums that are focused within local communities. Fostering a culture of social support,

Box 2.1
Antenatal Booking Interview – a breakdown in communication (with kind permission this true account has been detailed)

Yhala had arrived in England 23 weeks pregnant. After disclosing her pregnancy to the nurse in the emergency accommodation unit she arrived at the antenatal clinic to be booked for maternity care. The previously booked female interpreter failed to arrive so the on-line interpreting service was used. The available interpreter was male.

Midwife: What is the ethnic origin of the baby's father?
Yhala: I don't know.
Midwife: What do you mean?
Yhala: I don't know.
Midwife: You must know.
Yhala: [silence, no response, head bowed]
Midwife to interpreter: Can you ask Yhala if she has a relationship with the baby's father?
Yhala: No.
Midwife: What is the nationality of the baby's father?
Yhala: [silence, deliberation for several minutes – long talk with interpreter] I was forced to earn money to escape from my country; to do this I became a prostitute, the baby's father could be anybody.
Midwife: [stunned silence]

forging networks for the exchange of information, developing a culture that encourages health-related behaviour change and forging partnerships between the public and professional groups are key examples of the potential benefits of antenatal and postnatal education forums.

Reflection on practice

Reflect on your experiences of supporting vulnerable groups of women and their families. How can your service provide support that is flexible, adaptable, accessible and reflective of local cultural need? Where is the main area of service provision located?

POSTNATAL PERIOD

Depression antenatally increases the risk of postnatal depression (see section on postnatal depression below). Disturbing thoughts, images and nightmares about past events impact on the woman's mental well-being. Sleep disturbances, irritability, aggression and panic responses that occurred antenatally may continue into the postnatal period. It is suggested that asylum seekers may report physical symptoms only, which may lead to misunderstandings and misdiagnosis. Parent–infant attachment may be challenged in women who have conceived as a result of rape. The midwife needs to be vigilant in recognising verbal and non-verbal cues that may indicate potential problems in this area. Community postnatal support is essential in ensuring a smooth transition to parenthood.

Social isolation/exclusion, loneliness, fear, uncertainty and socio-economic disadvantage can impact negatively on postnatal health and well-being. McLeish (2002) highlighted the emotions experienced by asylum seekers and refugees during the postnatal period. Qualitative data revealed that once the baby was born, some women drew a degree of comfort from their love for the baby and the practical preoccupations of motherhood: this served to distract them from anxiety about their distress and situation. This only provided temporary relief for others who experienced uncontrollable sadness and loneliness that sometimes turned to hopelessness and despair.

REDUCING INEQUALITIES IN HEALTH AND HEALTH CARE PROVISION

The Government strategy to reduce inequality in health and health care provision is reflected in a programme for action that sets out plans to tackle health inequalities over the next 3 years. It sets out to establish the foundation to achieve the 2010 national target to reduce the gap in infant mortality across social groups and raise life expectancy in the most disadvantaged areas (DH 2003). To close the gap in infant mortality, key short-term interventions include improving the quality and accessibility of antenatal care and early years support in disadvantaged areas.

Maternity care provision straddles the primary and acute care sectors and constantly seeks to provide midwifery care that is sensitive, flexible, accessible and adaptable to meeting the needs of local communities and delivering high-quality, culturally sensitive health care. Midwives constantly seek ways to improve health care provision and work towards reducing inequalities in health, by working with local agencies and multidisciplinary groups (see Box 2.2). Sure Start is the Government's programme to deliver the best start in life for every child by bringing together early education, childcare, health and family support. The Sure Start programme aims to reduce health inequalities by making health services more accessible to the most disadvantaged children and families. The Government will invest almost £200 million over the next 4 years to support new projects. Midwifery services are integral to Sure Start projects nationally, focusing on areas of greatest need including drug and alcohol misuse, teenage pregnancy, single parents, socio-economically disadvantaged groups, domestic violence and refugees and asylum seekers.

An increasing number of focused specialist maternity care projects are developing to help meet the needs of pregnant asylum seekers. Several Sure Start programmes have included services to support the asylum seeker and refugee communities. They seek to enhance health care provision and reduce inequalities in access to health and community services. The main emphasis of a midwifery service to asylum seekers and refugees in South-East London is on:

- Reaching pregnant asylum seekers and refugees
- Providing early antenatal care regardless of whether the woman is registered with GP services or not
- Encouragement and support to register with a local GP
- Encouraging dialogue between maternity services in the dispersal area.

Box 2.2
Action points for midwives

- Support women in their rights to benefit, e.g. free NHS health care including the uptake of dental care and prescriptions
- Support women to register with a GP (The new General Medical Service contracts reward family doctors with significant additional income to provide a range of essential and additional services)
- Ensure that the application for the maternity grant has been processed
- Ensure appropriate interpreter services are employed
- Make timely links with mental health support services including local support for victims of torture
- Develop community groups both ante- and postnatal
- Collaborate with primary care colleagues and community support services including: Health visitors, Newpin, refugee organisations, refugee health teams, Home start, local Sure Start partners and workers
- Develop a referral network of specialist agencies who can offer added support on specific issues including: housing, welfare and immigration
- Remember women who are pregnant may now apply for an additional £3.00 towards the cost of healthy foods, and 4 weeks prior to birth and up to 2 weeks after the birth they may apply for the £300 cash maternity payment; a MAT B1 is required. Once the baby has been added as a dependent on the family's support application an additional £5.00 is issued for the baby until its first birthday

The Medical Foundation is a support agency for victims of torture. It is an independent charity that provides care and rehabilitation to survivors of torture and other forms of organised violence. Services include counselling, psychotherapy, marital and family therapy (British Medical Association 2001, Medical Foundation for the Care of Victims of Torture).

The National Service Framework for mental health sets down national standards for mental health (see below). It calls for the development of culturally sensitive services and goes on to identify that refugees and asylum seekers are a group vulnerable to suicide.

Midwifery services must continue to ensure that maternity care is sensitive, flexible, accessible, adaptable and reflective of the needs of local women. Maternity care for asylum seekers and refugees must remain high on the local, national and political agenda if inequality in health and health care provision for this group is to improve. Close liaison and collaboration with PCT colleagues is an essential part of this drive and will ensure that the greatest area of health care provision is allocated in areas of greatest need.

EMOTIONAL DISTURBANCES ACROSS THE CHILDBIRTH CONTINUUM

Emotional disturbances during pregnancy may be influenced by social, physical and psychological factors including unplanned pregnancy, single parenthood, unsupportive partner, marital conflict, fear of childbirth, previous traumatic delivery, homelessness, poor housing, inadequate finance and uncertainty about social circumstances. The provision of holistic health care that encompasses all dimensions of health including mental, physical, emotional, societal, sexual and spiritual health should serve to identify the woman's predisposition to emotional liability. Antenatal, intrapartum and postnatal care can then be planned ensuring that care and support are responsive to the needs of the woman and her infant. The mental health of the woman has the potential to influence the emotional and psychological health of the infant. With good communication and appropriate screening, pre-existing or existing mental ill health may be established in the early antenatal period. Previous history of postnatal depression or emotional lability may be confirmed, enabling the midwife to work in partnership with the woman toward ensuring optimum mental health.

POSTNATAL DEPRESSION

Postnatal depression refers to a non-psychotic depressive episode that begins or extends into the postpartum period. The clinical features of postnatal depression can be generalised to depression that occurs outside of the childbearing experience and includes: tearfulness, lethargy, irritability, anxiety, over-sensitivity, disturbed sleep patterns, low self-esteem and irrational fears. Conversely, it is suggested that the signs and symptoms described can be considered a normal response to the demands of becoming a mother (Paradice 1995). Episodes of postnatal depression may begin within 2–4 weeks after birth and may last for 2–6 months, usually resolving by 1 year. The United Kingdom Confidential Enquiry into Maternal Deaths reports that death resulting from mental illness is the second leading cause of maternal mortality. If all deaths in this category were accurately recorded, mental illness would be the leading cause of death. Psychiatric disorders are known to have caused or contributed to 12% of maternal deaths, 10% of which were due to suicide. The cases detailed in the Confidential Enquiry reveal that suicide was four times more likely to occur in the 9 months after childbirth than during pregnancy. Childbearing women who complete suicide expressed warning signs throughout pregnancy and had increased risk factors, including: previous history of self harm, depression, adverse life events, lack of social support and social isolation. In order to improve detection rates of mental ill health and thus influence early intervention, the recommendations from the confidential enquiries suggests that rigorous antenatal screening should be employed together with early management of identified postnatal psychiatric illness (DH 2001).

GOVERNMENT AGENDA

Mental health and well-being is one of the health priorities detailed in *Saving Lives: Our Healthier Nation* (DH 1999). The National Service Framework for mental health was therefore considered one of the priority frameworks for development. The framework sets national standards and defines service models for promoting mental health and treating mental illness. One of the milestones detailed in Standard 1 of the

Framework refers to maternity services working with health visitors to develop and implement protocols for the assessment and management of mental health during pregnancy and after delivery. Promoting a seamless service for care delivery is attractive for those who experience mental ill health. Good practice involves systems and foundations that support early antenatal referrals to health visitors and mental health services if the woman is identified as being at risk of developing postnatal depression. An early antenatal visit from the health visitor will provide complementary support to the woman, further identify areas of mental health need and encourage the establishment of the woman/health visitor relationship early. The midwife and the health visitor would have an opportunity to work collaboratively, employing other support services where deemed appropriate. This might involve social service referral and possible pre-birth conference participation.

ANTENATAL RECOGNITION

During the antenatal consultation, preferably at the booking visit, the midwife should establish the woman's previous history of mental ill health. This should include the nature of the illness, the severity, its clinical presentation, the timing of onset, the duration, medication taken and support services involved during this time. Postnatal depression should not be used as a generic term to describe other mental illness as this may lead to the severity of the recurrence being underestimated and opportunities for prevention missed. It is not uncommon for women who experience postnatal depression to start feeling depressed during pregnancy. It is suggested that an objective, psycho-social assessment during pregnancy improves recognition of women at risk (Webster et al 2000). Failure to recognise antenatal depression is a failure to address a major public health problem (Fawcett et al 1998).

A study sought to assess whether symptoms of depression were more common or severe after childbirth than during pregnancy. Researchers assessed the mood of mothers throughout pregnancy and after childbirth and reported symptoms of depression at each stage. More mothers moved above the threshold for depression between 18 and 32 weeks of pregnancy than between 32 weeks of pregnancy and 8 weeks postpartum. The study demonstrated that symptoms of depression are more common or severe during pregnancy than after childbirth. The researchers emphasise the need for research and clinical efforts to be moved towards understanding, recognising and treating antenatal depression (Evans et al 2001). Items displayed in Box 2.3 are currently used in a specialist midwifery community clinic in South-East London to explore issues related to mental health and well-being, once a mental health history has been established. The questions are used within the context of the woman's everyday life. Frequently during discussion, points are raised that reveal risk factors that are associated with postnatal depression and trigger therapeutic discussion related to, for example, marital conflict, single parenthood, dysfunctional family relationships and fears of failure (Dunkley-Bent 2004). Referral to and collaboration with psychological services is frequently initiated. The importance of routine enquiry at booking about previous psychiatric history should not be underestimated.

Box 2.3
One-to-one discussion or triggers for group discussion

- Antenatal experience to date
- Planned or unplanned pregnancy
- Labour hopes and fears
- Parenting hopes and fears
- Debriefing post delivery
- 'Bonding' issues, 'instant love'
- Support systems
- Coping mechanisms
- Social expectations
- Personal expectations

Action plan
- Influence the things you can
- Preparation: home/family/birth/baby
- Identify support person and involve in the discussion
- Set realistic goals

Reflection on practice

How can the items detailed in Box 2.3 be used to explore factors that may predispose to feelings of depression?
Think about the range of issues that could be explored for each point.

BABY BLUES

Postpartum baby blues is frequently described as a period of weepiness and mood instability. It may be characterised by feelings of anxiety, irritability, forgetfulness, lability of mood and fatigue, and occurs between the third and tenth postnatal days. The prevalence is reported to be 70–80% (Blackburn & Lopar 1992). There is no specific treatment but education and awareness is an important part of the midwives' health promotion strategy in encouraging early identification of symptoms that persist. It is well documented that there is a higher incidence of the blues among women who experience postnatal depression (Stowe & Nemeroff 1995, Dunkley-Bent 2004).

It may be useful to highlight the cocktail of events that surround the baby blues, that may present a physical challenge to most women. The following areas may be discussed during antenatal and postnatal education sessions.

- The settling of emotions after the euphoria frequently experienced after delivery
- Slight temperature increase frequently experienced with venous engorgement where some women experience breast tenderness
- Involuting uterus that may manifest as mild/moderate to severe uterine pain depending on the woman's parity
- Sore or painful perineum and/or caesarean section scar
- General aches and pains from different positions assumed during the childbirth process.

PUERPERAL PSYCHOSIS

This is the most severe form of postnatal mental ill health. It is characterised by delusions and hallucinations about self, the baby and/or others. It is a severe form of depression and may result in infanticide or suicide. The prevalence is one in 500 births. The onset is rapid, with reported cases occurring as early as 2 weeks post partum. Immediate psychiatric support is required as hospitalisation is usually necessary. The midwife's role involves early detection, including risk factors presented antenatally, and early referral to psychiatric support services.

SCREENING

Despite the drive to improve screening and recognition for postnatal depression, there is little evidence that this has resulted in improved care (DH 2001). The Edinburgh Postnatal Depression Scale provides a reliable basis for screening for postnatal depression. It was developed by Cox, Holden and Sagovsky in 1987, as a 10-point self-reporting scale about feelings in the past week. It is a reliable psychometric test rather than a diagnostic instrument. A large community study revealed a specificity of 92% and a sensitivity of 88% (Murray & Carothers 1990). The tool is currently used more widely by health visitors than general practitioners and midwives. Distribution of the tool varies in terms of timing. Randomised controlled trials have demonstrated that the variations in the administration times do not affect the scale's validity (Brown & Lumley 1998). The nature of the questions does not encourage the describing of symptoms fully, but they do provoke thought. Completion of the tool is frequently preceded by discussion, particularly for those women who score above the predetermined cut-off line of 12. Dunkley (2000) argues that people who cannot read English and/or are from different cultures may be excluded from completing the tool, or may be unable to respond to questions. This may be due to a cultural expression of psychological disorders into a language of signs, behaviour and physical symptoms that are not represented on the Edinburgh Postnatal Depression Scale. Helman (1990) refers to this as cross-cultural somatisation. As described above, the expression of symptoms may be misunderstood or misinterpreted, leading to poor identification in groups who are extremely vulnerable.

RISK FACTORS

Factors that predispose to postnatal depression include: history of psychiatric disorder, previous history of postnatal depression, and socioeconomic disadvantage. Midwives should be mindful of women who present with a history of severe mental illness, as the risk of recurrence is between one in two and one in three following delivery. The risk of recurrence is at its greatest in the first 30 days post partum (Wieck et al 1991). There has been a strong association between postnatal depression and absent partners or poor relationships with partners and marital conflict (Gallagher et al 1997, Beck 1998).

Obstetric risk factors during pregnancy and birth do not significantly increase the risk of depression. An Australian-based study sought to examine obstetric risk factors for postnatal depression in an urban and rural community sample. Obstetric information, personality, psychiatric history and life events information was obtained, and depression status was assessed at 8 weeks postpartum using the Edinburgh Postnatal Depression Scale. The results demonstrated that most obstetric risk factors during pregnancy and birth do not significantly increase the risk of postnatal depression. The researchers emphasised the importance of psycho-social risk factors and the association with postnatal depression (Johnstone et al 2001). The maternal and infant relationship plays an important role in infant behavioural and cognition development. Accumulating evidence suggests that postnatal depression is associated with disturbances in child cognition and emotional development in children aged between 4 and 5 years, particularly among children of socio-economically disadvantaged mothers (Murray & Cooper 1997). Midwives should discuss and encourage strategies that serve to enhance parent–infant attachment including early skin-to-skin contact, breastfeeding and baby massage. It is strongly recommended that health professionals, particularly midwives and GPs who are at the forefront of maternity care, strengthen risk assessment strategies used to identify women who are at risk of developing mental illness.

THE MIDWIFE'S ROLE

Antenatal education programmes can be effective in improving important aspects of psycho-social functioning (Barlow & Coren 2001). Midwives have a responsibility to raise awareness about postnatal depression in the antenatal period (see Box 2.4). It is important to emphasise that early detection of depressive symptoms with prompt reporting can reduce the severity of the illness. Okano et al (1998) found that women who attended antenatal education and suffered from postnatal depression were more likely to receive early psychiatric referral, with a subsequent reduction in the severity of the illness, than control counterparts. Raising awareness about the factors that predispose to postnatal

Box 2.4
Practical things that you can do in antenatal and postnatal groups

- Raise awareness about mental health and ill health
- Present health as an holistic concept and explore the influences of health deficit
- Foster an environment of social support by emphasising valuable learning that can take place within the group
- Introduce the idea of a telephone network or telephone tree
- Provide the environment for ongoing antenatal drop in classes once the mainstream classes have concluded
- At the postnatal reunion class, remind the group about the postnatal education/support classes
- Invite members of the multi-disciplinary team to attend, including the health visitor and a midwife/health visitor who can lead baby massage sessions to enhance parent–infant attachment
- Involve community support services including Newpin and family support workers
- Involve the local Sure Start partners and workers
- Allow the group to evolve as you remain the facilitator.

depression and the signs and symptoms are extremely important and integral to the midwife's role. An informal approach to raising awareness may be adopted by some, whilst others may choose a rather scientifically focused approach. The optimal timing of antenatal interventions to reduce the incidence of postnatal depression is still not established. Researchers sought to test whether an education intervention given to women in the antenatal period would reduce postnatal depression. The intervention was an education package designed to inform women of mood changes that occur in the prenatal and postpartum periods. The results demonstrated that the antenatal intervention made no difference to the reduction of postnatal depression (Hayes et al 2001). It is suggested however that until the aetiology of postnatal depression is better understood, early recognition and aggressive management may be a more feasible and effective goal than prediction or prevention, as demonstrated by Okano et al (1998). The physical and psychological benefits of continuity of carer are well documented (Green et al 2000, Hodnett 2002). A recent study sought to explore the prevention of postnatal depression by assessing the effect of continuity of midwifery care on rates of postnatal depression in high-risk women. The researchers found that while continuous midwifery care had no impact on psychiatric outcome, it was highly successful at engaging women in treatment. They concluded that continuity of carer has an important contribution to make in the care of childbearing women with mental health problems (Marks et al 2003).

CONCLUSION

The midwife plays an important role in contributing to the health of the nation through focused, individualised care of the woman and her family throughout the childbirth continuum. The potential for health enhancement through health promotion is unquestionable. Enhancing the health potential of asylum-seeking women is not a basic process and requires resource commitment and a multi-agency, multi-disciplinary approach. Health promotion can only be truly effective in this situation if the process is delivered within the context of the person's everyday life. Emotional disturbances exist across the childbirth continuum for all women. They may range from the euphoria and elation experienced by many women after childbirth, to depression or psychotic illness. It is important for midwives to embrace this aspect of health care as an integral part of midwifery practice, thereby helping to reduce the stigma associated with mental ill health. Good communication skills and robust assessment and screening tools will help midwives to explore mental health with the same rigour that underpins the assessment of physical well-being across the childbirth continuum. Collaboration and liaison with members of the multidisciplinary and multi-agency team are essential when supporting women and their families during a time in their lives that is frequently perceived to be the most challenging.

References

Barker D 1997 The long term outcome of retarded fetal growth. Clinical Obstetrics and Gynaecology 40(4):853–863

Barlow J, Coren E 2001 Parent-training programmes for improving maternal psycho-social health (Cochrane review) (update of most recent substantive update: 2 February 2001). In: The Cochrane Library, Oxford: Update Software, issue 2

Beck C T 1998 A check list to identify women at risk for developing postpartum depression. Journal of Obstetrics, Gynaecological and Neonatal Nursing 27(1):39–46

Blackburn S T, Lopar D L 1992 Maternal Fetal and Neonatal Physiology. A Clinical Perspective. Saunders, Philadelphia

Braveman P, Egerter S, Edmonston F, Verdon M 1995 Racial/ethnic differences in the likelihood of cesarean delivery, California. American Journal of Public Health 85:625–630

British Medical Association 2001 Asylum seekers and health: a BMA and Medical Foundation for the Care of Victims of Torture dossier. BMA, London

Brown S, Lumley J 1998 Maternal health after childbirth: results of an Australian population based survey. British Journal of Obstetrics and Gynaecology 105:156–161

Cefalo R, Bowes W, Moos M 1995 Preconception care: a means of prevention. Baillière's Clinical Obstetrics and Gynaecology 9(3):403–416

Centers for Disease Control and Prevention 2000 Entry into pre-natal care – United States 1989–1997. MMWR Morbidity Weekly Report 49:393–398

Cowen T 2001 Unequal Treatment: Findings from a Refugee Health Survey in Barnet. Refugee Health Access Project, London

Cox J L, Holden J M, Sagovsky R 1987 Detection of postnatal depression. Development of the 10-item Edinburgh Postnatal Depression Scale. British Journal of Psychiatry 150:782–786

Department of Health 1999 Saving Lives: Our Healthier Nation. DH, London

Department of Health 2001 CEMD. Why mothers die. Confidential Enquiry into Maternal Deaths, 1997–1999. TSO, London

Department of Health 2003 Tackling Health Inequalities – A Programme For Action. DH, London

Donaldson L J, Donaldson R J 2000 Essential Public Health Medicine, 2nd edn. Petroc Press, Newbury

Dunkley J 2000 Health Promotion in Midwifery: A Resource for Health Professionals. Baillière Tindall, Edinburgh

Dunkley-Bent J 2004 A consultant midwife's community clinic. British Journal of Midwifery 12(3):144–150, 171

Evans J, Heron J, Francomb H, Oke S, Golding J 2001 Cohort of depressed mood during pregnancy and after childbirth. British Medical Journal 323(7307):257–260

Fawcett J, Tulman L, Myers S 1998 Development of the inventory of functional status after childbirth. Journal of Nurse Midwifery 33:252–260

Gallagher R, Steven E, Ritter C, Ritter S, Lavin J 1997 Marriage, intimate support and depression during pregnancy. Journal of Health Psychology 2(4):457–469

Green J, Renfrew M, Curtis P 2000 Continuity of care: what matters to women. A review of the evidence. Midwifery 16:186–196

Hart T L 2000 Commentary: three decades of the inverse care law. British Medical Journal 320:18–19

Hayes B, Muller R, Bradley B 2001 Perinatal depression: a randomised controlled trial of an antenatal education intervention for primparas. Birth issues in perinatal care. Birth 28(1):28–35

Heath T, Jeffries R, Lloyd A 2003 Asylum Statistics in the UK. Home Office, London. Online. Available: www.homeoffice.gov.uk

Heller R F, Heller T D, Pattison S 2003 Putting the public back into public health. Part II: How can public health be accountable to the public? Public Health 117(1):66–71

Hellerstedt W, Pitie P, Lando H, Curry S, Mcbride C, Grothaus L, Nelson J 1998 Differences in preconceptional and prenatal behaviours in women with intended and unintended pregnancies. American Journal of Public Health 88(4):663–666

Helman C G 1990 Culture, Health and Illness. Butterworth-Heinemann, Oxford

Hodnett E D 2002 Continuity of caregivers for care during pregnancy and childbirth (Cochrane Review). In: The Cochrane Library, Issue 4. Update Software, Oxford. Last amended March 1998

Ibison J M 2005 Ethnicity and mode of delivery in 'low-risk' first-time mothers, East London, 1988–1997. European Journal of Obstetrics, Gynecology and Reproductive Biology 118(2):199–205

Ibison J, Swerdlow A, Whitehead J, Marmot M 1996 Maternal mortality in England and Wales: an analysis by country of birth. British Journal of Obstetrics and Gynaecology 103:973–980

Johnstone S J, Boyce P M, Hickey A R et al 2001 Obstetric risk factors for postnatal depression in urban and rural community samples. Australian and New Zealand Journal of Psychiatry 35(1):69–74

Kennedy P, Murphy-Lawless J 2001 The maternity care needs of refugee and asylum seeking women in Ireland. In: Treacher A et al (eds) 2003 Feminist Review 73(1):39–53

Kirkham M 2002 The inverse care law in antenatal midwifery care. British Journal of Midwifery 10(8):509–513

McLeish J 2002 Mothers in Exile: Maternity Experiences of Asylum Seekers in England. Maternity Alliance, London

Marks M N, Siddle K, Warwick C 2003 Can we prevent postnatal depression? A randomised controlled trial to assess the effect of continuity of midwifery care on rates of postnatal depression in high-risk women. Journal of Maternal–Fetal and Neonatal Medicine 13(2):119–127

Medical Foundation for the Care of Victims of Torture. Website www.torturecare.org.uk

Murray L, Carothers A D 1990 The validation of the Edinburgh Postnatal Depression scale on a community sample. British Journal of Psychiatry 157:288–290

Murray L, Cooper P 1997 Effects of postnatal depression on infant development. Archives of Diseases in Childhood 77:99–101

Okano T, Nagata S, Hasegawa M et al 1998 Effectiveness of antenatal education about postnatal depression: a comparison of two groups of Japanese mothers. Journal of Mental Health 7:191–198

Paradice K 1995 Postnatal depression: a normal response to motherhood? British Journal of Midwifery 3(12):632–635

Royal College of Midwives 2000 Vision 2000. RCM, London

Royal College of Obstetricians and Gynaecologists 2001 Caesarean section. Chapter 20 in: CEMD. Why mothers die. Confidential Enquiry into Maternal Deaths, 1997–1999. RCOG, London, p317

Sim S, Schiller G, Walters R 2002 Public Health Workforce Planning for London. DH, London

Stowe Z N, Nemeroff C B 1995 Women at risk for postpartum depression. American Journal of Obstetrics and Gynecology 173:639–645

US Department of Health 1990 Healthy People 2000: National Health Promotion and Disease Prevention Objectives. US Department of Health and Human Services, Public Health Service, Washington DC. DHHS publication 91-50213

Webster J, Linnane J W J, Dibley L M et al 2000 Improving antenatal recognition of women at risk for postnatal depression. Australian and New Zealand Journal of Obstetrics and Gynaecology 40(4):409–412

Wieck A, Kumar R, Hirst A D, Marks M N, Campbell I C, Checkley S A 1991 Increased sensitivity of dopamine receptors and recurrence of affective psychosis after childbirth. British Medical Journal 303:613–616

Chapter 3

Expanding horizons: developing a public health perspective in midwifery

Cindy Carlson

CHAPTER CONTENTS

INTRODUCTION

This chapter explores what public health actually means and its relevance to midwifery practice. Initially it considers definitions of public health that are common currency and attempts to unpick these, while also providing a historical perspective. From there, attention is given to part of the 'science' of public health, essential epidemiological terms that are of relevance to the understanding of the place of midwifery in improving population health. The definition of public health is then further refined by looking at what competencies or standard areas are used in different countries for describing what public health professionals need to be able to do. These are compared with midwifery competencies to examine how much public health practice is already integrated into the work of midwives, and key elements are explored in greater depth to consider the specific public health functions midwives might perform and the skills they need to do so.

UNDERSTANDING PUBLIC HEALTH

'Public health' is one of those terms that sometimes defies definition, and as such then takes on an aura of mystique, where practitioners are those initiated into the secret rites of the cult. The definitions put forward in recent years do not seem to do much to demystify what public health actually is. One of the more widely spread definitions of public health is: 'the science and art of presenting disease, prolonging life and promoting health through the organised efforts of society' (Acheson 1988). The US government defines public health as 'what we, as a society, do collectively to assure the conditions in which people can be healthy' (Centers for Disease Control 1999). These definitions, when unpicked, show 'public health' to be all those activities aimed at securing and promoting the health of a population that are the collective responsibility of some social organisation, for example the state or government. Our understanding of public health becomes clearer when we explore what types of functions or activities are covered under the rubric of public health, as we will see below.

Public health came into its own in the nineteenth century, when European and North American countries were undergoing rapid industrialisation, which brought with it both great wealth and great misery. Social reformers concerned themselves with the conditions of both workers and the destitute, and began to look at how to make changes in people's social, economic and environmental conditions as part of improving living conditions and well-being overall. Primary amongst these reformers was Edwin Chadwick, Secretary to the Poor Law Commission, whose Report on an Enquiry into the Sanitary Condition of the Labouring Population of Great Britain (Chadwick 1843) galvanised the social conscience of the middle classes of the day, and led to eventual changes in law to the advantage of those living in poverty. John Snow's powers of observation during a cholera epidemic in London in 1848 led to the first technical health protection intervention – the removal of the Broad Street pump from the source of cholera-contaminated water. Public health activists throughout the nineteenth century focused primarily on social and environmental conditions that impacted on health, and paved the way to major improvement in population health more generally through a reduction in infectious diseases. During most of the 1800s health care workers had little idea of what actually caused the diseases they were treating, as Box 3.1 illustrates. (Most continued to operate under the 'miasma' theory, that 'bad' air and 'bad' water were to blame – not completely without reason.)

It was only towards the end of the nineteenth century with the invention of the microscope and the identification of the first bacteria that 'germ theory' was born and action began to shift away from improving living conditions to developing medicines to prevent and treat diseases. 'Miasmists' aligned themselves with social radicals who continued to push for social reform as the best way to improve health and living conditions. 'Contagionists' were more politically conservative and pushed for medical solutions to health problems (Young 1999).

Box 3.1
Example – health protection in childbirth

Ignaz Semmelweis was a Viennese obstetrician in the 1800s, who developed a keen interest in trying to explain, and then reduce, puerperal fever among patients in his maternity hospital. The hospital had been divided into two wards to help improve the quality of training for health care professionals. One ward was attended to only by (all male) medical students while the other ward was attended by midwives. The medical student ward records showed consistently higher rates of puerperal fever than the midwives' ward, which excited Semmelweis's interest even more. On investigating practices in both wards, he observed that puerperal fever appeared to spread from bed to bed only on the medical student ward. After the unfortunate death of one of the pathology professors from a fever whose symptoms were very similar to puerperal fever (having been stuck by a student's autopsy knife), Semmelweis began to suspect that puerperal fever might be transmitted by the medical students themselves. On closer investigation he observed that medical students would go directly from the autopsy room in the mornings to ward rounds and examine all women in labour, with no hygienic precautions taken. Handwashing was unheard of in hospitals but Semmelweis instituted a regime whereby medical students had to wash their hands in chlorinated lime solution. This intervention led to a dramatic decline in morbidity and mortality by puerperal fever on the medical students' ward. Sadly the other doctors in the hospital ridiculed Semmelweis's ideas and he eventually went mad.

Public health may also be understood through an analysis of the determinants of health. Several models of health determinants have been put forward. One of the most commonly used is shown here in Figure 3.1, developed by Dahlgren and Whitehead in 1991.

The factors influencing health are multiple and multi-level, as indicated by Figure 3.1. While individual factors, such as age, gender and genetic

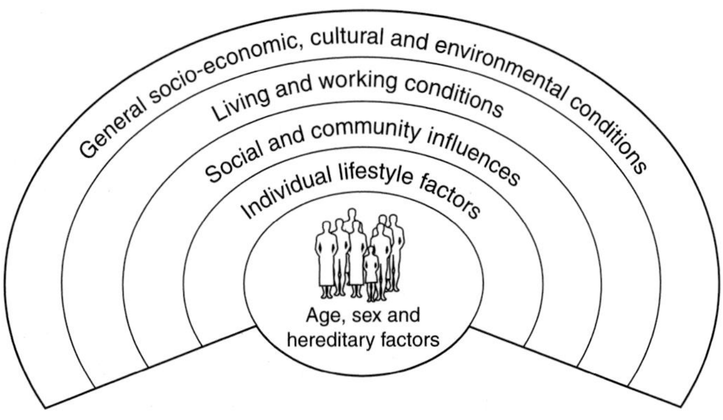

Fig. 3.1 Health determinants (reproduced with permission from Dahlgren & Whitehead 1991).

make-up create a predisposition to good or poor health, wider determinants of health have been shown to be as, or more, important in dictating an individual's or community's health status. The UK House of Commons Select Committee Report (2000) provides greater detail of the wider determinants, taken from the Public Health Green Paper Reducing Health Inequalities: An Action Report:

Fixed:	Genes, sex, ageing
Social and Economic:	Poverty, employment, social exclusion
Environment:	Air quality, housing, water quality, social environment
Lifestyle:	Diet, physical activity, smoking, alcohol, sexual behaviour, drugs
Access to services:	Education, National Health Service, social services, transport, leisure

Today, depending on the country, social policy dictates what determinants of health governments will and will not intervene in for protecting and improving the health of their populations. Health care is a major feature of public health policy and can absorb a large part of a country's health-related resources. Environmental health protection remains an important public health function, though in countries such as England, where the public health function sits within the National Health Service and environmental health sits with local governments, there have been structural barriers to a unified approach to protecting the public's health. Other traditional local government public health functions include such areas as support to families, community development and urban regeneration.

Midwives have an honourable tradition themselves in the public health arena. The health promotion work training women in 'mothering skills' carried out by midwives and health visitors in the first half of the twentieth century helped lead to a radical drop in infant mortality rates, from 150 per 1000 in 1900 to 55 per 1000 in 1940 (Williams et al 1994).

MEASURING MATERNAL HEALTH

One important area of public health is being able to assess the degree of a particular problem by measuring its extent in a population. The main aspect of a midwife's role is ensuring a positive outcome to pregnancy, measured through the health of mothers and their infants. Throughout the world numerous initiatives have been developed to tackle the problem of poor pregnancy outcomes and high infant death rates. In the 1960s the World Health Organization (WHO) reported its concerns about the much higher rates of mother and child mortality in developing countries. Its 1969 Expert Committee Report found that high mortality in both mothers and their children were caused mainly by poor nutrition and widespread infection, as well as dangerous and excessive childbearing related to poor access to health services (WHO 1992).

Sadly, little has changed since the Expert Committee first published its report thirty-plus years ago. Maternal and infant mortality rates remain unacceptably high in many developing countries, as well as within more socially excluded groups in developed countries. Before looking at the figures, it is worth spending some time reviewing definitions of mortality (death) and morbidity (illness) related to maternal health. The focus is primarily on mortality, perhaps a strange indicator of 'health'. Mortality is most often used for understanding the health of populations because there is no ambiguity about death, though there may be a great deal of controversy over the cause of death. In general death rates are seen as a useful way of measuring health status within populations and comparing these across populations. In public health, various measures of mortality and morbidity are used to describe what is happening in that population. A few of these are given here.

Crude birth rate

$$\frac{\text{the number of births in a given year}}{\text{the population total at the mid-point of that year}} \times 1000$$

Crude death rate

$$\frac{\text{the number of deaths in a given year}}{\text{the population total at the mid-point of that year}} \times 1000$$

Age-specific death rate

$$\frac{\text{the number of deaths in a specific age group}}{\text{the total population of that age group at the mid-point of the year}} \times 1000$$

Rates of disease can be measured in similar ways, by creating disease-specific rates for the whole population or within specific age groups. When measuring disease there are two key rates to understand: incidence and prevalence.

Incidence is the number of new cases of an 'event' or disease in a population, within a defined population. To determine the incidence rate the number of new cases is divided by the total population at risk of having this disease. For example, when calculating the incidence rate of eclampsia in a population, the numerator would be the number of new cases of eclampsia reported, divided by the total number of women of reproductive age (15 to 49) within the population. This is because only pregnant women can develop eclampsia. A more accurate denominator would be the total number of women who become pregnant within that particular year, but this may be harder to determine.

Prevalence is the number of existing cases of an 'event' or disease within a defined population. As with incidence rate, the prevalence rate is determined by counting the number of people with a particular condition, divided by the total population at risk for developing that condition within a population. Point prevalence is a measure of the number of people with the condition at a specific 'point' in time (e.g. 1 July), while

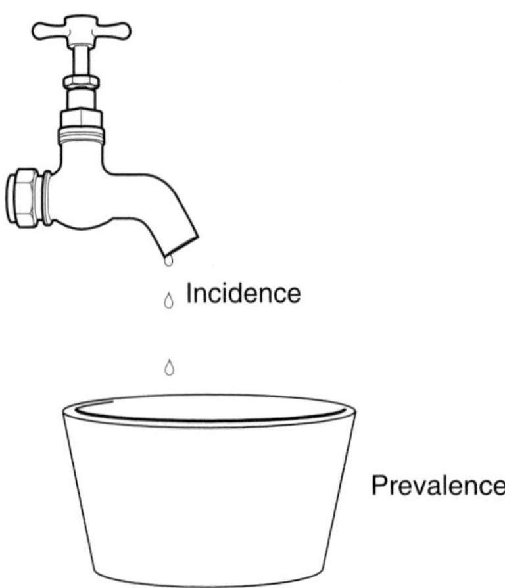

Fig. 3.2 The prevalence pot.

period prevalence is a measure of the number of people with the condition in a given time period.

The difference between incidence and prevalence can be understood as follows: incidence is about 'becoming' while prevalence is about 'being' (see Fig. 3.2). An example of this, when discussing pregnancy, is that the incidence of pregnancy = the number of women who become pregnant during a specific time period vs the number of women who are pregnant during a specific time period. Women who already are pregnant would not be included in the denominator for the incidence rate; they are not at risk of becoming pregnant since they already are pregnant!

A maternal death can be defined as: 'the death of a woman while pregnant or within 42 days of termination of pregnancy, regardless of the site or duration of pregnancy, from any cause related to or aggravated by the pregnancy or its management' (WHO 1999:9). This same WHO document goes on to identify two main types of maternal death: direct or indirect obstetric death. Direct obstetric death is any death arising from complications of pregnancy, labour or the postpartum period, usually due to haemorrhage, sepsis, eclampsia, obstructed labour or the complications of unsafe abortion. Other causes of direct obstetric death include dangerous obstetric interventions, omissions or incorrect treatment (WHO 1999). Indirect obstetric deaths result from pre-existing conditions, or conditions that arise as a result of the pregnancy (e.g. diabetes, malaria, HIV/AIDS, cardio-vascular disease).

There are three measures of maternal mortality that are most commonly used when trying to understand maternal death within a given population. These are maternal mortality ratio, maternal mortality rate, and lifetime risk of maternal death.

Maternal mortality ratio

This is the number of maternal deaths during a given year per 100,000 live births during the same period, or

$$\frac{\text{\# of maternal deaths during year x}}{\text{\# of live births during year x}} \times 100{,}000$$

The maternal mortality ratio gives an idea of the obstetric risk associated with each pregnancy.

Maternal mortality rate

This is the number of maternal deaths in a given period per 100,000 women of reproductive age (usually 15–49 years).

$$\frac{\text{\# of maternal deaths during year x}}{\text{\# of women of reproductive age in year x}} \times 100{,}000$$

The calculation measures both the obstetric risk and the frequency with which women are exposed to this risk.

Lifetime risk of maternal death

Lifetime risk of maternal death is estimated by multiplying the maternal mortality rate by the length of the reproductive period (average around 35 years). This allows planners to review both the probability of becoming pregnant and the probability of dying as a result of pregnancy, cumulated across a woman's reproductive years. Another way of calculating the lifetime risk of maternal death is by multiplying the total fertility rate by the maternal mortality rate. The total fertility rate can be calculated by taking the sum of the age-specific fertility rates for women of child-bearing age (15–49), as explained in Box 3.2.

There are numerous direct causes of maternal death, and these too differ between developed and developing countries. The pie charts (Figs 3.3

Box 3.2 Fertility rates and mortality rates/ratios: calculation

Age-specific fertility rate is the number of live births in women in a specific age group divided by all women in that same age group, multiplied by 1000. In the US in 1993, the age-specific fertility rates for women of all races were:

15–19:	60.7/1000
20–24:	114.6/1000
25–29:	117.4/1000
30–34:	80.2/1000
35–39:	32.5/1000
40–44:	5.9/1000
45–49:	0.3/1000

This information in itself provides useful facts about what is happening with births in a population. In order to calculate the total fertility rate (TFR), you take the sum of these rates, which comes to 411.6/1000. This then is multiplied by 5 (because each age band represents 5 years) to 2,058 births/1000 women, or 2.06 births per woman. The TFR therefore provides us with a snapshot of the average number of births per woman we can expect to see in a specific population. The TFR in many European countries is less than 2, while in some developing countries it is as high as 7 or more.

The **maternal mortality ratio** for this would be calculated as 2,200 maternal deaths divided by 17,480,250 live births multiplied by 100,000, which comes to 12.6 deaths per 100,000 live births. In most developed countries the maternal mortality ratio is around 27 maternal deaths per 100,000 live births. In developing countries the ratio is far higher, at 480 maternal deaths per 100,000 live births.

(continued)

Box 3.2 *Continued*

To take this example further, if the **maternal mortality rate** is calculated (hypothetically) as 2,200 maternal deaths in 1993 divided by 43,750,000 women of reproductive age in 1993 × 100,000, the result is a maternal mortality rate of 5 maternal deaths per 100,000 women of reproductive age. This is an average maternal mortality rate for a developed country. In many developing countries the maternal mortality rate can be 100 deaths (or more) per 100,000 women.

Finally, then, to calculate the lifetime risk of maternal death, you need to multiply the maternal mortality rate (5/100,000) by the number of reproductive years (35) to get a 0.17% lifetime risk of maternal death. In developing countries, with their far higher maternal mortality rate, the lifetime risk of dying, using the above figures, would be a 3.5% lifetime risk of maternal death.

Adapted from: Young (1999) and WHO (1999)

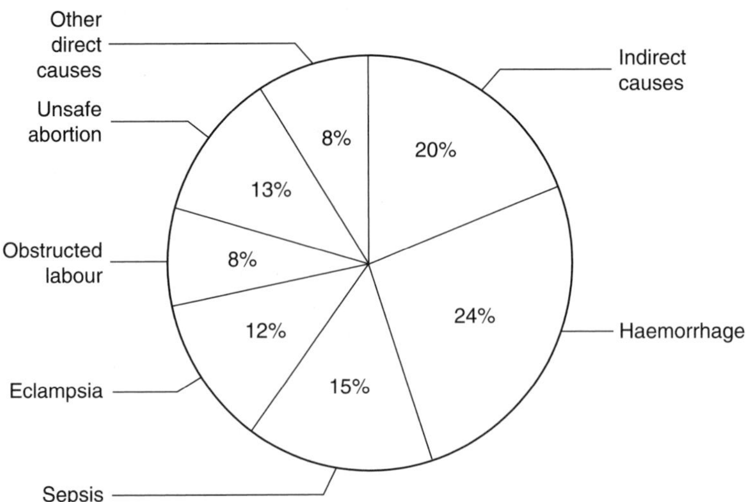

Fig. 3.3 Causes of maternal deaths: global estimates (WHO/UNFPA/UNICEF/ World Bank 1999:13).

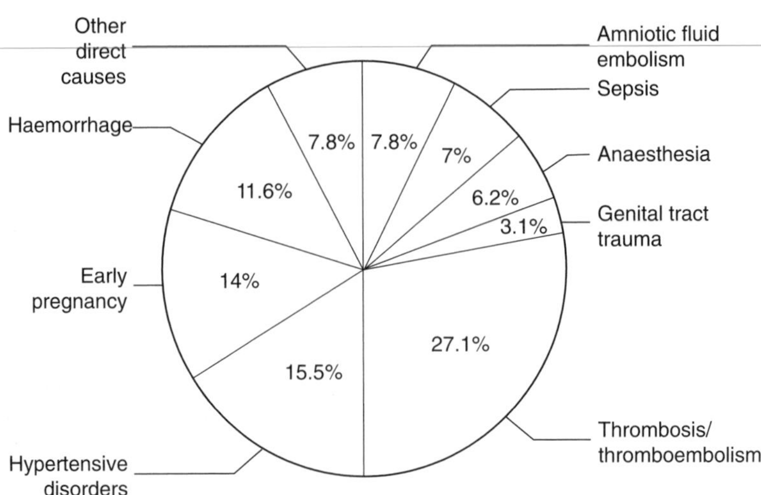

Fig. 3.4 Causes of direct maternal deaths, UK 1991–1993 (Reproduced with permission from Donaldson L J, Donaldson R J 2000:251).

and 3.4) illustrate the main direct causes of maternal death, comparing the global picture and the UK.

These measures give health workers some empirical evidence of the extent of a particular problem in their community. For example, if records indicate high rates of hypertension within a particular group it could be more resource-effective to try to tackle hypertension through group-wide interventions, as well as supporting individual women, especially if the causes of such high rates of hypertension are generally well understood. In the same way other psycho-social factors of keen interest to midwives can also be measured (e.g. rates of postnatal depression, breastfeeding, prenatal anxiety, etc.). We will now look at what midwives could do to *practise* public health and improve the health of their communities.

PRACTISING PUBLIC HEALTH

Having looked at what public health is, and the importance of being able to measure health and disease within a given population we now look at the midwife's role as a public health practitioner. During the end of the 1990s and early 2000s a number of countries reviewed their public health functions to try to modernise how public health operates. These exercises have included setting or revising standards and competency areas for public health. In England much effort has gone into reworking the essential paradigm of public health being within the medical domain to acknowledging the much greater contribution of other professional groups and opening up official public health organisations, such as the Faculty of Public Health Medicine, to non-medics. This particular concern has not been an issue in countries where public health has always been multi-disciplinary, such as the US, though the US has also revised its public health standards and public health curriculum. Table 3.1 compares how different countries have broken down the public health function into component areas.

In England the Chief Medical Officer recommended that the public health workforce be divided into three levels (DH 2001):

- **Public health specialists**: from a variety of disciplines who have a strategic influence on planning and co-ordinating the breadth of public health function for a population. This group includes Directors of Public Health, who may either be public health consultants or multi-disciplinary specialists. It has been suggested that there is a sub-group of specialists who may not have the breadth of function but who have highly-sought specialist technical functions (e.g. epidemiologists).
- **Public health practitioners**: professionals who practise public health by largely working with individuals or communities on public health issues. This group includes, for example, health visitors, midwives, school nurses, environmental health officers, health promotion officers and community development workers.
- **Public health wider workforce**: those whose roles have a strategic or general influence on the wider determinants of health. Within this group are included, for example, chief executives of NHS trusts, managers in local government and in the NHS, and teachers.

Table 3.1 Components of public health function: England, USA and Australia

England[1]	USA[2]	Australia[3]
Surveillance and assessment of the population health and well-being (including managing, analysing and interpreting information, knowledge and statistics)	Monitoring health status to identify and solve community health problems	Applying epidemiological and biostatistical skills to public health practice
Promoting and protecting the population's health and well-being	Diagnosing and investigating health problems and health hazards in the community Informing, educating and empowering people about health issues Enforcing laws and regulations that protect health and ensure safety	Managing the prevention, surveillance and control of infectious diseases Promoting the health of populations
Collaborative working for health	Linking people needed to personal health services and assuring the provision of health care when otherwise unavailable	Applying communication skills to meet public health objectives
Developing quality and risk management within an evaluative culture Developing health programmes and services and reducing inequalities	Evaluating effectiveness, accessibility, and quality of personal and population-based health services	Assessment and management of public health risks Evaluation of public health interventions Understanding the contribution of economic evaluation to public health interventions
Policy and strategy development and implementation	Developing policies and plans that support individual and community health efforts	Analysis and development of health policy
Working with and for communities	Mobilising community partnerships and action to identify and solve health problems	Promoting the health of populations
Research and development	Research for new insights and innovative solutions to health problems	
Strategic leadership for health Ethically managing self, people and resources (including education and continuing professional development)	Ensuring a competent public and personal health care workforce	Promoting and monitoring own professional practice Applying managerial skills to meet public health objectives

[1] Faculty of Public Health Medicine 2001
[2] United States Public Health Service 1997
[3] New South Wales Health Department 2000

As seen above, the midwifery role falls within the category of public health practitioner. Public health standard areas, as they are currently being developed for England, are identical for the specialist and practitioner role, with the difference being the degree of expertise and strategic direction required by the different levels. It is also argued that public health practitioners are likely to be more expert in some areas (e.g. promoting individual and community health) than public health specialists, while specialists will assure the overall strategic direction of public health interventions.

An exploration of the Nursing and Midwifery Council's midwifery competencies compared to England's public health standard areas (Table 3.2) gives a good view of how much public health work midwives are already expected to carry out (UKCC/NMC 2000).

In essence, midwifery competencies could easily be matched across most, if not all, of the public health competencies. So why do midwives not see themselves as public health practitioners? What are some of the structural or professional barriers to being part of a local public health team? It is up to midwives, educators and public health managers to work on overcoming those barriers that do exist. The last part of this chapter explores how midwives are, or could be, putting the above public health standards into practice, taking a wider, population-level perspective.

PUBLIC HEALTH INTO PRACTICE

This section examines the public health standard areas, as defined in England, and the detail of where midwives meet these standards in practice.

PROMOTING AND PROTECTING POPULATION HEALTH AND WELL-BEING

Midwives do an extensive amount of work in protecting and promoting individual and family health and well-being. Specific areas where midwives intervene include:

- **Screening**: There are numerous antenatal tests that midwives take a role in, or encourage mothers-to-be to participate in. In Britain, antenatal screening tests include: blood pressure screening, blood glucose levels, blood type, Down's Syndrome and most recently HIV testing. Each of these tests is important for ensuring the continued health of mothers and their unborn babies.
- **Breastfeeding**: Midwives are influential in a mother's decision whether or not to breastfeed, and the duration of breastfeeding. As breastfeeding is a critical component of ensuring a baby's health, the more women breastfeed, and the longer they breastfeed, improves babies' health and well-being.
- **Family planning**: Midwives can provide advice and support to women who wish to delay becoming pregnant again after the birth of a child, or who wish to stop childbearing altogether. As having large numbers of children can have a highly detrimental effect on a woman's health (and in some communities in developing countries, on the community as a whole), family planning promotion can be a vital public health role.
- **Health protection**: Other areas where midwives can play a role in protecting both the mother's and the baby's health is through advice on

Table 3.2 English public health standard areas and NMC competencies: comparison

FPHM standard areas	UKCC/NMC midwifery competencies
Surveillance and assessment of the population health and well-being (including managing, analysing and interpreting information, knowledge and statistics)	
Promoting and protecting the population's health and well-being	Caring for and monitoring women during the puerperium, offering the necessary evidence-based advice and support on the baby and self care Practice in accordance with relevant legislation Supporting the creation and maintenance of environments which promote the health, safety and well-being of women, babies and others
Collaborative working for health	Providing seamless care and interventions in partnership with women and other care providers during the antenatal and postnatal periods Demonstrating effective working across professional boundaries and developing professional networks
Developing quality and risk management within an evaluative culture	Applying relevant knowledge to the midwife's own practice in structured ways which are capable of evaluation Informing and developing the midwife's own practice and the practice of others through using the best available evidence and reflecting on practice Contributing to the audit of practice to review and optimise the care of women, babies and their families
Developing health programmes and services and reducing inequalities	Contributing to enhancing the health and social well-being of individuals and their communities, including: • Planning midwifery care within the context of public health policies • Contributing midwifery expertise to local strategies • Identifying and targeting care for groups with particular maternity needs • Involving users and local communities in service development and improvement
Working with and for communities	
Policy and strategy development and implementation	Contributing to the development and evaluation of guidelines and policies and making recommendations for change in the interests of women, babies and their families
Research and development	
Strategic leadership for health	
Ethically managing self, people and resources (including education and continuing professional development)	Practising in a way which respects and promotes individuals' rights, interests, preferences, beliefs and cultures Reviewing, developing and enhancing the midwife's own knowledge, skills and fitness to practise

nutrition and highlighting dietary, behavioural and environmental risks that have a harmful effect on mothers and babies. These could include concerns around eating food containing raw eggs (risk of salmonella infection), smoking cigarettes or drinking alcohol, and certain types of work or leisure environments that may be harmful. Here midwives can also serve as advocates to improve the living, working and leisure environments of women and young children.

The skills a midwife needs to develop to deliver the health protection and health promotion aspects of the public health function are:

- Health needs assessment and problem analysis skills to understand the problems faced by mothers and young children in the community. Community profiling is an important aspect of health needs assessment and is covered in more detail in Chapter 6
- Understanding and use of health promotion models for individuals and groups
- Understanding of screening, both in terms of what screening tests actually say and the technical aspects of carrying out valid and reliable tests.

COLLABORATIVE WORKING FOR HEALTH

Midwifery competencies already emphasise the need for midwives to collaborate across professional boundaries to ensure the best possible care for women. At a community level collaboration could involve midwives, school nurses, young people, family planning nurses, GPs, youth workers and social workers working in partnership to reduce teenage pregnancy in their area. The point of collaboration is to create synergy from the individual skills offered by different professional groups. Collaboration and partnership are words that are frequently used interchangeably, and reflect the sense of approaching a particular task or concern as equals, with each party respected for what they have to contribute.

Potential areas for collaborative working between midwives and others, besides teenage pregnancy, could include: improving the working environment in the local factory for pregnant women, offering parenting classes to new mothers and fathers, or providing reproductive health education in secondary schools and universities.

The skills a midwife needs to develop to deliver the collaborative working aspects of the public health function are reasonably generic and include:

- Communication skills
- Networking skills
- Planning skills.

DEVELOPING QUALITY AND RISK MANAGEMENT WITHIN AN EVALUATIVE CULTURE

This standard area crosses all professional boundaries, as it is an obligation of all health and social care professionals to evaluate risk and the quality of the services they offer. Midwives need to be up-to-date with what constitutes best practice, as well as what guidelines are in place to ensure high-quality services. Specific areas where midwives intervene in this context encompass:

- **Evidence-based practice**: midwives need to be able to ask appropriate clinical questions, search the research databases for relevant evidence, appraise research articles that they read, and put that evidence into practice. Other forms of evidence could include examining innovative programmes that appear to have a positive impact on community or health services, and looking at ways of adapting these to one's own area of work. Regular review of and reflection on clinical practice helps to ensure higher-quality services for women and infants.

- **Carrying out audit**: auditing one's own services is another way of ensuring a continuous feedback loop and supporting a learning culture within midwifery services. Audits could cover areas such as problematic versus non-problematic outcomes, women's satisfaction with services, or continuity of care to individual women.

The skills a midwife needs to develop, to deliver the quality management aspects of the public health function, include:

- **Critical appraisal skills**: evidence-based practice workshops and courses emphasise the combination of research skills, appraising research articles and reflecting on the usefulness of the findings for individual practice.
- **Audit/evaluation skills**: this includes determining what areas need auditing or evaluating, determining what data should and can be collected, undertaking data collection and analysis, and then being able to report this back to colleagues and other stakeholders.
- **Change management skills**: taking leadership for introducing changes in practice, based on research evidence and other sources of good practice, is becoming increasingly crucial for practitioners, no matter what level they work at. The field of change management embodies a complex range of skills in and of itself, which is worth exploring in more detail through change management literature (Handy 1994, Senior 2002).

DEVELOPING HEALTH PROGRAMMES AND SERVICES AND REDUCING INEQUALITIES

Developing programmes and services can be seen as strategic level activities (see Box 3.3), and it is important that all those involved in programme design and implementation, even as stakeholders, are well aware of the key elements of the programme management cycle, and community involvement. Developing programmes builds on many aspects of other standard areas and competencies, as individuals need to be able to assess the current situation and make plans for future, high-quality interventions. The key aspect here is setting up programmes that contribute to reductions in health (and social) inequalities. Much more will be said about this in Chapter 4, with examples of programmes that are striving to do just this.

The project management cycle is well described in many health promotion texts (Ewles & Simnett 1999, Naidoo & Wills 2000) and health management texts (Reinke 1988). The main steps include:

- **Problem analysis**: problem analysis includes aspects of health needs assessment and a review of other externalities, such as views of stakeholders, available resources, and an internal organisational analysis to determine how prepared one's own organisation is for taking on a particular project or programme.
- **Setting aims and objectives**: having defined the problem(s), the next step is to delineate where one wishes to get to in future – what will the

Box 3.3
Teenage Pregnancy Strategy, England

In June 1999 the Government produced a National Teenage Pregnancy Strategy to try to tackle what is felt to be a major health and social problem for the country. England has the highest teenage conception rate in Western Europe and the rates have remained static or increased, unlike in other countries in Europe where rates have declined. The strategy set three strategic goals:

- To halve the rate of conceptions among under 18-year-olds in England by 2010
- To set a firmly-established downward trend in the conception rate of under-16s by 2010
- To achieve a reduction in the risk of long-term social exclusion for teenage parents and their children.

Each Health Authority/Local Authority was required to develop their own local strategy based on local circumstances, though they were circumscribed by needing to contribute to the overall national goals. Developing local strategies has been complicated as well by the fact that there are many government initiatives that overlap with the Teenage Pregnancy Strategy that local co-ordinators had to take into account and work with. One area, Calderdale and Kirklees Health Authority and Kirklees Metropolitan Council, developed a thorough plan based on a rigorous analysis of the teenage pregnancy rates in their area and other local initiatives that could be drawn into the project. In 1998 teenage pregnancy rates in Kirklees were reported to be around 48.6 conceptions per 1000 under-18s on average, with even higher rates in more deprived areas. As such, it was agreed to set local targets as:

- A reduction of teenage conception rates by 15% by 2004
- A reduction of teenage conception rates by 50% to achieve a rate of 24.3 conceptions per 1000 under-18s by 2010.

Programme planners then looked at all relevant stakeholders' plans to see what aspects were appropriate to incorporate into the overall teenage pregnancy strategy plan, so as to not replicate work that was ongoing. For example, objectives from the Local Education Authority's sex education policy, the Youth Service's programmes for young men and Social Services' Social Housing plans, as well as Health Service plans, were all incorporated into the overall strategy. A multi-agency Teenage Pregnancy Implementation Team was set up to assist with continued collaboration across all the agencies whose work contributed to the TPS's goals. A Young People's Advisory Group was created to provide a forum for young people to feed their views into the Implementation Team, with one member of the group attending Implementation Team meetings. Local evaluation plans had to be developed by Teenage Pregnancy Co-ordinators along with their partners, while a national evaluation is being carried out by a university group.

Source: Kirklees Metropolitan Council and Calderdale and Kirklees Health Authority (2001)

future situation be as a result of your project? Programme or project aims are often aspirational (e.g. 'to improve women's health status within x years'), while objectives are often the results one hopes to achieve (e.g. 'reduce the incidence of pregnancy-related hypertension by y% in x years').

- **Defining options**: this step allows planners to consider all the options available to them for meeting the programme aim and objectives. What are the possible strategies and activities that could be employed? Which ones are the most realistic? Having done this thinking, planners then choose the option that appears most suited to their situation and most likely to achieve their objectives.
- **Implementation**: once the map of where the programme is going is defined, it is then time to put the plan into action. It is often helpful to set milestones or benchmarks to help with reviewing progress towards the programme's objectives. Here key elements of management come into play, such as managing the people and money relating to the project.
- **Monitoring and evaluation**: throughout the implementation of a programme or project it helps to collect data (both qualitative and quantitative) to help review progress on an ongoing basis. Evaluations are often quantitative in nature, particularly where large amounts of funding are concerned, as funders usually wish to see empirical evidence of the impact of the programme on the target population.
- **Review and revision**: this step happens at various times, since not all eventualities can be accounted for in the original project plan. Adjustments are invariably needed along the way to cope with unforeseen external events or unforeseen impacts being made by the programme's interventions (both positive and negative).

The skills a midwife needs to develop to achieve the programme delivery aspects of the public health function include:

- Problem analysis skills
- Planning skills
- Resource management skills
- Evaluation skills
- Reporting and communication skills.

WORKING WITH AND FOR COMMUNITIES

There is a large literature around working with and for communities that can only be touched on briefly here, and which is returned to in Chapter 4, when looking at how to address inequalities. At the forefront of the WHO's primary care policy since the late 1970s has been the paramount importance of community participation in health service decisions (WHO 1977). This was further reinforced in the Ottawa Charter for Health Promotion, which speaks of health promotion as empowering communities to take responsibility for their own health (WHO 1986). Debates continue to rage as to the degree that professionals or outsiders to particular communities are able to 'empower' others, as the concept inevitably involves giving up or giving over power to others. With more recent UK government policies that emphasise 'patient-centred' health services there has been renewed interest in patient and public involvement in health service delivery (DH 2000). This is, perhaps, a more honest way of describing how patients and the public interact with health services, rather than the idea that patients and the public participate on an equal basis with health professionals. There are a few roles that midwives and other public health practitioners can play to assist with generating greater community involvement in decision making about services.

Building and sustaining partnerships with groups and communities

This involves getting to know the views of community members, identifying their concerns and priorities. As the relationship develops, the midwife may also act as an advocate on behalf of the community in other forums to ensure that these concerns are heard and addressed.

Working in partnership with groups and communities to build and sustain their capacity for improving health and well-being

Here midwives would take on the more transformational aspects of health promotion, whereby individuals, groups and communities are enabled (through knowledge transfer and skills development) to improve their own and others' health and well-being. These concepts are based originally on the work of radical educationist Paolo Freire, who worked with very poor communities in Brazil in the 60s and 70s, and saw his own role as helping people to understand their own contexts and struggle to improve themselves and their communities (Freire 1972).

Midwives need a number of the skills already cited to fulfil this part of their work in public health, including:

- Understanding and use of health promotion models and processes
- Community profiling and health needs assessment skills
- Change agent skills (e.g. personal enthusiasm, interpersonal and communication skills, political awareness, team building and facilitation skills) (Senior 2002).

POLICY STRATEGY AND IMPLEMENTATION

As noted in Chapter 1, there has been a plethora of health policy in the last few years in Britain, focusing on improving the quality of health services provided and health improvement in general. The key policy affecting midwifery practice, *Changing Childbirth*, was legislated for in 1993 (DH 1993). The policy emphasised putting women first in decisions about childbirth, and a move away from medical models of childbirth. Midwives were instrumental in bringing this change of policy about, along with women in general, feminists and academics (Doyal 1995). Putting this policy into practice has been less successful, and parts of the midwifery profession remain disillusioned. In general, where obstetricians are relatively few and far between, midwives have been able to take on a more proactive role in involving women in making decisions about their care and delivery experience. This has not been the case in larger hospital environments (Brooks & Lomax 1999). However, the fact remains that the midwifery lobby does have a voice and can make important changes to health policy in favour of their clients and potential clients.

In the same way, midwives can help influence policy development to benefit the communities they work within. Midwives' input into local policy development and implementation of larger national initiatives such as the Teenage Pregnancy Strategy and Sure Start should be invaluable in keeping the concerns of women and their children at centre stage.

Table 3.3 A continuum for public health practice in primary care for nurses, midwives and health visitors

Leadership of public health programmes at community level ↔	Community development	Group work on health issues	Health promotion with families	Health promotion with individuals	The application of a public health approach within individual care ↔
Co-ordinating HNA, HImP/NSF implementation PCT liaison Lead midwifery team Work to public health objectives Inter-agency local planning Evaluation Regeneration work	Community involvement in HNA Community-based groups Support/run health projects Provide health information Lay worker projects	Parent support groups Smoking cessation Antenatal groups Health education groups Self-help groups	Family health plan Input to HNA Health education Access to health information	Immunisation Screening Health education Contribution to HNA Holistic assessment	Holistic assessment Input to HNA Health education Inter-agency care Information on health

HImP/NSF, Health Improvement Programme/National Service Framework; HNA, health needs assessment; PCT, primary care trust.

They should also, through links with their own health and social care community, and through national associations, be able to influence larger policy agendas.

The skills midwives need to be part of developing and implementing policy include:

- Knowing what current policies are
- Having a good grounding in policy analysis (Where is the policy derived from? Which stakeholders are for and against the policy? Who has the power to make decisions?)
- Communication skills for influencing others
- Networking skills to create wider momentum behind specific issues.

ETHICALLY MANAGING SELF AND OTHERS

Management skills required for public health practice are very similar to those described as competencies for midwifery practice.

Respect for professional codes of conduct

This involves knowing and following relevant legislation, respecting confidentiality and informed consent, as well as supporting women as autonomous individuals with individual needs.

Respect for clients and other professionals

As a good manager the midwife needs also to be a team player, with the ability to work across professional boundaries, and to break down profession–client boundaries where appropriate.

Resource management

Managers need to understand what their resource base is, financial, material and human, in order to put all to the most effective use. As staff retention in the health services continues to be problematic, sensitive and supportive human resource management becomes all the more critical. Midwives also need to understand the larger resource base in their organisations in order to be able to lobby for a greater share of those resources as necessary.

Skills needed to be an effective manager include:

- Strong sense of professional behaviour – confidentiality, working collaboratively, leading in one's own professional area
- Financial management skills – budgeting, financial reporting, reviewing accounts
- Human resource management skills – recruitment, performance management, team building.

Table 3.3 provides a useful model for considering the continuum of a midwife's public health role.

CONCLUSION

Midwifery, as it is currently practised in the UK, already contains several elements of public health. While many midwives are focused on individual patient care, there is scope for expanding their role to take on a greater population perspective. This can be by simply understanding the health of mothers-to-be within their socio-economic, cultural, environmental and policy contexts, building on social models of health that midwives are introduced to in their training. Or it can be taken further by applying this understanding to developing community projects targeting changes to identified problems in order to improve pregnancy outcomes in general. Greater knowledge of the interventions and programmes that might be possible to improve health, and the skills to put these in place, are vital for moving the public health agenda further. Midwives are called on to be more proactive in assisting with community health needs assessments, to work in partnership with other agencies and community women to resolve problems identified by needs assessments and to know the research evidence base to help ensure that actions put into place will be effective.

References

Acheson D 1988 Public Health in England: the report of the Committee of Enquiry into the future development of the public health function. HMSO, London

Brooks F, Lomax H 1999 Labouring bodies: mothers and maternity policy. In: Dean H, Ellis K, Campling J (eds) Social Policy and the Body: Transitions in Corporeal Discourse. Macmillan, Basingstoke

Centers for Disease Control (CDC) 1999 Essential Services of Public Health. Division of Public Health Systems, Centers for Disease Control, Atlanta, GA

Chadwick E 1843 Report on an Enquiry into the Sanitary Condition of the Labouring Population of Great Britain. Clowes, London

Dahlgren G, Whitehead M 1991 Policies and Strategies to Promote Social Equity in Health. Institute for Futures Studies, Stockholm

Department of Health 1993 Changing Childbirth. Report of the Expert Maternity Group, Part 1. HMSO, London

Department of Health 2000 The NHS Plan. TSO, London

Department of Health 2001 The Report of the Chief Medical Officer's Project to Strengthen the Public Health Function. DH, London

Donaldson L J, Donaldson R J 2000 Essential Public Health, 2nd edn. LibraPharma Press, Newbury

Doyal L 1995 What Makes Women Sick: Gender and the Political Economy of Health. Macmillan, Basingstoke

Ewles L, Simnett I 1999 Promoting Health: A Practical Guide. Baillière Tindall/RCN, Edinburgh

Faculty of Public Health Medicine 2001 Good Public Health Practice. Faculty of Public Health, London

Freire P 1972 Pedagogy of the Oppressed. Penguin, Harmondsworth

Handy C 1994 Understanding Organisations. Penguin, London

House of Commons Select Committee for Health 2000 Public Health. TSO, London

Kirklees Metropolitan Council and Calderdale and Kirklees Health Authority 2001 Teenage Pregnancy Strategy. Kirklees Metropolitan Council

Latcham S 2001 A Review of Public Health Skills of Nurses, Midwives and Health Visitors. Health Development Agency, London (unpublished report)

Naidoo J, Wills J 2000 Health Promotion: Foundations for Practice. Baillière Tindall/RCN, Edinburgh

New South Wales Health Department 2000 Informing Public Health Practice – Competencies of the Graduate Diploma of Applied Epidemiology. Department of Health, New South Wales, Sydney

Reinke W 1988 Health Planning for Effective Management. Oxford University Press, Oxford

Senior B 2002 Organisational Change. Financial Times–Prentice Hall, Harlow

UKCC/NMC 2000 Requirements for Pre-registration Midwifery Programmes. Nursing and Midwifery Council, London

United States Public Health Service 1997 The Public Health Workforce: An Agenda for the 21st Century – Full Report of the Public Health Functions Project. Public Health Service, Washington DC

Williams C, Baumslag N, Jelliffe D 1994 Mother and Child Health. Oxford University Press, Oxford

World Health Organization 1977 Health for All by the Year 2000. World Health Organization, Geneva

World Health Organization 1986 Ottawa Charter for Health Promotion. WHO, Geneva

World Health Organization 1992 Women's Health: Across Age and Frontier. WHO, Geneva

World Health Organization 1999 Reduction of Maternal Mortality: A Joint WHO/UNFPA/UNICEF/World Bank Statement. WHO, Geneva

Young T K 1999 Population Health: Concepts and Methods, 2nd edn. Oxford University Press, Oxford

SECTION 2

Developing ideas and opportunities: key themes and concepts

SECTION CONTENTS

Chapter 4

Tackling health inequalities: a midwifery challenge

Stephen Peckham and Cindy Carlson

CHAPTER CONTENTS

SUMMARY

This chapter opens by examining health inequalities as they relate to maternal and child health. It provides information on the range of inequalities that exist within an international context. The chapter then examines theories of health inequalities and how these relate to debates about the causes of such inequalities and the social impact that they have. In particular it examines how wider social inequalities impact on health. The chapter then goes on to examine how policy has been developed to tackle health inequalities and the types of response that have been developed at an international level by the United Nations and World Health Organization as well as in the UK. The last part of the chapter focuses on policy and practice. It outlines key UK and international developments relevant to tackling health inequalities relating to midwives. This section discusses what approaches midwives can take to tackle health inequalities and includes examples of good practice.

INTRODUCTION

The health of the world's population has improved faster in the last 50 years than at any other point in human history. When reviewing measures of human health, such as life expectancy or disease-specific mortality rates, we see remarkable increases in longevity alongside a rapid decline in rates of what used to be killer diseases, such as smallpox or cholera. However, while gross statistics show what great progress has been made, they also hide highly variable pictures within countries. The health status gap between the richest and poorest nations, and the richest and poorest communities within nations, has expanded in the last 30 years, leading policymakers in many countries to turn their attentions to health inequalities. But what action should be taken? The concept of health inequalities is highly contested, precisely because of debates around what should be measured, how to measure it and what is causing health inequalities in the first place. This chapter reviews the debates and considers the practical implications for midwifery practice in the short and long term.

UNDERSTANDING HEALTH INEQUALITIES

What do we mean when we talk about 'health inequalities'? One need only look at national and international statistics on maternal and child health to understand that there is great variation within and between populations, and that, therefore, the concept of health inequalities should be relatively straightforward. During the 1800s in Britain, when vital statistics such as births and deaths were being systematically recorded for the first time, the country's first public health officers noted large variations in the health of different populations. William Farr worked as 'Compiler of Abstracts' for the General Register Office in the mid-1800s and reported stunning differences in birth and mortality rates by area (according to population density) and by social class. Table 4.1 is taken from his report *Life and Death in England* (Humphreys 1885).

When we look at international data we find that the maternal mortality ratio in Eritrea for the period 1990–1998 was 1000/100,000 compared to the UK's 7/100,000 (World Bank 2001). In 1998 the World Health Organization identified maternal mortality, and the stark inequalities in maternal mortality between developing and developed countries, as a major health issue (see Box 4.1) with women's risk of dying in pregnancy or childbirth as much as 40 times greater in developing countries than in developed countries (World Health Organization 1998). Within the UK, life expectancy for women varies from 82.26 years in Kensington and Chelsea (a relatively prosperous area) to 76.58 years in Manchester. Infant mortality rates in Manchester are double the rates in Kensington and Chelsea (9.2 per 1000 live births versus 4.1) (ONS 2002). These rates in themselves mask variation within local areas and between different

Table 4.1 1861–70: density of population, death-rate, birth-rate, excess of births over deaths and increase of population per 1000 persons living in seven groups of districts arranged in the Order of Mortality

			1861–70 (To 1,000 persons living)			
Number of districts	Range of mortality rates per 1,000 living	Persons to a square mile	Average annual deaths	Average annual births	Average annual excess of births over deaths	Average annual increase of population in middle of period
England and Wales 616	15–39	307	22.4	35.1	12.6	12.4
51	15–17	171	16.7	30.1	13.4	15.8
349	18–20	193	19.8	32.2	13.0	8.8
142	21–23	447	22.0	35.6	13.6	16.2
56	24–26	2,183	25.1	38.1	13.0	15.3
16	27–30	6,871	27.8	39.1	11.3	8.9
1	32	12,172	32.5	37.3	4.8	3.2
1	39	65,834	38.6	37.6	−1.0	−12.3

Box 4.1
Maternal mortality
(WHO 1998:1)

Every day, at least 1600 women die from the complications of pregnancy and childbirth. That is 585,000 women – at a minimum – dying every year. The majority of these deaths – almost 90% – occur in Asia and sub-Saharan Africa; approximately 10% in other developing regions; and less than 1% in the developed world. Between 25% and 33% of all deaths of women of reproductive age in many developing countries are the result of complications of pregnancy or childbirth.

Of all the health statistics monitored by the World Health Organization, maternal mortality is the one with the largest discrepancy between developed and developing countries. While infant mortality, for example, is almost seven times higher in the developing world, maternal mortality is on average 18 times higher. In addition to the number of deaths each year, over 50 million more women suffer from maternal morbidity – acute complications from pregnancy. For at least 18 million women, these morbidities are long term and often debilitating.

The goal of the Safe Motherhood Initiative is to cut maternal mortality by half by the year 2000. We know what to do to reduce the tragedy of maternal mortality; what we need is the political will and strong, concerted action.

groups in local areas. In the US, where health statistics are kept by ethnic origin, infant mortality rates within large cities can vary as much as 300% between whites and ethnic minorities. For example, in Chicago, the infant mortality rate in the non-hispanic white population is 7 per 1000 live births, while for the non-hispanic black population it is 17.8 per 1000 live births (CDC 2002).

Any discussion of equity or equality, and thus inequality, needs to define the equality of what and between whom. The term 'health inequalities' encompasses two very loaded words – 'health' and 'inequalities'. Both need definition in order to understand the overall term itself. This area is well explored in 'The Black Report' (Townsend et al 1988), which considers the thorny issues of defining 'health' and 'inequalities' and then considers what indicators to use for measuring both (see Box 4.2). The writers of the Black Report opt for using the World Health Organization (WHO) definition of health, 'a state of complete physical, mental and social well-being and not merely the absence of disease or infirmity' (WHO 1985). This definition allows the inclusion of indicators that reflect social, economic and environmental as well as biological determinants of health. When defining inequalities, the authors of the Black Report place emphasis on those differences between people that are social constructs, such as social class or income levels, as opposed to differences that are part of one's natural physiology, such as gender or age. The indicators of inequalities used by the Black Report are social class, which they define as 'segments of the population sharing broadly similar types and levels of resources with broadly similar styles of living and some shared perception of their collective condition' (Townsend et al 1988:39). This view of health inequalities is summarised by John McKinlay who wrote, 'While still largely overlooked in epidemiologic thinking, social system influences … may account for as much (if not more) of the variation in health and/or illness statistics as do environmental influences, or even the attributes and lifestyles of individuals' (McKinlay 1995:2).

Box 4.2
The Black Report 1988

The controversial nature of discussing health inequalities is depicted by the history of the Black Report. A study of national and international evidence on inequalities was commissioned by a Labour Government in the UK in the late 1970s and the report presented in 1980 to a (by then) Conservative administration. The main policy recommendations featured in the report were:

- A call for a total and not merely service-oriented approach to the problems of health
- A call for a radical overhaul in the balance of activity and proportionate distribution of resources within the health and associated services, all in favour of those who are most disadvantaged in British society.

The report was promptly buried by the Conservative Government, who could not marry up its redistributive thrust and their own free-market agenda. The report was published 2 years later by Penguin Books and generated tremendous interest beyond Britain's borders, where it influenced the World Health Organization's European office as it developed its own health promotion strategy focusing on reducing health inequalities.

Since the publication of the Black Report numerous researchers have taken up the challenge of identifying the 'best' indicators for understanding the relationship between socially constructed inequalities and health, and it is widely recognised that there are inequalities in health status between deprived and affluent communities, confirmed by numerous studies, and inequalities exist not only in mortality but in morbidity (Davey Smith et al 1994, Blane et al 1996, Eachus et al 1996, Kaplan et al 1996, Kennedy et al 1996). However, the precise causal relationship between deprivation and health inequalities is unclear: both individual characteristics and geographical and social factors are implicated (Duncan et al 1993). The relative effect of these will vary according to specific circumstances, and interventions to reduce health inequalities will therefore require a range of approaches tailored to societies, communities and individuals. It has also been suggested that early life factors and/or the cumulative effects of life events, including the effects of deprivation on social cohesion, play a significant role (Davey Smith et al 1997, Kawachi et al 1997).

A further debate has centred around whether attention should be given to health *inequality* or to health *inequity*. Those who concern themselves with health inequalities wish to see the closure of the health gap between rich and poor, while those focusing on health inequity wish to tackle the injustice of the most disadvantaged populations having the poorest health. Gwatkin (2000) considers the main arguments in this debate and writes, 'the distinction between poverty, equality and equity is often of limited practical importance' where policy is concerned, though in specific situations understanding the differences in meaning could take on greater significance.

INCOME INEQUALITY

Some argue that the key inequality that needs exploring, and tackling, is income inequality (Kaplan et al 1996, Wilkinson 1996, Lynch et al 1998). Richard Wilkinson has pulled together impressive amounts of economic and health indicators to demonstrate a direct relationship between levels of income inequality and health across more developed countries. In his book *Unhealthy Societies* Wilkinson pulls together 'a growing body of new evidence which shows that life expectancy in different countries is dramatically improved where income differences are smaller and societies are more socially cohesive' (1996:1), where life expectancy becomes his indicator for health. In so doing he explores data on relative income levels within countries and compares these with life expectancy. In countries such as Japan and the Netherlands where income disparities are relatively small, life expectancies are indeed higher than in countries where income disparities are much wider, such as the United Kingdom and the United States. Wilkinson goes on to posit that the absolute income poverty of less developed countries accounts for their appalling health statistics. However, for further health improvement in more developed countries, rather than focusing on increasing economic growth or improving living standards, the policy focus now needs to be on reducing the income gap between the highest and lowest paid in any given country. The policy implications of accepting the arguments around income inequality lead to a need for redistribution of income in any given population so as to narrow the gulf between the highest and lowest earners in society.

CLASS INEQUALITY

Other authors argue that indicators of income inequality are not sufficient for explaining the differences in life expectancy and other indicators of health status. Instead the focus should be social class and the differences in relative and perceived social status between classes (Muntaner & Lynch 1999, Coburn 2000). These authors argue that it is important to study the social mechanisms that create income inequality in the first place – in other words, social class – if policy makers are to genuinely work towards reducing inequalities. The nub of this line of thinking is that concentrating on income levels doesn't adequately explain other research findings that link different social *position* with differing health status. The relative effect of being of a certain social class can, in itself, influence an individual's health. Marxists and neo-Marxists consider the importance of class relations and exploitation of one class by another as a key feature explaining differences in income levels and other social welfare indicators. For example Wright (1997), writing on class exploitation, suggests that class exploitation occurs when a) the wealth of a social group causally depends on the deprivation of another; b) the causal relation in (a) involves a disproportionate exclusion of those who are exploited from access to certain resources, usually backed by structures that limit property ownership, and c) the causal mechanism that translates exclusion in (b) into differential health and welfare outcomes involves the disproportionate allocation of the benefits of production by owners and managers to the detriment of workers. Or, more simply, that those who own the means of production (e.g. chief executives and senior managers of large corporations) enjoy greater health because they can control how the wealth that is generated is then distributed. The policy implications of following this line of thinking would be to work on breaking down class structures so that there can be greater social mobility and a greater sense of control for all parts of society.

INEQUALITY IN INDIVIDUAL HEALTH CONDITION

Murray et al (1999) define health inequality as 'composite measure of variation in health status across individuals in a population' (p.537). The same group of authors grapple with defining indicators for measuring health inequalities in Gakidou et al (2000). By asking themselves 'Equality of what?' they go on to consider whether they should focus on equality of 'healthy lifespan' (the number of years one lives in a state of good health) or equality of 'health risk' (the level of health risks an individual faces in the course of life) or 'health expectancy' (which measures expected levels of morbidity and mortality in individuals based on health risk). They dismiss the usefulness of social class as an indicator of inequality, arguing that health should be considered as much of a 'commodity' as any economic commodity, and that therefore inequalities in health between individuals are valid to measure in and of themselves. While interesting, this argument does tend to leave aside the complexity of the interactions between an individual's social world and personal responses to it that are better captured in both the social class and income inequality schools of thought. Further, the implications of concentrating on health aspects alone might lead to inattention to wider societal determinants that lead to health inequalities (Acheson 2000).

INEQUALITIES IN LIFE COURSE

While there is concern about focusing on individual health factors, there is evidence to suggest that individual life course factors can and do play an important role (Ben-Shlomo & Davey Smith, 1991, Elford et al 1991, Davey Smith et al 1997, Kawachi et al 1997). Research on birth weight has found that the risk for coronary heart disease and stroke falls with increasing birth weight (Frankel et al 1996, Barker 1998). Similar observations have been made in relation to insulin resistance syndrome, accelerated ageing and the increased likelihood of a woman born under weight giving birth to an under-weight baby (Barker 1998).

Similarly, nutrition in early years is also associated with life-course health. Nutritional deficiency in early years is associated with many adult diseases such as cardio-vascular disease, diabetes, cataracts and lower hearing acuity (Kuh & Ben-Shlomo 1997, Barker 1998). It is not surprising therefore that the World Health Organization has highlighted the need to address such areas in its approach to well-being in later life (Stein & Moritz 1999). While such an approach does not negate the importance of wider social determinants on health, it is thought that the interaction of life-course and social determinants experienced in life are important factors when considering health inequalities (Stein & Moritz 1999).

EXPLAINING THE IMPACT OF SOCIAL INEQUALITIES ON HEALTH

Besides the debates around what are in fact the most significant causal social mechanisms with regard to health inequalities, there has also been a fair degree of debate around how these mechanisms interact to create better or poorer health. A great deal of research has gone into explaining the nexus of social and health inequalities, with some interesting findings. The Whitehall Study followed a group of 17,000 civil servants working in government offices over a period of time, and found that the employment grade of individuals proved to be far more important as a risk factor for coronary heart disease than the combination of 'class' risk factors, such as cigarette smoking, blood pressure or serum cholesterol levels (Marmot et al 1984). Social epidemiologists, using the results of this and other long-term studies, speculate that there is an interweaving of psychosocial and biological factors that link social status with health. Figure 4.1 provides one such model that has developed out of this work.

There are several other factors associated with poorer health status that have an important bearing on the health inequality–health inequity debate. Besides income, education, occupation, gender and ethnicity have been shown to correlate positively with health status (Gwatkin 2000). Table 4.2 provides an international comparison of the impact of mothers' education levels on under-5 mortality.

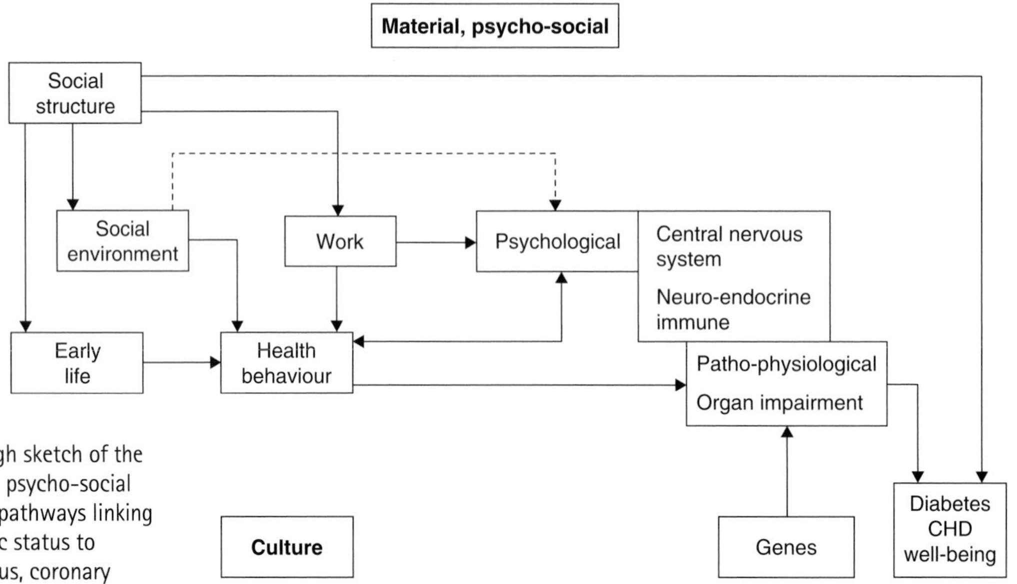

Fig. 4.1 Rough sketch of the environmental, psycho-social and biological pathways linking socio-economic status to diabetes mellitus, coronary heart disease (CHD) and well-being (Marmot 2000:354).

Table 4.2 Under-5 mortality according to mother's education (expressed in terms of number of deaths per 1000 live births)

Country	Mother's educational status	
	No education	Secondary/Higher education
Asia/Near East		
Indonesia	111	51
Pakistan	128	65
Turkey	109	30
Latin America		
Peru	150	45
Dominican Republic	91	31
Sub-Saharan Africa		
Burkina Faso	212	87
Kenya	100	54
Niger	334	106
Rwanda	177	94

From: Bicego & Ahmed (1996) in Gwatkin (2000)

Again, the exact triggers within each of these areas that can lead to differential health status are contentious, though social status provides an important link for all. What is remarkable is in poorer countries where income levels are far lower than in the UK or other European countries, but where investments have been made in education, and especially girls' education (e.g. Kerala State in India or Sri Lanka), health status indicators are impressive. A leading economist on development issues concludes from his own research that *support-led* economic processes, that focus on 'skilful social support of health care, education and other relevant social arrangements' (Sen 1999:46) have led to rapid reductions in mortality rates in countries such as India's Kerala State, Costa Rica and Sri Lanka, without any of these countries experiencing much economic growth. Sen also cites research that shows that survival rates within some African–American communities in the US are lower than survival rates of people born in developing countries, e.g. China, Costa Rica, and indeed Kerala State (Sen 2001).

INEQUALITIES IN ACCESS

One further dimension of inequalities in relation to health is access to services. In relation to midwifery services, equity has traditionally been viewed as an access or service distribution issue – particularly at an international level (World Health Organization 1998, 2002). Concern here is, for example, with the 'inverse care law' (Tudor-Hart 1988), the distribution of health care professionals being inversely related to the need for health services. For example while women in developing countries are at up to 40 times the risk of dying in pregnancy and childbirth compared with women in developed countries, only 53% of the 60 million deliveries in developing countries take place with the assistance of a skilled birth attendant, compared with 98% in Europe (WHO 1998).

Most maternal deaths could be prevented if women had access to basic medical care during pregnancy, childbirth and the postpartum period. This implies strengthening health systems and linking communities, health centres and hospitals to provide care when and where women need it (WHO 1998:2).

However, concerns regarding access to relevant services is not just an issue in developing countries, although clearly this is where the worst inequalities of access occur. For example in developed countries there are concerns about whether specific groups of the population have the same level of access. In the UK there have been increasing concerns about differential access to pregnancy, maternity and postpartum support services between different age groups, different socio-economic classes and different cultural and ethnic groups (Social Exclusion Unit 1999, Bailey & Pain 2001, Davies & Bath 2001). This would suggest that the absolute provision of midwives and skilled birthing attendants, their availability and accessibility, and the way in which they work are all important in addressing inequalities in access for women.

TACKLING HEALTH INEQUALITIES – POLICY RESPONSES

Inequalities in health are amenable to direct policy interventions on four levels: strengthening individuals; strengthening communities; improving access to services; macro-economic change (Whitehead 1995). In recent years most policy initiatives have fallen into the first category, but with the emphasis within the World Health Organization's Health For All programme many countries have begun to place more emphasis on the last three categories. For example, in the UK proposals contained in *Saving Lives: Our Healthier Nation* (DH 1999a) place a greater emphasis on a broader strategic approach. This fits with calls for new approaches to tackling inequalities that move away from the disease model towards the promotion of social support and the development of family and community strengths (Wilkinson 1997, Campbell & Aggleton 1999). The focus of much of this debate is on local areas and communities, with a strong emphasis on collaboration and participation. Within the current UK policy context the focus of developments at this level will be the new primary care organisations (DH 2002a) but the wider societal context is at the heart of the UK's approach to tackling health inequalities (DH 1998, 1999a, 2002b). However, the UK's policy approach does reflect a wider international agenda as well.

The World Health Organization formally adopted a programme to address health inequalities within the Health For All 2000 programme (WHO 1985), although equity has long been seen as an important element of health policy and is one of the key pillars of primary health care (WHO/UNICEF 1978, Macdonald 1992). Internationally midwives, often working as part of the primary health care service, but also within secondary care centres, are seen as playing an important role in tackling health inequalities. The World Health Organization has identified a number of key roles for midwives and nurses in response to the United Nations Millennium Development Goals to eliminate world poverty (UN 2001):

- Monitoring poverty, by documenting the prevalence of under-weight children
- Promoting gender equality, by educating girls and women about health
- Reducing child and maternal mortality, by delivering maternal and child health services
- Combating HIV/AIDS, malaria and other diseases, by lowering their prevalence through activities directed towards prevention and treatment (WHO 2002:3).

These roles are central to both addressing inequalities and providing a new framework for midwives and, in an international context, other skilled birth attendants. They clearly develop a strong public health role that focuses on inequalities in socio-economic circumstances, inequalities in access and inequalities in health.

UK POLICY

One key theme of the government's approach to public health has been the renewed emphasis on tackling health inequalities. Public health policy during the 1980s ignored the findings of key reports on structural influences on health, and in particular the Black and Whitehead Reports (Townsend et al 1988) on inequality and health. Until 1995 the then Conservative governments made no explicit recognition of socio-economic issues relating to variations in health or health inequalities. In the mid 1990s the government went some way to addressing these shortcomings with the acknowledgement that there are variations in health, and a national research programme on variations in health was established (DH 1995, NHS CRD 1995). However, this only related to the contribution that can be made by the NHS and DH and specifically avoids addressing the role of other areas of government policy such as the environment, transport, employment and welfare benefits.

Since 1997, the Labour government has taken various steps associated with tackling health inequalities. One of its first actions was to commission an Independent Inquiry into Inequalities in Health, chaired by Sir Donald Acheson, the former Chief Medical Officer. The inquiry reported in November 1998 (DH 1998). The inquiry reviewed the research evidence related to health inequalities and made 39 recommendations. Only three of the recommendations were directed to the NHS, thereby underlining the relative contribution of health care services to tackling health inequality, compared to poverty, education, employment, housing, transport and nutrition. However, one key recommendation was of direct relevance to midwifery:

> We recommend a high priority is given to policies aimed at improving health and reducing health inequalities in women of childbearing age, expectant mothers and young children.
>
> (DH 1998:1)

The government's commitment to public health and tackling health inequality was also encapsulated in early policy documents such as *The New NHS* (DH 1997) in which it was proposed to renew the NHS and to tackle the 'unfairness', 'unacceptable variations' and 'two-tierism' of the Conservative internal market (Powell & Exworthy 2000). However, the White Paper on public health *Saving Lives: Our Healthier Nation* (DH 1999a), while acknowledging the importance of tackling health inequalities, fell short of setting specific targets on health inequalities or maternal and neonatal health. This emphasis on addressing inequality is central to a key government policy document aimed at the nursing profession. *Making a Difference* (DH 1999b) places an emphasis on the role of nurses, midwives and health visitors in tackling inequalities in health, stressing the need for midwives, for example, to take on a health promotion role with 'disadvantaged' women – although as Hart and Lockey (2002) have argued there is no clear definition in the document of what this means. Central to *Making a Difference* is the idea that midwives should be working with the wider community and across organisational boundaries undertaking health promotion activities. This represents a shift from previous policy on midwifery, such as *Changing Childbirth* (DH 1993), that emphasises one to one contact as being central to midwifery practice. Such a view of an enhanced role is shared by the Royal College of Midwives in their document *Vision 2000* with its emphasis on the midwife working '… as a public health practitioner, promoting community well-being and reducing inequalities in health …' (RCM 2000:14).

In the same year the government published *The NHS Plan* for England which specifically mentioned midwives and the need to develop their role in public health and family well-being and announced the intention to have national targets on health inequalities (DH 2000):

- Starting with children under 1 year, by 2010 to reduce by at least 10% the gap in mortality between manual groups and the population as a whole
- Starting with health authorities, by 2010 to reduce by at least 10% the gap between the fifth of areas with the lowest life expectancy at birth and the population as a whole.

These targets were added to in the *Priorities and Planning Framework 2003–2006* (DH 2002c) and include targets on reducing smoking amongst pregnant women, focusing on smokers from disadvantaged groups, and increasing breastfeeding rates by 2 percentage points per year, especially amongst women from disadvantaged groups. There are also additional targets in respect of teenage pregnancy, to reduce conception rates of under 18-year-olds by 15% by 2004 and 50% by 2010. The health inequalities targets make certain workforce capacity assumptions, including more trained health care professionals providing antenatal and child health services in deprived areas.

Two recent reports have also highlighted inequities in maternity service provision in the UK. In 2001 the Department of Health report, *Why Mothers Die 1997–99* (Lewis & Drife 2001), produced by the Confidential Enquiry into Maternal Deaths, found that women from families where neither they nor their partners held down a job were 20 times more likely to die than those from the two highest social classes. In addition, babies born to women from disadvantaged groups were more likely to have a low birth weight, so continuing these health inequalities into the next generation. These issues were further examined by the Parliamentary Health Select Committee whose findings were published in a report, *Inequalities in Access to Maternity Services* (House of Commons 2003). It found that women from a range of backgrounds, including those on a low income, asylum seekers, those who are homeless, women from black and minority ethnic (BME) groups and travellers are unlikely either to demand – or receive – the attention they need to see them through pregnancy, labour and the postnatal period (see Box 4.3).

In September 2004 the government published the National Service Framework for Children's Services, also covering maternity services. National Service Frameworks are a key plank in the UK government's approach to developing national standards for health care, and areas already covered include mental health, coronary heart disease, older people and diabetes. Within existing frameworks there is already an emphasis on public health and addressing health inequalities. As in previous National Service Frameworks there are specific guidelines on inequalities and access in the Children's Services National Service Framework, as these are core themes underpinning its development. The Expert Working Group for Maternity Services, that developed this strand of the new framework, has a subgroup on inequalities and access that has midwifery membership.

The UK government has, then, adopted a range of policy responses which address both the inequalities in health status between specific

Box 4.3
Findings from the Parliamentary Health Select Committee Report (House of Commons 2003)

Disadvantaged women faced a number of barriers when accessing maternity services, including:

- Prejudice in relation to class, race or disability
- Lack of advocacy and interpreting services
- Lack of continuity of care, particularly for homeless women and dispersed asylum seekers
- Little support for mothers with disabilities
- Lack of consultation – maternity services liaison committees do not always encompass women from disadvantaged backgrounds
- An insufficient number of mother and baby units for women suffering from severe mental health problems
- The dispersal system exacerbates the barriers to maternity services faced by women seeking asylum.

groups of the population (social class, geographic location) focusing particularly on area-based initiatives in deprived areas, and also a life-course approach with initiatives such as Sure Start (discussed in the information Box 4.4 and in Chapter 10) and more recently Sure Start Plus, and strategies to address teenage pregnancy and smoking. All of these have a particular relevance to midwives and are discussed in more detail below. What is clear within the UK context, however, is the changing nature of midwifery with a shift from a focus on one-to-one relationships in assisting and supporting childbirth to a broader public health role with a direct focus on addressing health inequalities.

Much of UK and international policy is increasingly being built upon the foundations of the three pillars of primary health care – equity, collaboration and participation (Macdonald 1992). In particular the primary health care approach binds these pillars together and recent research on public health and primary care in the UK (Taylor et al 1998, Turton et al 1999) would suggest that to tackle inequalities it is necessary to adopt collaborative and participative approaches. These can also be seen to underpin much of the development of policies to address inequalities, and in defining the new public health role of midwives in UK programmes such as *Making a Difference* (DH 1999b) and the recent Royal College guidelines *Vision 2000* (RCM 2000). Internationally similar tenets are encapsulated in *Safe Motherhood* (WHO 1998) and *Strategic Directions for Strengthening Nursing and Midwifery Services* (WHO 2002). The next sections therefore explore such approaches that involve midwives within a UK and international context.

SUPPORTING INDIVIDUAL MOTHERS AND BABIES

Midwives can undertake health promotion approaches at individual, community or group, and strategic levels. Individual approaches may include working with women to address issues such as smoking, diet, breastfeeding, malaria, HIV/AIDS and family planning. Midwives can also play a role in promoting gender equality by educating women about health, and identify and support women who suffer from violence, abuse and socio-economic deprivation. All these factors can lead to higher morbidity and mortality rates (Standing 1997). Midwives also play an important role in ensuring that women have access to support during pregnancy, during childbirth and in the immediate postpartum period. Finally they can provide support for individuals through support groups such as mother and baby clinics, antenatal and parenting classes, and breast-feeding groups.

In relation to health promotion, midwives provide information on diet during pregnancy, provide parenting classes, and they have an important role to play in tackling smoking reduction. Smoking is linked to miscarriage, lower birth weights and higher rates of perinatal death. Midwives have also played key roles in supporting particularly vulnerable women such as teenagers who are pregnant, where rates of smoking are likely to be higher than for older women. Midwives also play an important role in the identification, prevention and treatment of mental health problems, particularly postnatal depression which can affect as many as 10–15% of women who give birth (Hampshire 2002).

Another recent UK government initiative aimed at teenage mothers and parents is Sure Start Plus, which currently operates in 15 target locations within existing Health Action Zone areas. This scheme works directly with parents to provide support packages covering health care, education and jobs, childcare, housing and benefits. A key aim is to try to lift teenage parents out of poverty and thus improve the life chances for the parents and their children. Midwives will be involved in a variety of ways including supporting teenage mothers, identifying families at risk, providing parenting skills support and working in partnership with other professionals, community organisations and teenage parents in running local programmes. This programme is focused on individual families and is an extension to the broader-based Sure Start community programme discussed below.

STRENGTHENING COMMUNITIES

To address inequalities in mortality and morbidity the government has funded a range of community-based initiatives aimed at improving the life chances of young children as well as supporting their families. As a result of these initiatives and the wider growth of community-based approaches in the UK there are increasing opportunities for midwives to work with other local practitioners, parents, families and community organisations.

The largest programme is Sure Start (see Box 4.4). In many areas midwives are active in projects running services for pregnant women and new mothers. For example, in Bristol a local midwife runs community-based pregnancy and breastfeeding clubs in deprived areas, aimed at

Box 4.4
Sure Start

In 2000 the then Secretary of State for Health, Alan Milburn, highlighted Sure Start as making one of the most important contributions to health improvement in the UK (Milburn 2000). Sure Start is one of many community partnership approaches being developed in many areas around the country which seeks to address individual problems through community-based responses, but by working with the local communities involved. Sure Start is based on a similar approach pioneered in the USA and has a strong neighbourhood focus, with each programme serving the local community 'within "pram pushing" distance'. The programme is targeted on children and families in deprived circumstances. It is being delivered through local partnerships with the aim of providing a range of support services, including childcare, early learning and play opportunities, and support with parenting skills, as well as improved access to primary health care. By the summer of 2003 there were 522 schemes up and running with the aim to reach 400,000 children by 2004 including a third of all under-4s living in poverty.

women who are isolated or suffering from depression. The clubs have crèche facilities and provide a setting for women to talk about things they feel are important to them as well as providing access to wider health, education, social and financial services (Hampshire 2002). The project in Bristol has improved breastfeeding rates at 6–8 weeks and thus provides an important approach to achieving improved child health and potentially adult health. In Southampton an important development of Sure Start is the funding of community midwives in deprived areas of the city. No formal evaluation has been undertaken of this service, but there were three times as many emergency caesareans in a similarly deprived area, where traditional services were being used, than in the targeted area and the number of babies born with a low birth weight was also five times higher in the traditional service area (Thorp 2003).

Another community-based project is Newpin, a national charity, that has 15 centres working with mothers and children. These are based mainly in Greater London, together with one centre in Chesterfield and two in Northern Ireland. Additionally, in Southwark they run a Fathers' Project, an Ante/Post Natal Project, a Young Mums' Project, and hold a variety of training courses. Centres normally accommodate between 25 and 30 families at any one time, and operate with a strong ethos of participation from user families working in partnership with practitioners, including midwives. With the support of staff, parents are responsible for their children and when receiving counselling or attending groups, childcare is shared between other user members. A significant degree of emotional and practical support between user members is also encouraged, including outside centre hours. Each centre has its own local management committee which includes representatives of those using the centre and representatives from local health and social care agencies. Many referrals for Newpin come from health care workers, including midwives, and there are midwives working alongside these projects.

There are, however, debates about the effectiveness of such programmes improving family health. In particular, concerns have been raised about whether programmes such as Newpin can reach those families most at risk (Oakley et al 1998). It is too early to know whether the Sure Start programmes have had similar problems, as the national evaluation only commenced in 2002. Thus while those receiving the service are often enthusiastic, little impact may be made on health inequalities.

IMPROVING ACCESS TO SERVICES

Internationally improving access to skilled birth attendants is a key World Health Organization objective. The Safe Motherhood programme aims to raise awareness of the problems of inequity in access to skilled birth attendants for mothers from less developed countries. The programme aims to achieve more services that are free to mothers and which meet their needs. This is a complex task, particularly in poor rural areas where transport is scarce and facilities are normally accessed on foot. Access to health care facilities is also associated with improved health and outcomes for mothers and their children. Poor maternal health is directly linked to poverty and in response to the United Nations Millennium Targets the World Health Organization has highlighted the important role of midwives in improving maternal health to reduce family poverty (WHO 2002). Midwives, like other health care practitioners, also have a key role in challenging gender discrimination in health care services.

SAFE MOTHERHOOD

The global Safe Motherhood Initiative started in 1987 with the aims of improving maternal health and cutting the number of maternal deaths in half by the year 2000. In the years following the tenth anniversary of the Initiative's launch the Inter-Agency Group that co-ordinates the Initiative has worked on drawing together lessons learned from field experience to date. A series of 'action messages' have been put out by the Inter-Agency Group (Safe Motherhood, Inter-Agency Group 2003), and include:

1. Advance Safe Motherhood Through Human Rights
2. Empower Women: Ensure Choices
3. Safe Motherhood is a Vital Economic and Social Investment
4. Delay Marriage and First Birth
5. Every Pregnancy Faces Risks
6. Ensure Skilled Attendance at Delivery
7. Improve Access to Quality Reproductive Health Services
8. Prevent Unwanted Pregnancy and Address Unsafe Abortion
9. Measure Progress
10. The Power of Partnership.

In the UK and other developed countries the debate relating to access focuses more on choice and place of delivery. The government's *Changing Childbirth* policy (DH 2003) places the choices of women at the centre of maternity care. There are also concerns in Western countries about the over-provision of medicalised maternity care with a higher degree of medical intervention – such as forceps deliveries and caesarean sections.

MACRO-ECONOMIC CHANGE

The Safe Motherhood programme is also linked to socio-economic goals and recent World Health Organization policy on developing nursing and midwifery services as part of the United Nations Millennium Development Goals programme to reduce poverty (UN 2001). The World Health Organization argues that improved maternal and postpartum care has a positive impact on poverty reduction. The subordinate status of women and their poor health status is seen as one of the key obstacles to poverty reduction. Health problems occurring during pregnancy, childbirth and post partum can, therefore, have significant socio-economic consequences for women (Wagstaff 2001). Midwives and other skilled birth attendants have an important role in monitoring poverty by documenting the prevalence of under-weight babies (WHO 2002).

CONCLUSION: MIDWIVES AND HEALTH INEQUALITIES

In this chapter we have demonstrated that many aspects of health inequalities for women and children are linked to pregnancy, maternity and postpartum care. Wider social determinants such as poverty and social status play an important role in structuring health inequalities, but the evidence also shows that differential access and the quantity and quality of care are important factors as well. Internationally there are gross inequalities in the risk of maternal death, and mother and child morbidity and mortality (WHO 1998). Inequalities during pregnancy, at childbirth and during early years may also play an important role in creating health problems in later life, and even in later generations (Barker 1998). Health systems also entrench gender inequalities in provision of services and in less developed and developed countries poor maternal health is linked to poverty.

It is clear therefore that midwives can and should play an important role in tackling such inequalities. The provision of skilled birth attendants would be fundamental in improving care for women and reducing inequalities in maternal mortality. We should, therefore, be concerned about the movement of trained birth attendants and midwives between nations, where developed countries may create worse inequalities in access and provision by employing staff from developing countries.

Midwives are also well placed to provide health promotion interventions to women at an individual and community level through individual, group and community-based initiatives and health promotion activities. However, this may challenge the traditional role of midwives as supporters of individual women (e.g. in *Changing Childbirth*), and some writers have also questioned whether midwives are appropriate as a 'patient friend' (Hart & Lockey 2002). Many of the roles of midwives incorporate roles of monitoring and controlling women, reporting to health and social care authorities, etc. Thus midwives may be placed in a dual role which can be difficult to follow. However, many of the approaches outlined in this chapter would suggest that developing a broader public health role to tackle health inequalities provides benefits both to women and to midwives in pursuing their support for women in pregnancy and childbirth. As such these developments may establish a new and enhanced role for midwives, providing important health benefits and, in time, reducing health inequalities.

References

Acheson D 2000 Health inequalities impact assessment. Bulletin of the World Health Organization 78(1):75–76

Bailey C, Pain R 2001 Geographies of infant feeding and access to primary health-care. Health and Social Care in the Community 9(5):309–317

Barker D J 1998 Mothers, Babies and Health in Later Life. Churchill Livingstone, Edinburgh

Ben-Shlomo Y, Davey Smith G 1991 Deprivation in infancy or adult life: which is more important for mortality risk? Lancet 337:530–534

Bicego G, Ahmed O B 1996 Infant and Child Mortality. DHS Comparative Studies 20. Macro International, Calverton, MD

Blane D, Brunner E, Wilkinson R (eds) 1996 Health and Social Organisation. Toward a Health Policy for the Twenty-First Century. Routledge, London

Campbell C, Aggleton P 1999 Young people's sexual health: a framework for policy debate. Canadian Journal of Human Sexuality 8(4):249–263

Centers for Disease Control 2002 (Infant mortality data by ethnicity). Online. Available: http://www.cdc.gov/nchs/data/nvsr/nvsr53/nvsr53_05.pdf

Coburn D 2000 Income inequality, social cohesion and the health status of populations: the role of neo-liberalism. Social Science and Medicine 51:135–146

Davey Smith G, Blane D, Bartley M 1994 Explanations for socio-economic differentials in mortality. Evidence from Britain and elsewhere. European Journal of Public Health 4:131–144

Davey Smith G, Hart C, Blane D, Gillis C, Hawthorne V 1997 Lifetime socio-economic differentials in mortality: prospective observational study British Medical Journal 314:547–552

Davies M M, Bath P A 2001 The maternity information concerns of Somali women in the United Kingdom. Journal of Advanced Nursing 36(2):237–245

Department of Health 1993 Changing Childbirth. HMSO, London

Department of Health 1995 The Health of the Nation: Variations in Health. What can the Department of Health and the NHS do? HMSO, London

Department of Health 1997 The New NHS. DH, London

Department of Health 1998 Independent Inquiry into Inequalities in Health Report (Chaired by Sir Donald Acheson). TSO, London

Department of Health 1999a Saving Lives: Our Healthier Nation. Cmd. TSO, London

Department of Health 1999b Making a Difference: Strengthening the Nursing, Midwifery and Health Visiting Contribution to Health and Healthcare. TSO, London

Department of Health 2000 The NHS Plan. TSO, London

Department of Health 2002a Shifting the Balance of Power: Next Steps. DH, London

Department of Health/Treasury 2002b Tackling Health Inequalities: Cross-Cutting Review. DH, London

Department of Health 2002c Improvement, Expansion and Reform: The Next 3 years. Priorities and Planning Framework 2003–2006. TSO, London

Duncan C, Jones K, Moon G 1993 Do places matter? A multi-level analysis of variations in health-related behaviour in Britain. Social Science and Medicine 37:725–733

Eachus J, Williams M, Chan P, Davey Smith G, Grainge M, Donovan J, Frankel S 1996 Deprivation and cause specific morbidity: evidence from the Somerset and Avon survey of health. British Medical Journal 312:287–292

Elford J, Whinchup P, Shaper A G 1991 Early life experience and cardiovascular disease – longitudinal and case-control studies. International Journal of Epidemiology 20:833–844

Frankel S, Elwood P, Sweetnam P, Yarnell J, Davey Smith G 1996 Birthweight, body-mass index in middle-age, and incident coronary heart disease. Lancet 346:1478–1480

Gakidou E E, Murray C J, Frenk J 2000 Defining and measuring health inequality: an approach based on the distribution of health expectancy. Bulletin of the World Health Organisation 78(1):42–54

Gwatkin D 2000 Health inequalities and the health of the poor: what do we know? What can we do? Bulletin of the World Health Organization 78(1):3–18

Hampshire M 2002 The bigger picture. Health Development Today 10:8–10

Hart A, Lockey R 2002 Inequalities in health care provision: the relationship between contemporary policy and contemporary practice in maternity services in England. Journal of Advanced Nursing 37(5):485–493

House of Commons 2003 Inequalities in Access to Maternity Services. Eighth Report of Session 2002–03 Hc 696. TSO, London

Humphreys N A 1885 in Preface to: Vital statistics: A memorial volume of selections from the reports and writings of William Farr. The Sanitary Institute of Great Britain, London

Kaplan G A, Pamuk E R, Lynch J W, Cohen R D, Balfour J L 1996 Inequality in income and mortality in the United States: analysis of mortality and potential pathways. British Medical Journal 312:999–1003 (erratum 31, 1253)

Kawachi I, Kennedy B P, Lochner K, Prothrow-Smith D 1997 Social capital, income inequality and mortality. American Journal of Public Health 87(9):1491–1498

Kennedy B P, Kawachi I, Prothrow-Smith D 1996 Income distribution and mortality: cross-sectional ecological study of the Robin Hood Index in United States. British Medical Journal 312:1004–1007

Kuh D, Ben-Shlomo Y (eds) 1997 A Life Course Approach to Chronic Disease Epidemiology: Tracing the Origins of Ill-health from Early to Adult Life. Oxford Medical Publications, Oxford

Lewis G, Drife J 2001 Why Mothers Die 1997–1999. The Confidential Enquiries into Maternal Deaths in the United Kingdom. RCOG Press, London

Lynch J W, Kaplan G A, Pamuk E F, Cohen R D, Heck K E, Balfour J L, Yen I H 1998 Income inequality and mortality in metropolitan areas of the United States. American Journal of Public Health 88(7):1074–1080

Macdonald J 1992 Primary Health Care. Earthscan, London

McKinlay J B 1995 Bringing the Social System back in: An Essay on the Epidemiological Imagination. New England Research Institute, Boston

Marmot M 2000 Multilevel Approaches to Understanding Social Determinants. In: Berkman L, Kawachi I (eds) Social Epidemiology. Oxford University Press, Oxford

Marmot M, Shipley M, Rose G 1984 Inequalities in death: specific explanations of a general pattern. Lancet 1:1003–1006

Milburn A 2000 A Healthier Nation and Healthier Economy: the contribution of a modern NHS. LSE Health Annual Lecture, 8 March, London

Muntaner C, Lynch J 1999 Income inequality, social cohesion and class relations: a critique of Wilkinson's neo-Durkheimian research program. International Journal of Health Services 29(1):59–81

Murray C J, Gakidou E E, Frenk J 1999 Health inequalities and social group differences: what should we measure? Bulletin of the World Health Organization 77(7):537–543

NHS Centre for Reviews and Dissemination 1995 Review of the Research on the Effectiveness of Health Service Interventions to Reduce Variations in Health. University of York, York

Oakley A, Rajan L, Turner H 1998 Evaluating parent support initiatives: lessons from two case studies. Health and Social Care in the Community 6(5):318–330

Office for National Statistics 2002 Infant Mortality Rates by District. Online. Available: http://www.statistics.gov.uk/STATBASE/Source.asp?vlnk=548. Accessed March 2002

Powell M, Exworthy M 2000 Variations on a theme: New Labour, health inequalities and policy failure. Chapter 4. In: Hann A (ed) Analysing Health Policy. Ashgate, Aldershot

Royal College of Midwives 2000 Vision 2000. RCM, London

Safe Motherhood Inter-Agency Group 2003 Priorities for Safe Motherhood. Viewed January 2005 at www.safemotherhood.org/smpriorities

Sen A 1999 Development as Freedom. Oxford University Press, Oxford

Sen A 2001 Economic progress and health. In: Leon D, Walt G (eds) Poverty, Inequality and Health. Oxford University Press, Oxford

Social Exclusion Unit 1999 Teenage Pregnancy. Cm 4342. TSO, London

Standing H 1997 Gender and equity in health sector reform programs: a review. Health Policy and Planning 12:1–18

Stein C, Moritz I 1999 A Life Course Perspective of Maintaining Independence in Older Age. WHO, Geneva

Taylor P, Peckham S, Turton P 1998 A Public Health Model of Primary Care: From Concept to Reality. Public Health Alliance, Birmingham

Thorp S 2003 Born equal. Health Development Today 18:21–23

Townsend P, Davidson N, Whitehead M 1988 Inequalities in Health, 2nd edn. Penguin, London

Tudor-Hart J 1988 A New Kind of Doctor. Merlin Press, London

Turton P, Peckham S, Taylor P 1999 Integrating primary care and public health. In: Lindsay G, Craig P (eds) Nursing for Public Health: Population-based Care. Churchill Livingstone, Edinburgh

United Nations 2001 Millennium Development Goals. United Nations, New York

Wagstaff A 2001 Economics, health and development: some ethical dilemmas facing the World Bank and the

international community. Journal of Medical Ethics 27(4):262–267
Whitehead M 1995 Tackling inequalities: a review of policy initiatives. In Benzeval M, Judge K, Whitehead M (eds) Tackling Inequalities in Health. An Agenda for Action. King's Fund, London
Wilkinson R G 1996 Unhealthy Societies: The Afflictions of Inequalities. Routledge, London
Wilkinson R G 1997 Health inequalities: relative or absolute material standards? British Medical Journal 314:591–595
World Bank 2001 Attacking Poverty: World Development Report 2000/2001. Oxford University Press, Oxford
World Health Organization 1985 Targets for Health for All: Targets in Support of the European Regional Strategy for Health for All by the year 2000. WHO European Regional Office, Copenhagen
World Health Organization 1998 World Health Day: Safe Motherhood. Pregnancy is Special: Let's make it safe. WHO, Geneva
World Health Organization 2002 Strategic Directions for Strengthening Nursing and Midwifery Services. WHO, Geneva
World Health Organization/UNICEF 1978 Alma Ata Declaration. WHO, Geneva
Wright E O 1997 Class Counts: Comparative Studies in Class Analysis. Cambridge University Press, Cambridge

Chapter 5

Celebrating diversity: meeting needs

Claire Chambers

CHAPTER CONTENTS

SUMMARY

Celebration of diversity and meeting needs are often cited as important concepts of midwifery practice, but what is actually meant by meeting diverse needs? What is diversity and how does that relate to current midwifery practice?

In this chapter these questions will be answered and the importance of raising awareness of diversity within midwifery practice will be discussed and various approaches explored in relation to this. In order for a service to meet the diverse needs of society there needs to be a heightened awareness of diversity issues and a non-discriminatory culture which is central to the philosophy of the service and organisation. This involves appropriate marketing and selection of staff, and clear management philosophy and policies. However, it also involves every practitioner being culturally aware and culturally competent and this often requires educational opportunities to challenge norms and assumptions and bring about change in the practice environment.

All of these concepts will be discussed in this chapter, building on the discussion on inequalities in health in Chapter 4 and using midwifery case studies to illustrate the points made. Midwives need to encourage an inclusive environment where their views and ways of thinking are challenged in order to challenge complacency and reduce discrimination, and thereby encourage an environment where non-discriminatory and antidiscriminatory practice, non-stigmatised care and non-judgemental practice are the norm. All of these issues will be discussed in relation to midwifery practice, and ways of developing cultural empowerment and intercultural communication strategies will be identified.

Key themes include:

- Celebration of diversity
- Awareness of diversity
- Cultural awareness
- Cultural competence
- Challenging norms and assumptions
- Inclusive environment
- Challenging complacency
- Discrimination
- Non-discriminatory practice
- Antidiscriminatory practice
- Non-stigmatisation
- Non-judgemental approach
- Cultural empowerment
- Intercultural communication.

WHAT IS DIVERSITY AND HOW DOES IT IMPACT ON MIDWIFERY PRACTICE?

> Diversity is a term increasingly being used to emphasise the differences between individuals and across groups and the fact that such differences are best seen as assets to be valued and affirmed, rather than as problems to be solved.
>
> (Thompson 2001:34)

Society is made up of people of different cultures, races, nationalities, abilities, ages, sexual identities, religions, beliefs and lifestyles, all of whom should have equal opportunity for achieving their potential in relation to health, employment, education, housing, civil rights and self actualisation. However, it is obvious from health statistics and data that this is not the case. There has been discussion in earlier chapters concerning widespread health inequality and how the most disadvantaged suffer most from ill health (DH 1999). Black (cited in Robinson & Elkan 1996) said that some individuals can suffer double or triple disadvantage and can be discriminated against in terms of race, lifestyle, gender and disability. This is a serious public health issue and as health professionals we should be doing all within our capability to address this issue and work towards reducing inequalities in health. After all, the Nursing and Midwifery Council Code of Professional Conduct in the UK says:

> You are personally accountable for ensuring that you promote and protect the interests and dignity of patients and clients, irrespective of gender,

> age, race, ability, sexuality, economic status, lifestyle, culture and religious or political beliefs.
>
> (NMC 2002)

We live and work in a multicultural and multifaceted society and this does and should influence the way we deliver care to patients and clients. In the case of midwifery this involves working with women and their partners and families in a concordant way to meet their differing and diverse needs. Concordance is a term that has been brought to the fore in the context of nurse prescribing, and refers to the way in which decisions are made jointly and in partnership in a mutually agreeable manner (Long & Baxter 2002) and Sanz (2003) discusses this in relation to children's needs. This replaces the outdated concept of compliance whereby the patient is expected merely to follow the doctor's instructions despite the impracticality of the advice in relation to the way that they live their lives. The following case study gives an example.

CASE STUDY

Mandy feels misunderstood by many people. They don't understand the many problems she faces just trying to live her life and bring up her children. Her partner Barry is in prison again and she really thinks that he has an easier time of it than she does. After all, he doesn't have to bring up six children on his own. On his last brief spell in between prison stays she managed to get pregnant again, which is the last thing she needed but he refuses to let her do anything to prevent future pregnancies. She really doesn't know what her GP will say, he wasn't very impressed when she got pregnant last time, and Natalie is only 3 months old now. He thinks she has got too much on her plate, and she thinks that he is right.

She plucked up the courage to see the midwife, Jenny, today and was pleasantly surprised by how it went. The appointment started badly, she was a bit late and had to take all six kids with her, which is never a good idea as it's difficult to keep them quiet in a strange environment with nothing to do. She feels that everyone else looks down on her, with their happy smiles and 'happy to be pregnant' looks and doting husbands, while she just feels desperate. She is happy for them but it just isn't the same for her.

Jenny actually seemed pleased to see her again but was concerned by how tired she looked. She really seemed interested in how she was and how she was coping with it all. They had discussed the best way for Mandy to have appointments with the midwife, and Jenny seemed to understand the difficulties Mandy had just coming for an appointment.

Overall Mandy left the clinic feeling as if what she needed was important to Jenny, rather than feeling as if she was viewed as a problem which had happened often before.

At first glance it can appear, as Mandy's ethnic background is not known and there is no reason to suggest that she has a disability and she appears to be heterosexual, that diversity issues are not relevant here. However, anyone can be discriminated against, because they smoke or indulge in health damaging behaviour, because they are overweight or lacking in education, or because they live their lives differently from the way that we live ours, whether through choice or lack of choice. Mandy has 'chosen' to bring her children to an antenatal clinic, which has undoubtedly made it more difficult for the midwife to assess her health needs and communicate with her. Her partner is in prison and she is undoubtedly suffering the consequences of this in terms of poverty and unemployment. Therefore she is in a position of disadvantage which will impact on her health, as can be seen in Chapter 1 in relation to the key determinants of health outcome and the worsened outcomes for maternal and child health. She might not have had the opportunity to fulfil her educational potential, and could be illiterate. She might also smoke and be unable to eat a nutritious diet, which would also impact on the health of her unborn baby, as can again be seen in Chapter 1. All of these factors might cause health professionals to act in a judgemental or patronising way towards her. However, she was treated with courtesy and respect and the midwife involved also made her feel important, valued and liked as an individual.

Mandy was treated as an individual by the midwife, and she was consulted about the care involved. Too often a judgemental attitude is adopted when individuals do not attend for appointments or do not follow health advice, when no attempts have been made to understand the situation from the client's viewpoint and therefore falling at the first hurdle is understandable and predictable. In terms of diversity this is important. Thompson (2001:34) says that the word diversity is becoming more popular because it is a positive term and 'emphasises the differences between individuals and across groups and the fact that such differences are best seen as assets to be valued and affirmed, rather than as problems to be solved'. In this way diversity is celebrated. This point about difference often being perceived as a problem is key to individuals feeling undervalued. The 'asset approach' is advocated in relation to this where individuals are seen as an asset rather than a problem. The opportunity to see Mandy at the antenatal clinic and become involved in her care is an asset, because it allows the midwife to become involved with her at an early stage of her pregnancy and to be involved with a complex range of needs. However, in a stretched service it is understandable why it would not always be seen in that way and Mandy would then be blamed for not fitting in with a service that seems to work for most pregnant women. Meeting the needs of those whose needs are often greater and who are often perceived as victims of the health inequalities divide is essential for midwives and other health professionals in order to address the public health agenda.

Reflection on practice

- Think about a situation when you judged someone because of their circumstances
- Reflect on how you delivered care to this mother and the way you gave health advice
- How do you think that this felt to her?
- How could you start to understand her situation better?
- Would you change anything about your practice in the future?

RAISING AWARENESS OF DIVERSITY

In order for midwives and other health professionals to meet the diverse needs of a diverse population they need to understand both the nature of diversity and how it manifests itself in practice situations. There are many different ways in which this awareness can be instigated and encouraged through initial education and subsequent formal education, study days or clinical supervision sessions.

CASE STUDY

Penny felt a little out of her depth during the first month of her midwifery course. She was already a qualified nurse and had worked on an acute medical ward before deciding that she wanted to be a midwife. It was becoming obvious that this course was very different from her initial nursing training. For one thing, patients were no longer patients: they were well women who wanted some control over their care and where it would take place. Secondly the hospital where she was now based was right in the middle of a city where there seemed to be a great deal of poverty and families from many different ethnic groups, many of whom did not speak English as a first language. She didn't know where to start in terms of assessing their needs, even less in trying to meet them.

However, in sessions within the course and out in the practice environment she was encouraged to think about needs from the individual's perspective and also to think about what options were actually possible for that family before she tried to discuss what they might want to do to increase the health potential of both themselves and the expected baby. This was new to her, and she began to see how when she gave advice on discharging a patient from the ward in her old role she had not really taken the patient's home circumstances or health beliefs into account. It wasn't surprising really that the same people came back again and again because she could see now how difficult it would be for some people to follow the advice that she and her colleagues were giving.

Penny's experience is very common. It can be extremely difficult to gain a full picture of the reality of patients' lives when you only see them in a hospital environment. Therefore tailoring health advice to their needs and their circumstances can be almost impossible. This is an area that professional education needs to address. Boi (2000) highlights the detrimental effect that a language barrier, exacerbated by a lack of knowledge of a patient's culture, can have on patient care and states that post-registration courses need to address the issues of different cultures, health beliefs and practices within the curricula. However, as this piece of research clearly states that nurses felt under-prepared for caring for patients from different cultural backgrounds, this would also need to take place in initial pre-registration training. Professional education and development has a responsibility to act as a catalyst in this area.

Duffy (2001) discusses the need for transformative cultural education whereby learning takes place through interaction between members of the group and is based on the assumption of shared power between different cultures. This approach uses Mezirow's (1990) perception of perspective transformation whereby individuals become aware of how their assumptions and beliefs constrain understanding of the world, and in the case of health professionals how this has a detrimental effect on client care. This approach requires risk taking and critical reflection, where individuals have to move outside their comfort zones and become vulnerable and question their values, beliefs and behaviours. Hannerz (1996) cited in Duffy (2001) says that this can be accomplished in various ways:

- Accentuating contradictions and misunderstandings
- Highlighting connections between cultures
- Refusing to generalise.

All individuals tend to be socialised to think that their ways of being are normal, which then creates the belief that others' ways are not. This ethnocentricism can result in the belief that a certain group is superior. Sutherland (2002) discusses this superiority of one's own group and says that it leads to a contempt for other cultural groups and a tendency to view other cultures in terms of one's own. Andrews (1992:7) goes further and says that:

> Ethnocentric beliefs by health care providers have resulted in misdiagnosis, alienation of patients, failure to adequately provide pain relief, and arrest of parents accused of child abuse because of culturally based practices.

An awareness of this is obviously essential for midwifery practice if care is to be carried out in a manner which is acceptable to all users of the service, and midwives need to be proactive in taking their service forward in a manner which explores all possibilities of culturally competent care. The concept of cultural competence will be discussed in greater detail later.

Reflection on practice

- Think about a situation when you made assumptions about a mother's ability to change her health behaviour
- How would you introduce more opportunities to develop cultural awareness into your practice?
- How would you encourage others to increase their cultural awareness in clinical supervision sessions?

CASE STUDY

Michelle was an extremely experienced midwife working in a rural environment where it was very rare to meet someone of a non-Caucasian ethnic group. However, she had lately had her beliefs and professional practice challenged by a woman who had recently given birth. Joyce was a teenage African asylum seeker with whom Michelle had to communicate via a translator. She was very vocal in expressing her pain throughout the labour, and other health professionals became dismissive of her cries for pain relief. However, Michelle took the time to sit with her, make eye contact and try to reassure her with words and therapeutic touch. By building this relationship she could see that Joyce was experiencing severe pain but she was also frightened, and Michelle was aware that pain is a personal perception and that comparing pain tolerance levels of other women was unhelpful in helping Joyce through the labour. She was able to use therapeutic touch to reduce her anxiety, together with increased analgesia, and Joyce became more able to cope with the pain and follow her advice.

The needs of asylum seekers have been thoroughly discussed in Chapter 2, and this chapter gives very detailed information about their needs and how midwives need to be aware of the traumatic lives that mothers have possibly experienced. Joyce is still very young and therefore has needs in relation to teenage pregnancies, discussed in previous chapters, but the immediacy of the situation, the language barrier and the lack of a clear history make it impossible for Michelle to know what trauma she may have endured. However, she took the time to build a relationship with Joyce and try to reduce her fear of both the birth and being in an alien environment, and Joyce became less frightened and more able to cope with her labour.

Reflection on practice

- Have you ever been in a situation where you were not sure why someone was behaving in the way that they were?
- What non-verbal communication strategies have you used when verbal communication is difficult?
- Do you change the way you communicate when the mother is very young or when the mother is finding it difficult to communicate with you?
- How would you pass these strategies on to others?

Example

Students undertaking Community Specialist Practitioner Award programmes in a particular university have been asked to use critical incidents within their competency achievement documentation to highlight whether the care that has been given would be appropriate to all patients and clients. This has increased their knowledge and awareness of diversity to a great extent, and the number of examples of competencies that address these issues, across all pathways, can be seen in Figures 5.1, 5.2 and 5.3, as can the range of client needs that have been used to highlight diversity.

For example, a competency addressing prescribing from a designated formulary, otherwise known as nurse prescribing, might also discuss

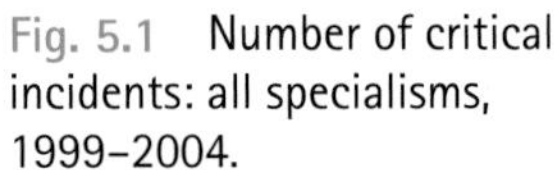

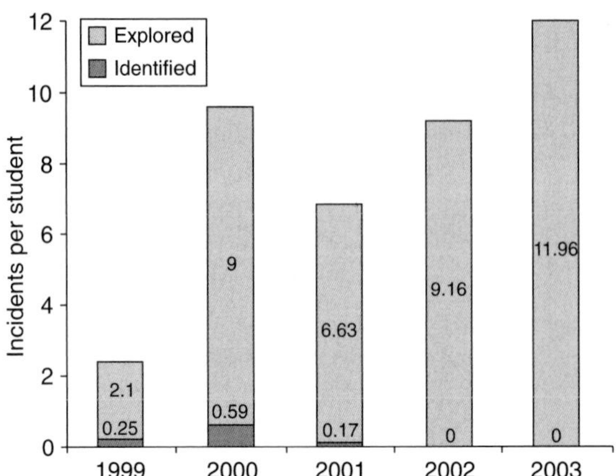

Fig. 5.1 Number of critical incidents: all specialisms, 1999–2004.

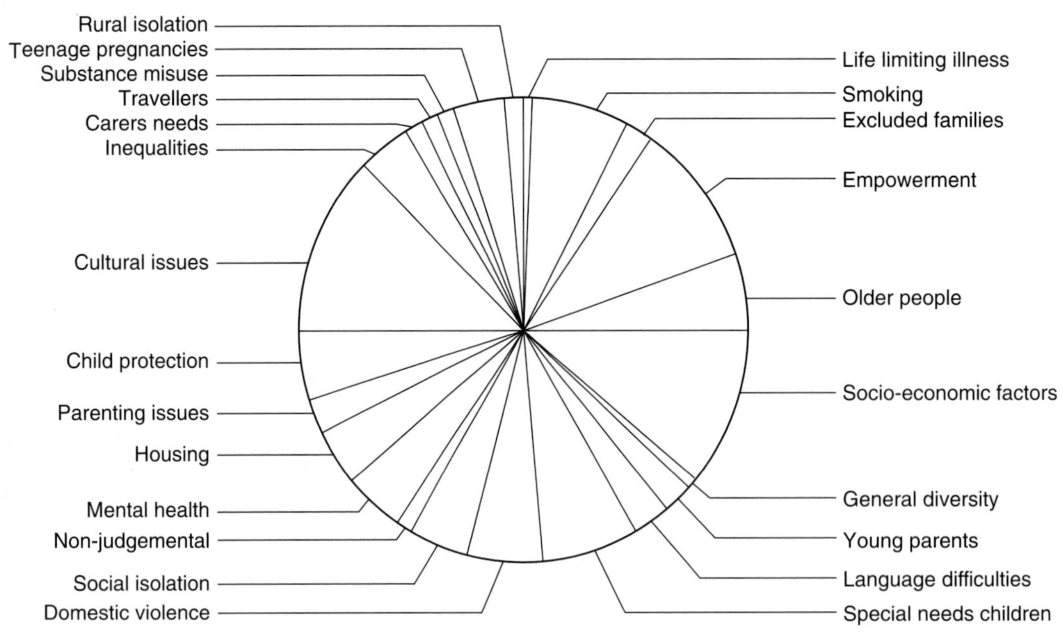

Fig. 5.2 Range of critical incidents: Health Visitors, 2004.

how the intervention might have changed in terms of documentation if the client had been illiterate or in terms of the whole prescribing process if English was not the client's first language and communication was limited by language difficulties.

Other examples might highlight when care would be carried out differently if the client had any form of disability, was geographically or socially isolated, or was living in multi-occupancy housing. In addition many incidents would describe and analyse situations where there were concerns about child protection or domestic violence or where parenting was far from ideal. The discussion would highlight how non-judgemental and

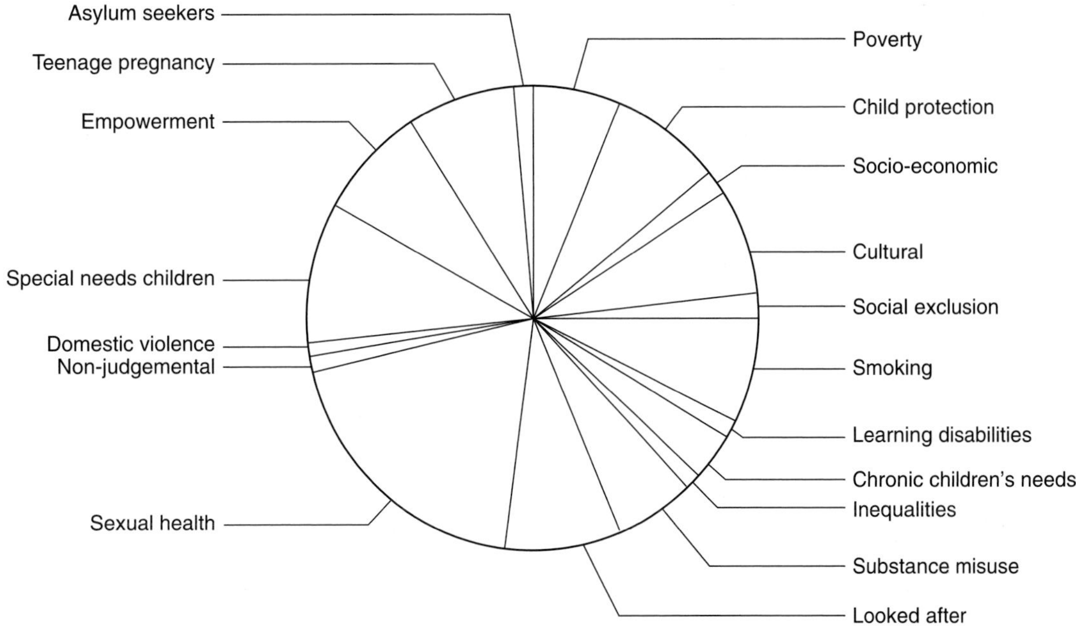

Fig. 5.3 Range of critical incidents: School Nurses, 2004.

client-focused care was carried out and what knowledge and skills had been utilised to provide effective care.

This approach could also work in midwifery education and in clinical supervision sessions, where students or practitioners could be encouraged to think about how care might have differed if circumstances had been slightly different, or alternatively if diversity issues were actually present, whether enough had been done to give client-centred care in that particular situation.

Some recommendations for education, staff development and clinical supervision sessions are as follows:

- Learning, teaching and assessment strategies which encourage exploration of the needs of the communities in which professional practice operates
- Assessment which identifies non-discriminatory practice and encourages antidiscriminatory practice
- The use of culturally appropriate case studies to develop practice and challenge norms and assumptions
- Literature sources and websites available to all staff, and time in which to read, discuss and apply this knowledge
- Culturally aware and non-ethnocentric practice environments
- Teaching and practice areas where all students feel comfortable and valued
- Opportunities to challenge ethnocentric beliefs, values and norms
- Role play which both accentuates contradictions and misunderstandings and highlights the connections between cultures.

Reflection on practice

- What other strategies could you use to encourage students and colleagues to increase their cultural awareness?
- Do you use case discussions as a tool to think about how care would have changed in different circumstances?
- Are culturally-appropriate case studies used to discuss care where appropriate?
- Do parents, students and colleagues from all ethnic backgrounds feel comfortable in your working environment?

CULTURAL COMPETENCE AS A BASIS FOR PROFESSIONAL PRACTICE

Having discussed how to raise awareness of diversity, it is now important to discuss how this awareness can be transformed into cultural competence. Cultural awareness, according to Jandt (2001), is being competent in intercultural communication and this involves individuals understanding the social customs and beliefs of the culture involved. In terms of midwifery practice this involves being aware of that culture's health beliefs and social structures and practices. Jandt goes on to say that 'understanding how people think and behave is essential for effective communication with them'. He goes on to say that three barriers to intercultural communication are high anxiety, assuming similarity instead of difference, and ethnocentrism. Ethnocentrism has been discussed earlier but the other two barriers to communication have many implications for midwifery practice.

CASE STUDY

Suri had seen the same midwife at all her antenatal appointments so far and was impressed by how he was really trying to find out her views about her pregnancy and labour. She had had reservations about having a male midwife but it was working out very well. When she had been pregnant with her previous daughter the midwife where she had lived before had tried to hide her lack of knowledge of Suri's cultural background by making sweeping statements about what she assumed Suri might want, based on other women who had given birth in the past. Didn't she know that her views were her own, and not totally determined by her ethnic background? The midwife never seemed relaxed with Suri and seemed constantly worried about saying the wrong thing, and this made Suri feel on edge too.

In comparison Dave started off by saying that he was recently qualified and had not met many women of her ethnic background, and would like to make sure that Suri's pregnancy and birth went as she would want them to. He offered to change with a female colleague if she was not comfortable with having a male midwife. He also said that he would welcome the opportunity to gain some insight into if and when her cultural background influenced her choices. He seemed comfortable and open with her and she felt relaxed from the start.

Campinha-Bacote (2002) states that cultural competence is a process and not an event, and Dave is recognising this by showing that he has some cultural awareness but would like to develop his cultural knowledge and skill further by capitalising on his cultural encounters. Through this he is demonstrating a desire to be more culturally competent. These are the five constructs of cultural competence according to Campinha-Bacote (2002), and the point is also made that there is more variation within ethnic groups than across them, a point that many people ignore when making sweeping assumptions based on ethnic group alone. Dave is clearly demonstrating to Suri that he has a strong motivation to provide ethnically sensitive and individualised care, and that he is entering a professional partnership with her which is based on mutual respect and increased knowledge on both sides.

It is easy to make assumptions and generalise care when this is not the intention. For example there is usually an assumption that women will attend antenatal appointments outside the home, or that visits in certain circumstances can be arranged by phone. Hilgenberg and Schlickau (2002) however give the example of Amish families where care had to be structured in different ways. Making appointments by phone, or appointments which necessitated families using cars or watching health promotional videos, was not part of their culture. If there was a large Amish community living locally then it would be assumed that midwives were aware of how such cultural norms might affect their planning of care, but if an Amish woman was living in an area where she was culturally isolated her care might be compromised by a lack of knowledge of cultural variations.

Reflection on practice

- Do you think that you have ever made assumptions on a mother's health beliefs based on experiences with others of her ethnic group?
- Do you ever feel uncomfortable about your lack of knowledge of certain ethnic groups?
- How do you deal with this situation?
- Do you think that there is room for a greater degree of cultural knowledge in how you or your colleagues practice?

THE IMPORTANCE OF INTERCULTURAL COMMUNICATION AND THE NEED TO CHALLENGE DISCRIMINATION

Jandt (2001) confirms that intercultural communication is interaction between people of diverse cultures. However, he says that stereotyping and prejudice can impede the communication that takes place. Stereotyping he defines as 'negative or positive judgements made about individuals based on any observable or believed group membership' (2001:45). This point about positive stereotyping also being harmful is a sensitive issue, as many people believe that positive stereotyping is not a problem. However, it allows individuals to be perceived as merely members of a group and not as individuals. Furthermore, the more visible their allegiance to a group, the more this can lead to prejudice. Prejudice, according to Jandt, is an 'irrational suspicion or hatred of a particular group, race, religion or orientation. Persons within the group are viewed not in terms of their individual merit, but according to the superficial characteristics that make them part of the group' (2001:45).

Thompson (2001) says 'there is no middle ground: intervention either adds to oppression (or at least condones it) or goes some small way towards easing or breaking such oppression'. He goes on to say that 'in short, practice which does not take account of oppression and discrimination cannot be seen as good practice, no matter how high its standards may be in other respects. For example a social work intervention with a disabled person which fails to recognise the marginalized position of disabled people in society runs the risk of doing the client more of a disservice than a service' (2001:11).

This is an important point. If health professionals do not take into account how individuals, ethnic groups and communities are marginalised within society and how their life chances and choices are limited by the way that the world perceives them or by their financial or social status, then it is not possible to deliver client- or patient-focused care. Midwives could find themselves in the position of giving advice which is impractical or impossible for the women in their care. This would then possibly lead to potential judgemental attitudes and behaviour when the women were not able to follow the advice.

CASE STUDY

Anita really couldn't understand why the student midwife kept going on at her about her diet and her smoking. She kept talking about eating fresh fruit and vegetables as if they grew in her garden. As she lived on the twelfth floor of her block of flats, that was clearly not an option. Didn't she realise that they were expensive and they didn't last long? She only managed to get to the out-of-town supermarket every few weeks and fruit cost so much and it was bulky and heavy to carry home. Even having made it to the bottom of her building she often found that the lift wasn't working. It made shopping locally in smaller amounts much easier. She tended to shop at the end of the week when at least some money was there. The corner shop was much more expensive, though, and the fruit never looked fresh.

As for the smoking. She'd tried to give up so many times, she really had, but other people didn't realise that they calmed her down and she had nothing else that she did just for herself. It was just too hard to give up the only thing in life that made things bearable.

Sue, the student midwife, couldn't see why Anita couldn't understand the importance of fresh fruit and vegetables in her diet. She had a responsibility to provide a balanced diet for her young family, and how hard could that be? The smoking was another factor in the family's health problems. The twins both had asthma and Anita seemed to have a bad cough every time she saw her. Didn't Anita care about her family's health at all?

She discussed the situation with Gloria, her mentor, hoping that she would help her with ways to convince Anita to give her family a healthy diet and give up smoking. However, Gloria took her down to the shop that Anita used and Sue was shocked at the poor quality of the fresh produce. She then took her to the building where Anita lived and she couldn't believe the state of the front entrance. The walls were covered in graffiti and the whole lift area smelt of urine. One lift was out of order and the other was dirty and smelly. Sue could not imagine living in such a place, and in her reflection session with Gloria later in the day she started to explore how her expectations were unrealistic as she had no idea of Anita's home circumstances and therefore the health advice she gave was totally impossible for Anita to follow. They then discussed ways in which health promotional advice could be more realistic and less victim blaming.

This situation highlights important public health issues, and in some areas practitioners are working with communities to change the environments where they live and to work towards improving the circumstances in which they live their lives. Midwives can play an active part in encouraging communities to change their circumstances and in changing the ways that women and their families are perceived by health professionals.

Gloria was practising in an antidiscriminatory manner, in that she was not only trying to eradicate discrimination in her own practice, but challenging this in the practice of others. Thompson (2001) refers to this as a type of emancipatory practice and this also involves challenging the organisational structures in which we practice. If there are ways of working which unfairly disadvantage some clients or patients, then we have a responsibility as health professionals to challenge these and act as agents of change and advocates for those in our care.

This leads to a cultural empowerment where 'discriminatory assumptions and stereotypes can be challenged in an attempt to break down an oppressive culture in which the values and interests of dominant groups are presented as normal and natural' (Thompson 1998:73). There are many examples of client groups who are systematically and persistently discriminated against and nurses, midwives and health visitors have an important role as advocates where this is the case. Misener et al (1977) discuss this role in relation to homophobia but discrimination can also take place against those who are homeless, survivors of domestic violence and those with mental health problems (Holmstrom 2001) and many other situations that bring about specific health or social problems of their own.

Jandt (2001) says that intercultural communication competence has various different components, namely: personality strength, communication skills, psychological adjustment and cultural awareness. Cultural awareness has been discussed already, and communication skills, comprising verbal and non-verbal skills and empathy, are an essential component of any nursing, midwifery or health visiting practice. However, the concepts of personality strength and psychological adjustment in intercultural communication are probably new to many practitioners.

Personality strength, according to Jandt (2001), involves having a positive self-concept, the ability to self-disclose and self-monitor, self-awareness, a friendly personality and the ability to initiate positive attitudes as well as being able to reveal little anxiety in communication, which he refers to as social relaxation. This, together with psychological adjustment, which involves the ability to acclimatise to new environments and handle 'culture shock' such as frustration or stress caused by new environments, is seen as central to being competent at intercultural communication.

Reflection on practice

- How would you start to understand the life experiences of the women and families in your care?
- How would you help a student gain this awareness?
- Would you be able to challenge the discriminatory practice of others?

CASE STUDY

Sue was starting to think that she was getting to grips with the reality of community midwifery practice, and was grateful to Gloria who was helping her to understand how women were not necessarily able to make healthy choices in their lifestyles and that life seemed to be stacked unfairly against some individuals and groups within society. However, she was constantly surprised at Gloria's ability to appear accepting of a woman's social environment and non-judgemental of her lifestyle, whilst still giving advice and support and encouraging her to take some control over her life. Gloria had explained that if a child was at risk and child protection issues were suspected, then it was important to maintain an honest relationship and express concerns and take action where appropriate whilst still demonstrating respect for those caring for that child. These were skills that Sue thought that she would find hard to develop, but she recognised that she was learning a great deal from Gloria's relaxed and professional approach and how she interacted with families from different backgrounds. She was also learning that by trying to understand the life experiences of the parents she could see why they had never had the opportunity to gain effective parenting skills or that they had experienced abuse in their childhoods which was becoming a cycle of abuse for future generations. Understanding this was helping her to become less judgemental and therefore more honest with parents, whilst still identifying when intervention was required to safeguard the safety or well-being of their children.

It is important that midwives are able to adopt this honest and relaxed communication with families, and this is even more important when problems are starting to arise that make this more difficult. Encouraging this approach through effective mentoring and clinical supervision is an important role for all midwives to adopt.

Reflection on practice

- How would you encourage an open and honest dialogue when standards of parenting were far from ideal?
- How would you maintain a trusting relationship with families?
- Would you find it difficult to respect parents in these situations?
- What would help you to do this?

CONCLUSION

In this chapter the topic of diversity has been explored from the midwife's and the mother's perspective, drawing on case study examples to analyse the points that have been raised. Inequalities in health are a particular challenge to public health practice today, and for midwifery there are clearly-evidenced worse outcomes for socially excluded individuals and families within our society. These have been discussed in various chapters within this book and Chapter 1 identified key determinants of health outcome where maternal and child health are compromised. Some midwifery scenarios have been chosen from some of these areas of health deprivation, for example, asylum seekers, those from ethnic minorities, teenagers and those living in deprived circumstances. However, there are many other individuals who can feel discriminated against – for example mothers with disabilities or who have same-sex partnerships. All health professionals have a role to play in ensuring that all individuals feel included and accepted rather than excluded and discriminated against.

In order for this to be the case in terms of midwifery practice, midwives have to ensure that they are culturally aware and culturally competent, that they adopt a non-stigmatising and non-judgemental approach to all families in their care. In addition midwives must challenge complacency and their own assumptions and norms and those of others, to ensure that the diverse needs of society are met. Diversity should be celebrated rather than berated and reflective discussion and clinical supervision sessions can help to enhance midwifery practice and reduce inequalities in health in the future.

References

Andrews M 1992 Cultural perspectives on nursing in the 21st century. Journal of Professional Nursing 8(1):7–15

Boi S 2000 Nurses' experiences in caring for patients from different cultural backgrounds. NT Research 5(5):382–389

Campinha-Bacote J 2002 The process of cultural competence in the delivery of health care services: a model of care. Journal of Transcultural Nursing 13(3):181–184

Department of Health 1999 Saving Lives: Our Healthier Nation. TSO, London

Duffy M 2001 A critique of cultural education in nursing. Journal of Advanced Nursing 36(4):487–495

Hannerz U 1996 Transnational Connections: Culture, People, Places. Routledge, New York. Cited in Duffy M 2001 A critique of cultural education in nursing. Journal of Advanced Nursing 36(4):487–495

Hilgenberg E, Schlickau J 2002 Building transcultural knowledge through intercollegiate collaboration. Journal of Transcultural Nursing 13(3): 241–247

Holmstrom R 2001 Celebrating diversity. Community Practitioner 74(10):377–379

Jandt F 2001 Intercultural Communication: An Introduction, 3rd edn. Sage, London

Long A, Baxter R 2002 Nurse prescribing: promoting concordance. Nursing in Practice 7:39–41. Also published by Royal College of General Practitioners Reference Books. Campden, London, 39–42

Mezirow J et al 1990 Fostering Critical Reflection in Adulthood: A Guide to Transformative and Emancipatory Learning. Jossey-Bass, San Francisco

Misener T, Sowell R, Phillips K, Harris C 1977 Sexual orientation: a cultural diversity issue for nursing. Nursing Outlook 45(4):178–181

Nursing and Midwifery Council 2002 Code of Professional Conduct. NMC, London

Robinson J, Elkan R 1996 Health Needs Assessment: Theory and Practice. Churchill Livingstone, Edinburgh

Sanz E 2003 Concordance on children's use of medicines. British Medical Journal 327:858–860

Sutherland L 2002 Ethnocentrism in a pluralistic society: a concept analysis. Journal of Transcultural Nursing 13(4):274–281

Thompson N 1998 Promoting Equality. Macmillan, London

Thompson N 2001 Anti-discriminatory Practice, 3rd edn. Palgrave, Basingstoke

Chapter 6

Community spirit: looking beyond the obvious

Pádraig Ó Lúanaigh

CHAPTER CONTENTS

SUMMARY

This chapter explores the key components and elements relating to health needs assessment and community profiling. Following discussion around the problems associated in defining what a community is, the area of needs assessment will be explored. An argument is put forward for midwives to play a much greater role in conducting community profiles and to have input into the planning and commissioning of local health services.

The process of community profiling is examined and explained, and a number of possible frameworks are discussed. Practical advice is then provided around actually planning and carrying out a community profile.

INTRODUCTION

This chapter will provide guidance on examining and assessing communities, with the aim of allowing midwives to play a much greater role in supporting and having input into community health needs assessment and the identification of health needs related to maternal, child and family health. When trying to see where this activity 'fits' within a public health approach to health care provision, it may be helpful to refer back to the continuum provided in Chapter 3 (Table 3.3). The diagram indicates that health needs assessment and community profiling are distant from the immediate activities and involvement with individuals. This can be a challenge to traditional midwifery practice since it may call for an approach which differs from traditional working boundaries.

For many midwives their client population or 'patch' may be very familiar to them, but the following discussion and debate will challenge you to look beyond the obvious and asks that we listen to and explore in greater detail the communities we work with.

Once we have discussed what in fact communities are, or indeed what they are not, we can focus on looking at how one can define, describe and measure a particular community in a way that informs health care practice. Once armed with the skills to measure communities and produce community profiles, one can then make real progress in starting to identify health and social needs within your particular practice area or community.

COMMUNITY – A KEY ASSUMPTION

The concept of a 'community', like so many other words such as 'health' and 'care', can have many different meanings and these are loaded words since they have a powerful ability to conjure up images and emotions when used.

Frequently you may hear people say that there is no sense of community these days, or how they want to live in a small village so that they can be part of a community. From this example it is clear that the term and concept of community is used to describe or imply a range of ideas and emotions such as belonging to, safety, something that no longer exists and something that can be identified or described.

Before trying to assess a community it is crucial to try to gain some agreement and understanding about what actually constitutes a community. It is generally agreed that communities have some form of social dimension to them – a common bond or shared interest. When we think about the concept of a community as a location, then the common bond tends to be the geographical area, for example a town, street of houses or a housing estate. It is also possible to have institution-based or defined communities such as schools, universities or work places. We also define ourselves within cultural or religious communities, and finally there can be communities of interest such as professional communities, pressure groups or leisure communities. McMurray (1999) offered an interesting perspective when describing an ecological view of community which she defined as 'an interdependent group of plants and animals inhabiting a common space' (1999:6). This definition highlights some key areas for consideration, the issue of a common bond or interdependence and the fact that there tends often to be a geographical or land-based association is an important idea to be aware of.

Reflection on practice

Think about the area where you *live* and list five words that you feel best describe this area.

Geographically how did you define your home community, was it by town or suburb or more locally defined such as your estate or street?

Repeat the exercise based on the community where you *work* or where your main client group live.

Did you list any of the same words when describing both areas?

What kinds of words did you use in both your descriptions?

Did you tend to describe the physical environment, e.g. urban, built-up, rural, or did you concentrate on the individuals living there, e.g. mostly young middle-class families, or did you use emotive descriptions such as 'nice/safe' or 'grotty/rough'?

How easy was it to describe your home and client communities?

What sort of information did you use to inform your descriptions?

The exercises in the 'Reflection' box may highlight to you that we tend to use a very narrow range of information when describing areas. Some may struggle to find five words to describe where they live or work, and often these descriptions can represent perceptions rather than any real, tangible facts about the area. You may also have struck difficulty in identifying the boundaries of your area or community. Would your neighbour or your client population agree with the terms you identified to describe both areas?

The key aspect to defining a community is the need for members of any particular community to recognise that they have something in common to be a community. The factors that may support group or community cohesion are diverse, and may include: occupation, unemployment, religion, culture, socio-economic grouping, education and language spoken.

As a midwife you may work with clients from a defined geographical community or area. Clearly you will work with a specific community within society – pregnant women and their families.

IDENTIFYING NEEDS – A KEY CHALLENGE

The question of need is a fascinating one. Just as we can struggle to untangle what it means to describe a community, the concept of need is equally problematic and needs careful consideration. It is important to acknowledge that frequently, reviews of health services tend to review the services that are currently provided and fail to explore what is actually needed and how best to address these needs. It is vital to a successful profile that you constantly remind yourself of the need to focus on unmet or unrecognised needs, rather than critiquing what is currently offered.

Health needs assessment and the identification of unmet needs is a key component or strategy in attempting to address health inequalities. The issues relating to health inequalities are discussed in Chapter 4.

A key target in the *Tackling Health Inequalities* document (DH 2003) is to improve early antenatal booking and take-up rates for women from low-income families and black and minority ethnic groups. Midwives were one of the key professional groups identified to work with communities to 'identify their needs, ensuring services are culturally appropriate and accessible, providing better information' (2003:25).

The document goes on to suggest (p. 28) that future practice and policy should ensure that 'local people are involved in identifying local needs, influencing decision making and evaluating local services'.

Bradshaw (1972) outlined four types of need as follows:

Normative need – defined by professionals according to professional standards
Felt need – individual or community perceived wants, desires and wishes
Expressed need – when felt need is made clear to others or expressed as demands
Comparative need – a need identified in relation to others (equity or access for example).

This attempt to classify need has been criticised, but this detailing of differing approach to need identification serves as a good indicator and reminder that perceptions of need can be greatly influenced depending on who is setting the need and how need identification is approached.

A differing approach to exploring need was provided by Gough (1992) and is outlined in Box 6.1 – this overview of need is clearly much more aligned to physical and psychological needs and identifies needs in a staircase fashion. For example, the need for adequate food and nutrition comes before all else, and once this need is met the next dominant need is that of adequate shelter or housing. In Western societies these needs may seem far removed from your experience; however, in examining the needs of homeless people, for example, this approach does not seem quite so unrealistic.

Box 6.1
Classification of needs (Gough 1992)

Intermediate needs
Adequate nutritional food and water
Adequate protective housing
A non-hazardous physical environment
Appropriate health care
Security in childhood
Significant primary relationships
Physical security
Economic security
Safe birth control and child-bearing
Basic education

Reflection on practice

> If you were asked about the main needs of your client group – how would you describe them?
>
> What types of need have you identified, based on Bradshaw's taxonomy of needs?
>
> With the same group, where are the identified needs in relation to the areas identified in the box above?
>
> It is worth exploring the differing types of need and how these are defined with your colleagues.

Can you in fact determine the needs of an antenatal mother or newborn in isolation or without consultation with those your decisions impact upon? Need assessment cannot be explored in isolation, and again it is key to successful needs identification that you are aware of and acknowledge the influences acting on need identification. These influences may include political, differing professional approaches, and those with a strong voice within a community, for example a pressure or residents' group.

As such, community health needs assessment can be described as the issues or factors that need to be solved or addressed to improve the health of a defined population group.

The issue of health need identification can be a potential source of personal and professional conflict, given that most countries struggle to try and provide and fund the range and type of health care services that the general public now expect. There needs to be caution when trying to address and set health priorities, by recognising the need to accommodate what should be done, while acknowledging what can be done realistically from a clinical perspective against what can be afforded at the time.

COMMUNITY PROFILING – A KEY SKILL

Having explored community structures and the identification of health needs, our focus now shifts towards actually assessing a community with the aim of identifying health needs. Community profiling (Box 6.2) is a skill that needs to be developed and does take time and effort on the part of the participants. Many practitioners may question the value of conducting or having involvement in a profiling exercise, and this section will examine the key reasons why midwives must ensure that they are equipped and able to support community profiling activities.

A health needs assessment may be an outcome of community profiling, and as such a community profile can be an important resource in identifying and more importantly gaining resources for unmet community needs.

Despite the range of health reform and policy changes implemented over the past 14 years, two common themes have been maintained (Payne 1999):

- That the allocation and funding of health services and clinical interventions should be informed by the best information and evidence available

Box 6.2
Possible positive outcomes from conducting a community profile

- Allows community members and individuals to have a voice and possible influence on health and social care service planning locally
- Recognises the input and role that midwives have in promoting individual well-being and how this contributes to the wider public health agenda
- Offers the potential for midwives to gain new skills and knowledge
- Promotes and provides opportunities for inter-professional and multi-agency working
- Provides a more structured and measurable account of local health needs and a baseline from which to gauge future levels of health needs and health outcomes
- Allows for more focused and, possibly, achievable health promotion targets
- May change service provision to reflect a much more needs-led approach.

- That health care 'consumers' should have a much greater role in the planning and rationing of services through meaningful consultation and involvement by health care commissioners or providers.

It is interesting that from the early nineties, it was clearly indicated that the midwife 'has an important task in health counselling and education, not only for women, but also within the family and the community' (ICM 1990, FIGO & WHO 1992)*.

Despite this clear indication for midwives to play a key role in promoting community and public health, in general the profession has had a limited and unrecognised role.

Chapter 1 identified the many political, social and health policy drivers which have placed and continue to place a greater emphasis on a reduction in health inequalities and longer-term improvement of the public health of women, their babies and families.

The National Service Framework (NSF) for children, young people and maternity services, published in September 2004, details the priorities for maternity service development in England. It is anticipated that the focus for maternity services will be on access and equity of maternity service provision, quality and appropriate and acceptable maternity care provision (Thomas 2003).

Unless those planning and prioritising maternity service provision have accurate and reliable information about the needs of the communities

*The definition of a midwife was adopted by the International Confederation of Midwives (ICM), International Federation of Gynaecology and Obstetrics (FIGO), in 1972 and 1973 respectively and later adopted by the World Health Organization (WHO). This definition was amended by the ICM in 1990 and the amendment ratified by the FIGO and WHO in 1991 and 1992 respectively.

they are planning for, any service provided will invariably fall short of any expectation the women and their families will have.

Prime Minister Blair wrote in the foreword to *Tackling Health Inequalities: A Programme for Action* of 'diverse, rather than identical, solutions which can only come from giving communities and front-line staff the power to redesign, refocus and reprioritise programmes to tackle local need' (DH 2003:1).

Many readers will be aware of the findings outlined in the fifth maternal mortality report which indicated that our current models and maternity services dramatically disadvantage those women suffering from social isolation and poverty, and that teenage pregnancy and mental illness are key issues in higher incidences of maternal and infant morbidity and mortality (Lewis & Drife 2001).

There are, however, some serious potential risks associated with community profiling which need to be given careful consideration; in the process of stigmatising an area:

- Identified needs may not receive the support or funding required
- The health needs identified may not be accepted as the priority by the community and may indicate a possible failure of a professional group or service.

The process of conducting a community profile or assessment was described as the 'systematic collection of data to identify the health needs of a defined population, and the analysis of that data to assess and prioritise strategies in health promotion' (Twinn et al 1990:2). It should be recognised that community profiling is not easy and is far from being an exact science. Community profiles can be as difficult to plan and define as the complex communities they are intended to represent and measure. Reflecting on her own experience, Lock (1999:158) argued that profiling and health needs assessment is a challenge and as such 'does not have to be perfect to be good enough'.

ACCESSING AND USING INFORMATION

To be of any real value a community profile needs to reflect a range of data sources and styles. Traditionally public health assessments have relied on quantitative hard data such as lives lost, mortality and morbidity statistics. Chapter 3 provides further information on how this information is defined and measured. While these data are an important source of information, a profile, which is based solely on quantitative, statistical data, is unlikely to capture much of the hidden life of a community. Returning to the earlier discussion about community composition, it should be clear that no community could realistically be reduced to a series of numbers or graphs.

Demographic information is readily available and census data are a good starting place. In the UK a census was conducted in 2001 and national and ward data based on the returns are accessible via the

Box 6.3
Planning a community profile

Step One: decide the purpose of the profile
Step Two: decide and define the boundaries for the profile
Step Three: find, collect and analyse the information gained
Step Four: disseminate and form an action plan based on the findings.

Internet (www.statistics.gov.uk/census2001/default.asp). Websites for other countries are provided under On-line resources on page 239.

There are some long-standing assessment scales such as the Jarman index, Townsend scale and ACORN classification. These ratings are generally based around a GP practice population or geographical/population area. Their rating is based on key variables influencing need, such as: children under 5 years, unemployment rates, overcrowded housing, ethnic minority groups, elderly living alone, single parent homes, percentage of households without a car. As part of your review of an area it would be beneficial to identify any recognised assessments that are available such as a Jarman index. While it will not provide you with all the answers, it may prove useful in identifying some key areas to explore.

For most individuals thinking about conducting a community profile the obvious question is, where do I start? As with any activity there are some key steps that can be followed, and Box 6.3 outlines one useful approach to planning a profile.

It is worth highlighting now that a key indication of the value of the outcomes identified in a community profile is the degree and range of collaborative partnerships used to conduct the profile. It is unlikely that any single agency or practitioner will have insight and access to all areas and components of a community, and while you may decide to conduct a small-scale profile, it is advisable to undertake profiles as part of a larger team or group.

The first step outlined in Box 6.3 is worth spending time thinking about since it will generally determine the amount of resource, such as time, and the scale of the profile that you will undertake. Box 6.4 should be of use in helping you to start defining the boundaries and start thinking about possible information sources for your work. I suggest you use the four titles Who, Where, Health trends and Services as headings and try to fill in as much detailed information as you can, and then look at possible relationships between each of the sections. This approach will also allow you to identify positive resources within your identified area.

COMMUNITY PROFILE FRAMEWORKS

There are developed frameworks to support community profiling, and an overview of two common approaches – the rapid appraisal and the life cycle – are provided. While both these frameworks are quite structured, you could for example build your profile around government and local health targets as an alternative approach. There can be no right approach,

Box 6.4
Planning a community profile: defining boundaries and sources of information (adapted from McMurray 1999)

WHO
Lives in the community?
What are the dominant age groups?
What is their relationship to the community/land?
Who are the recognised leaders/spokespeople?
What types of family unit exist, e.g. lone parent?

WHERE
What is the history of the community?
How is the community defined geographically?
What are the physical links and networks?
What is the type of environment?
Are there identified industrial or environmental hazards?

HEALTH TRENDS and BEHAVIOURS
What are the identified health and social issues?
What is the prevalence of chronic disease, e.g. diabetes and coronary heart disease?
What are the public health data indicating in relation to health behaviour, e.g. smoking, obesity, substance abuse?

SERVICES/POLICY
What services are available, e.g. housing, health, education?
What are the local policies?
Who sets and determines the services/policy?
What is the recorded information about health and social issues, e.g. local reports, minutes, newsletters, community groups?

but you need to give some thought to the approach, which will allow you to achieve your aim.

RAPID APPRAISAL FRAMEWORK

The rapid appraisal framework is popular due to the focus on a multidisciplinary approach. The approach is named since it was designed to be conducted in a relatively short period of time. Ideally the rapid appraisal should be set up as a co-ordinated multi-agency project with each group feeding into the assessment. However, it is feasible to carry out a profile using this approach without having the direct involvement of a range of services or agencies.

One of the more important aspects is that the framework does provide a list of key areas that need to be considered and consulted as part of the assessment. This overview provides a useful checklist to ensure that your profile is comprehensive and inclusive. The process resembles a pyramid, with your assessment building upon each layer. The base and starting point of the assessment explores the community composition, community organisation and structures and the physical environment. Building upon this gathered information, you can then move to the next layer of assessment and explore the socio-economic environment and levels and rates of disease and disability. The next layer explores services in the community, for example, health, social and educational provision. It is important to stress that this process is much more than information gathering or reviewing official statistics. As identified earlier, to be of true value, a community profile needs to draw on a range of information sources and from a range of informants, most importantly those living in the community. To be successful you will need to draw on your interviewing and group facilitation skills as much as the ability to read graphs.

The rapid appraisal approach has been demonstrated to be effective in assessing both health and social needs in urban areas where high levels of deprivation and poverty exist (Murray et al 1994). I particularly like the emphasis placed on using 'key informants' and the valuing of the input of local voluntary agencies and self-help groups (Ong 1991).

LIFE CYCLE FRAMEWORK

The life cycle framework could have a certain appeal to midwives since the lived experience of health is viewed as transitionary and is broken into different life stages.

There are nine stages within the framework: late pregnancy to 1 week after birth, 1 week of age to 1 year old, 1 year to 4 years old, 5–14, 15–24, 25–44, 45–64, 65–74, and finally 75 plus years.

The framework identifies and recognises that there are key health and lifestyle issues and needs that are particularly important at various stages of our lifespan. For example, if you identified a large population of 15–24-year-olds living in a particular community, there are key areas you may want to explore in terms of a needs assessment. These areas include: substance abuse, sexual health, homelessness and managing relationships.

Midwives clearly have a focus on the stages relating to pregnancy and the reproductive years. In a collaborative approach it may well be useful and appropriate for midwives to lead the assessment of these stages. However, there is value in exploring professional input across the age span and I would encourage midwives to explore other age groups where we do not traditionally have input. The life cycle framework provides a logical approach to assessing health needs and attempts to explain and make sense of a population's health rather than simply to identify and describe it. If you are interested in this approach I strongly suggest you read the text by Pickin and St Leger (1993) outlined in Further reading at the end of this chapter.

The first two frameworks discussed provided approaches which were quite structured and offer a clear approach to needs assessment. Another more direct and policy-focused method is to conduct a needs assessment based on a key national or local target. There may, for example, be a local target set by your health agency to increase the number of women choosing to breastfeed. Your needs assessment may target an area to explore the uptake of breastfeeding and try to explore issues that may impact on breastfeeding rates. Such an approach will require you to examine the range of factors that impact on health just as the rapid appraisal or life cycle frameworks do.

CONCLUSION

Without doubt there is a clear national and local government drive towards collecting meaningful and accurate information on local community and population health needs. The earlier discussion highlighted that the process of collecting data which are useful, let alone meaningful, is not without difficulty. There is always the very real possibility that those who are most at risk or disadvantaged within our communities will remain silent or be silenced, and unless we can support all groups and individuals in the profiling process then no amount of political goodwill or funding will have any real impact on addressing health inequalities.

As midwifery practitioners we need to find ways of recording and measuring our experiences of working with women and families. We need to reflect on our practice and examine the ways services are structured and provided, and continue moving towards more user-led rather than service-led maternity care.

Midwives need to work flexibly to ensure that our practice and services are delivered in ways which are accessible, and appropriate to the communities we work with. We need to move beyond working solely with individual women and explore how maternity services can be expanded or adapted to address wider public health needs. There are a number of real-life clinical examples of how midwives have done just this throughout the rest of this book.

You are challenged to discuss the potential to conduct a community profile with your colleagues and midwifery leader or manager, to look at possible opportunities to ensure that the knowledge can be captured and fed into health improvement plans and strategies.

References

Bradshaw J 1972 The concept of social need. New Society 30:640–643

Department of Health 2003 Tackling Health Inequalities: A Programme for Action. DH, London

Gough I 1992 What are human needs? Percy-Smith J, Sanderson I (eds) Understanding Local Needs. Institute of Public Policy Research, London, Ch. 1

International Confederation of Midwives 1990 Definition of a Midwife. ICM, London

Lewis G, Drife J (eds) 2001 Why mothers die 1997–1999: the fifth report of the confidential enquiries into maternal deaths in the United Kingdom. RCOG Press, London

Lock K 1999 Meeting the need. Community Practitioner 72(6):157–158

McMurray A 1999 Community Health and Wellness: a Sociological Approach. Harcourt, Sydney

Murray S A, Tapson J, Turnbull L, McCallum J, Little A 1994 Listening to local voices: adapting rapid appraisal to assess health and social needs in general practice. British Medical Journal 308:698–700

Ong B N 1991 Rapid appraisal in an urban setting – an example from the developed world. Social Science Medicine 32(8):909–915

Payne J 1999 Researching Health Needs. Sage, London

Thomas M 2003 The crest of a wave – will midwives ride it? MIDIRS Midwifery Digest 13(3):295–300

Twinn S, Dauncey J, Carnell J 1990 The process of health profiling. Health Visitors' Association, London

World Health Organization 1992 Definition of the Midwife as stated in the recently-released document Reproductive Health Care: Midwifery – its role in safe motherhood and beyond. WHO, Geneva

Further reading

Hawtin M, Hughes G, Percy-Smith J 1999 Community Profiling: Auditing Social Needs. Open University Press, Buckingham

Pickin C, St Leger S 1993 Assessing Health Need using the Life Cycle Framework. Open University Press, Buckingham

Robinson J, Elkan R 1999 Health Needs Assessment: Theory and Practice. Churchill Livingstone, Edinburgh

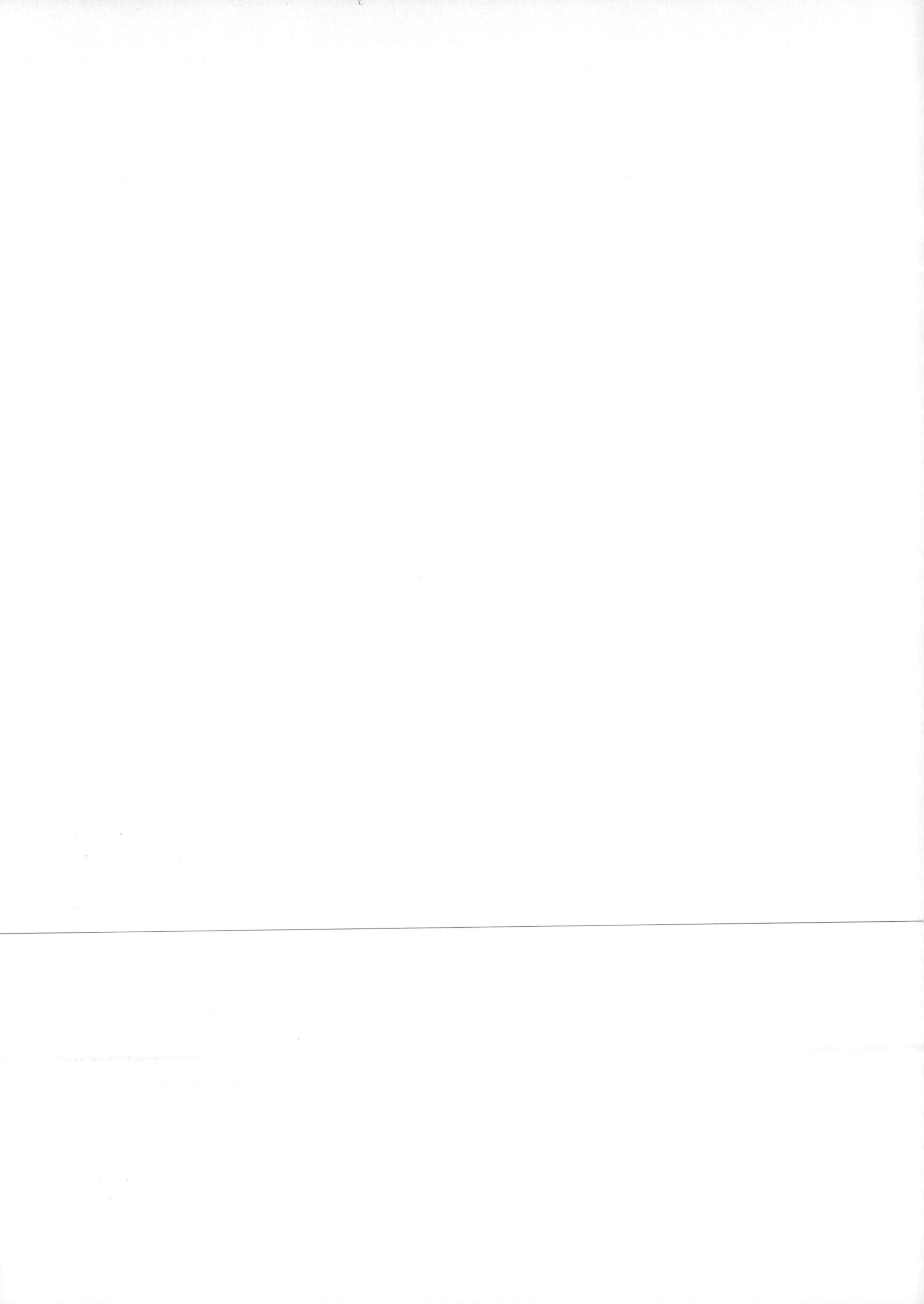

Chapter 7

Being with women: public policy and private experience

Tina Miller

CHAPTER CONTENTS

SUMMARY

This chapter explores the ways in which societal changes, together with policy and organisational shifts, have led to new challenges for midwives. Using data from a study on transition to motherhood, women's accounts of their experiences of becoming mothers are set against a backdrop of policy and care delivery.

Women becoming mothers in western societies do so within the context of changing and increasingly diverse social and familial circumstances. Patterns within women's lives have shifted, with many women having children either much earlier or later in life, combining work and mothering, mothering alone, or choosing to remain childless. These changes mean that many women come to motherhood without having served an 'apprenticeship' of mothering in a traditional family context, and they will mother in more diverse circumstances.

Policy responses to these wider structural changes have focused on promoting greater social inclusion through economic mechanisms as well as the professional support of families (for example, Sure Start). In relation to the delivery of maternity care, these policy shifts follow earlier initiatives, which sought to meet the needs of childbearing women in more effective and efficient ways (Winterton Report 1992, DH Expert Maternity Group 1993 *Changing Childbirth*). Being with and supporting women throughout the childbearing period has always been a defining feature of midwifery practice, and more recently partnership with women has been emphasised as part of improving service delivery (DH 2003 *Delivering the Best*). However, wider societal changes, together with policy and organisational shifts, offer new possibilities – and raise new challenges – for midwifery practice and care delivery. This chapter will focus on the interplay and tensions that arise from care, which is shaped by wider policy concerns and grounded in professional, normative practices, and personal experiences that are private, individual and increasingly diverse. This focus interweaves empirical data – women's accounts of first-time motherhood – with consideration of current midwifery practices and future developments. In the following section the changing context in which contemporary motherhood is experienced is outlined.

THE CHANGING CONTEXT

At an individual level, becoming a mother changes lives in all sorts of ways. Journeys into motherhood have implications for our sense of who we are, as our old recognisable selves can become subsumed within the new identities associated with being a mother and motherhood. The enormity of the changes that transition to motherhood can reap should not be underestimated, and often require adjustments on the part of all family members (Miller 2000a). At a wider level, social changes have translated into mothering occurring in different places and at different times in women's lives. Family size has also been reduced, and over a third of births occur outside marriage. The significance of mothering to women's lives, within the context of changed educational opportunities for (some) women and the resulting shifts in patterns of employment, also has implications for the ways in which we think about mothering and motherhood. There has been an increase in the number of single mothers and others who follow 'non-traditional' ways of living and parenting, as well as an increase in the number of women choosing to remain childless (McRae 1999). In all post-industrial societies, contemporary mothering arrangements are more diverse, yet often remain unrecognised in areas of family policy and practice, which continue to assume traditional family types (Duncan & Edwards 1999). This is apparent in relation to mothers whose mothering challenges stereotypes. The experiences of mothers who have found themselves to be marginalised have been studied in recent years – teen mothers, immigrant mothers, lesbian mothers, homeless mothers, welfare mothers and incarcerated mothers (Garcia Coll et al 1998). These 'types' of mothers serve to emphasise the way in which particular ideas about 'good' mothering and who constitute 'good' mothers are reinforced. This morally charged context can make it difficult for mothers experiencing 'normal' difficulties associated with pregnancy and early mothering to speak out, and so needs may remain unvoiced. Yet, although feminist and other research has pointed to the diversity of contemporary mothering experiences, services around childbirth in many western countries continue to be provided in particularly uniform ways (Treichler 1990, Glenn et al 1994, Barclay et al 1997, Garcia Coll et al 1998, Chase & Rogers 2001).

A further feature of contemporary society in which mothering is experienced and midwifery services provided is linked to perceptions of risk. Social scientists have argued that changes in late modern societies have led to increased perceptions of risk as a result of old traditions and habits no longer providing the certainties for us that they once did (Giddens 1991, Beck 1992, Beck & Beck-Gernsheim 1995, Lupton 1999). In relation to reproduction and childbearing, perceptions of risk have led women increasingly to look to those with expert knowledge – doctors, midwives and other health professionals – to provide guidance (Lupton 1999). In this rapidly changing context, the childbearing experiences of previous generations have become less relevant as trust is placed in those with professional, expert skills. Clearly, increased perceptions of risk, together with other changes such as those in family formations, have implications both for women's expectations and experiences of pregnancy and childbearing and for midwives supporting and meeting their needs. This 'moral minefield' provides a powerful backdrop against which women take reproductive decisions and make 'choices' (Murphy 1999). The changing context, then, in which reproduction and childbearing take place is culturally, morally and socially shaped and experienced by women in different ways: experiences are far from universal (Davis-Floyd & Sargent 1997).

BEING WITH WOMEN: MIDWIFERY PRACTICES

Historically midwives have had the main responsibility for providing care to childbearing women: to be 'with woman' (Kitzinger 1988:1). However, in recent times the development of more formal and regulated health services in the West, together with the medicalisation of childbirth, has led the midwife's role – and areas of practice – to shift. According to Kitzinger, 'in childbirth today the Obstetrician usually stands centre-stage' (1988:1). Although there have been more recent changes in relation to where and how services are provided to childbearing women, with an increased emphasis on team work and community-based service provision, perceptions vary of the autonomy of midwives as independent practitioners. In a study by Sikorski et al (1995) it was reported that obstetricians did not tend to regard midwives as independent practitioners – whilst most midwives did in fact see themselves in this way. In many ways midwives can find themselves in the difficult position of being both with women and providing care and support whilst at the same time negotiating the contours of medicalisation and hierarchical working structures. The midwife's independence as an autonomous practitioner can be hard to assert in this challenging context.

In terms of service planning and provision, the early 1990s in the UK were characterised by a series of investigations, reviews and reports into the delivery of maternity services (National Audit Office 1990, Winterton Report 1992, DH Expert Maternity Group 1993 *Changing Childbirth*, National Health Service Management Executive 1994). These resulted in policy shifts that emphasised greater autonomy for midwives, hand in hand with more community-based 'woman-centred participatory care, accessible and appropriate services and effective and efficient care' (Dowswell et al 2001, Wrede et al 2001:32). Recent policy changes have called for the delivery of maternity services that promote continuity of care and meet women's needs in a way that encourages participation and more recently partnership (DH 2003, *Delivering the Best*). For midwives, being with women in recent years has increasingly involved practice that is evidence based, and focused on meeting women's needs in the community. Although widely welcomed, in practice the implementation of such policy recommendations has not been straightforward. Policy recommendations do not always map neatly onto existing working structures or individual lives. For example, as Wrede et al have observed (2001:33), 'continuity of care has not always resulted from the establishment of midwife schemes because team midwifery is more popular among midwives than is caseload midwifery'. And whilst there have been real attempts to change and improve service delivery, Page and Sandall have recently noted (2000:673) that 'standard maternity care still consists of fragmented relationships between caregivers and families, confusion about the role of the midwife in relationship to the obstetrician and GP, and an increasing series of screening tests throughout pregnancy, labour and the postnatal period'. Unfortunately this confusion is also evident in some of the accounts of women receiving maternity care (Miller 2000a). In the following section the research approach that provides the empirical data for this chapter is outlined.

MAKING SENSE OF BECOMING A MOTHER

It has recently been noted that 'despite the large volume of literature on maternity care, the amount that is known about midwives' contribution to care and what women think about it is limited' (Dowswell et al 2001:99). The small-scale, longitudinal qualitative study reported here makes a small contribution to placing women's experiences of receiving care in the academic and professional arena. The study explored the ways in which women experience and construct narratives of their transition to first-time motherhood (Miller 1998, 2000b). The 17 participants in this study were all white, first-time mothers-to-be, who were in employment at the time of confirmation of their pregnancy. The sample was accessed away from formal health services, initially using the researcher's own social networks and then snowballing techniques. In-depth interviews were carried out on three separate occasions; at 7–8 months antenatally, 6–8 weeks postnatally and finally 8–9 months postnatally. A total of 49 interviews were undertaken and these were followed up by a short postal questionnaire. The mean age of the participants was 30 years at the time of the first interview. Analysis of the data focused on the ways in which individuals make sense of their experiences through narrative construction (Miller 2000b). The research approach did not set out to generate findings from which generalisations could be made, but rather to produce rich data from which theory could be generated. The findings add to a limited but growing body of qualitative research on women's experiences of reproduction and childbirth. In many ways this sample conforms to stereotypes that are held in wider society about those who are positioned as 'good mothers'; these women were white, predominantly middle-class and either married or in partnerships. Yet the data reveal how diverse and complex their experiences of becoming mothers were. In the following sections lengthy extracts from the antenatal and early postnatal interviews will be used to show the ways in which this group of women construct their needs and experience care. The tensions that can arise from care which is shaped by wider policy concerns, and grounded in sometimes entrenched professional practices – often task-based and routine – and personal experiences which are individual and increasingly diverse, are explored below.

PRACTICES AND PERSONAL EXPERIENCES: THE ANTENATAL PERIOD

In the UK, preparation for motherhood continues to be located within a highly developed system of antenatal care that is located within a formalised, medical context: the clinic and the hospital (Tew 1990, Oakley 1993, Miller 1995). Indeed it could be argued that the hospital is now culturally accepted as the 'natural' place to give birth in many developed societies where everyday aspects of life are increasingly medicalised and expert, authoritative knowledge sought (Foster 1995, Davis-Floyd & Sargent 1997). Technological advances have also contributed to claims of expertise and provided practitioners with the tools to monitor progress during pregnancy and childbirth, for example screening. It is interesting then, but perhaps not surprising, to note that attempts to redefine women as consumers of maternity care with a right to choice, control and continuity, have faltered. Indeed one conclusion from a recent review of the literature on midwifery and community-based care was that in the antenatal period 'offering women choices about care may be problematic', and this was because women 'may not be aware of what different options put to them entail' (Dowswell et al 2001:98). Supervision and medical regulation continue to characterise service delivery in some areas, rather than more participatory styles of care that some policy initiatives had called for. But this 'supervision' is largely welcomed by women who derive reassurance from, and want, expert guidance and do not feel competent in making choices about something they know very little about. For most women expecting a child – especially a first child – making use of antenatal services and seeking professional advice is regarded as the appropriate way to diminish risk and to prepare responsibly and safely. There is some irony then that the antenatal period is experienced as less certain and more complex at a time when biomedical, expert knowledge has apparently provided greater scientific certainty than at any time before (Lupton 1999).

A key part of the midwife's role involves supporting women in their preparation for childbearing. In relation to information giving and care in the antenatal period, the findings from the qualitative study confirmed that women expected this to be provided by those they perceived to be expert. The women's antenatal accounts were characterised by engagement with, or in some cases the handing over to, doctors and midwives. For example, whilst the women all referred to gathering information about pregnancy and childbirth from relatives and friends, these were regarded as less reliable – less expert – than that provided by health professionals, as the following extract shows. (All names and any other identifying features have been changed.)

> I don't like getting information from other people because it's always so subjective and they always want to harp on about their little story, and so I have actually avoided other people … I've steered away from those, those are the most unhelpful, personal experiences that I've steered away from. But I think the books, and the midwives and my doctor, my doctor's been good …
>
> (Rebecca)

Similarly, this theme of wanting, and seeking out, expert advice is continued in the following extract in which Angela talks of her wishes in relation to feeding, but within the context of having to seek *confirmation* from the midwife.

> … there's things like … 'cos I can't make up my mind whether I'm breastfeeding or bottle feeding. So, I'd like to have a go at breastfeeding but you've got to know all the bits and bobs that go with it, like I didn't find out until the other day that, I want to go half and half so that my husband will be involved, and what I was going to do was do half formula and half breast, but I found out that if you've got eczema or asthma in the family, they don't like you doing a mixture, well, I only found that out Monday … so looks like I'm going to do totally breast but I can't confirm that with the midwife until I see her.
>
> (Angela)

The perceived power of professional knowledge is implicit within the extract '*they* don't like you doing a mixture'. In the following example, Wendy also talks positively of her encounter with the midwife.

> I'm going for the breast first to see how I get on. I did actually say to the midwife that I wanted to do both, I wanted the bottle and … but she said you can't actually do that … (but) it's been good. They just tell you everything.
>
> (Wendy)

Clearly, the policy aims of delivering maternity services based on choice, participation and partnership for and with women may be difficult to achieve when women perceive their needs differently, wanting and prioritising 'expert' information and advice. Indeed, this may be a consequence of changed family formations and different ways of living. Women no longer serve an 'apprenticeship' of mothering, and so come to motherhood with little or no first-hand experience of its dimensions (Oakley 1980). And it can be profoundly felt:

> Don't keep giving me decisions to make, I don't know, I've not done this before.
>
> (Peggy)

The findings from the study also showed that establishing a relationship with members of the health care team was seen as an important part of the antenatal preparation. Anticipating and preparing to become a mother was not a solitary endeavour but was expected to involve regular interaction with different experts – predominantly midwives during the antenatal period – at different times. The women produced accounts that showed their particular expectations of the relationship, which later interviews in the postnatal period revealed were not always met. In the following extract from an antenatal interview, Rebecca talks of her expectations of the relationship she had anticipated she would have with a midwife, and her confusion when this was not (initially) forthcoming:

> The midwife came round the very first time when I'd just found out I was pregnant and I was very, as I said, confused and very unsettled and she was not that interested. They're very good now, they're very interested and they keep a tab on everything, but at the very beginning, I suppose because people miscarry in the first three months so they don't spend a lot of time with you then in case it's all for no reason. But I did feel very left on my own. They saw me once and then they didn't see me for a month and I didn't know when I was supposed to book up for classes, the antenatal parent classes, and I didn't know when I was meant to see them and how often and what I was supposed to be doing, and that kind of thing, and I just felt at the beginning I could have done with more support because I really needed it then. Not so much physically, but emotionally.
>
> (Rebecca)

The above extract is interesting because it shows how, when initial expectations were not met, the participant was able to make sense of this by focusing on the possibility of miscarriage and this not being thought to be relevant to the job of a midwife. Having anticipated interaction with the midwife once her pregnancy had been confirmed, Rebecca describes her confusion when this was not forthcoming in the ways she had anticipated, that without them she didn't know 'what [she] was supposed to be doing'. In the past it might have been the case that mothers and other family members would have had a more significant role in providing the support and care that Rebecca now looks to midwives for. In all the accounts the women regarded themselves as novice and non-expert, and this could lead to confusion with the routine practices that characterise formal antenatal care and that are often taken for granted by those providing the service. This sense of confusion is captured in the following extract from Philippa:

> I did feel very confused to start with because I think they assumed … There was also, there was kind of confusion over just very silly things like, I remember where you had to sort of take your notes with you and they kind of assumed things like you knew you had to take a urine sample with you and stuff and there was a bit of kind of … and I didn't on the first occasion and they said, oh I can tell it's your first baby, and I thought no-one ever told me. I don't know, there were just little things like that that I just found irritating, this kind of assumption that it was … you were kind of stepping in to something and you'd automatically know where to go and who to see, and what sort of … And I got a note from [hospital]

> saying come for your booking in, and I thought, 'what's a booking in?' And I had no idea. So there was, I think that was, there was a lack of kind of explanation of the process that I'd be going through in terms of the healthcare I'd be receiving, but once I kind of got my head round it and asked questions, that was fine. And actually the healthcare itself was not the problem, it was more kind of procedural.
>
> (Philippa)

As well as taking account of the knowledge levels and differing needs of (new) mothers, midwives need to be sensitive to the ways in which aspects of antenatal care might be differently perceived. In the following extract taken from earlier research, which focused on take-up of antenatal services amongst British Bangladeshi women (Miller 1995), different cultural perceptions of need are clearly expressed. In the extract Munia, a British Bangladeshi woman, has been asked about attendance at antenatal parent-craft classes and she replies:

> That is what most mother-in-laws doesn't like, they said 'why so much bothering?' you have to go and practise … I think that's not necessary, because our culture is so different, we do learn so much from our mum.
>
> (Munia, in Miller 1995:307)

CARE IN THE HOSPITAL

Clearly factors such as cultural location, social class, age and partnership status will all affect women's perceptions of their care needs during pregnancy and beyond. The challenge for midwives is to take account sensitively of these increasingly diverse needs within working structures that may appear to offer flexibility but in practice often do not.

Although changes in policy and practice mean that most antenatal care is now community based, the vast majority of women in the UK continue to give birth in hospital. For example in 2001 98% of women gave birth in hospital, and this is a trend which is echoed across many other industrialised countries (Office for National Statistics 2001). All the women in the study 'chose' to give birth in hospital, their decisions based on concerns such as those expressed in Philippa's account below.

> I mean partly because I don't know what to expect. I think I'd rather have everything on tap at the hospital if necessary because you don't really know the shape … or anything, so I just think I'd rather, especially for a first baby, I'd rather have the care on hand if I need it … I do think I'd rather come back to my house as something that is kind of sorted out, to some extent quite clean and what have you, rather than where this kind of event takes place … I can't see the benefit of having it at home. I just think I'd rather go away, do it somewhere else and then come back.
>
> (Philippa)

All the births were different from what the women had expected, and in the early postnatal interviews the women reflected back on the preparation they had received. In the following extracts Diana, Rebecca and Faye acknowledge the difficulties for midwives of providing information regarding the birth when individual experiences will be diverse.

> I just think they could do with being a bit more realistic without frightening you, you know, because I know that they don't want to tell you what it's really like because it can sound quite terrifying if you try to say you know the pain is like indescribable and it is, but you forget, you do forget, I know that it was horrible but I can't really remember how horrible.
>
> (Diana)

> Yes I suppose looking back on the antenatal care, it was as good as I suppose it could be, given the fact that the midwife who was leading it had no idea basically of what we were all going to go through. She knew the kind of experiences that can be gone through.
>
> (Rebecca)

> Everybody was saying that they don't tell you enough about the birth and what it's like.
>
> (Faye)

Felicity also felt that the midwives could provide more helpful parameters in order to help her think about the birth:

> I'd be much happier if they actually said you know well I expect it's going to hurt like hell, how long it's going to take, sort of maximum and minimum, what they're going to do, but they haven't.
>
> (Felicity)

Of the 17 women in the study, 15 had 'normal' deliveries – although this was not how they would describe them – whilst one had an elective caesarean and another an unplanned caesarean. As noted above, all the births were different from what the participants had expected. In the following extracts Clare and Abigail reflect on their birth experiences.

> I wanted to have a water birth originally and because I was induced I couldn't, that's why I was stuck on this bed. And I had like … I had everything in the end, I had an epidural … I knew that … you know … originally they examined me and they said you're only three centimetres, you can't have an epidural yet, and I was absolutely desperate … and they made me hang on for another two hours, and I was like … I just thought I was going to die.
>
> (Clare)

> It got hideously painful, but it wasn't what I was expecting.
>
> (Abigail)

Most of the women spoke of handing over, at some point during their labour, to others (midwives, obstetricians, anaesthetists) who they wanted to take control. This was in stark contrast to their earlier antenatal accounts where they had spoken of their desire to retain control during the birth, and had listed a range of drugs and procedures they would use if necessary in order to achieve this. In the following extracts, the unexpected experiences of birth led to control being handed over.

> Yes, well because they were worried about her, although she showed no signs of distress at any point, but meconium in the waters means you've got to have what they say which is … the drip … well I don't know if …

> much choice. But by that time I was thinking I want her out and whatever you think is best and get on with it.
>
> (Gillian)

> And I was desperately trying to breathe in and that, and I just couldn't, lost it totally. And I had the epidural, told the anaesthetist he was god … Because I tried gas and air, revolting, disgusting, let's throw up, it was obscenely revolting. And the TENS machine was well, a total waste of time I think, but it felt as if you were in control, and so I had no pain relief at all basically, other than the epidural when I eventually succumbed …
>
> (Abigail)

> When he [obstetrician] said to me I think we should do such and such, and I just said yes, whatever, you know best. I just took … gave it totally over to him … I knew that I would just want somebody to take control and take over from me.
>
> (Sheila)

Following the safe delivery of their babies the women spent varying lengths of time in hospital before going home, and again experiences were varied. In the extract below, Felicity talks of her experiences in hospital following the birth of her baby and the way in which particular practices only served to reinforce her sense of failure.

> In the hospital – I mean this is another thing about the isolating experiences – they stuck me in a ward with four beds in it and I was the only one there. So I'd had this horrible experience and then I was stuck in this room on my own and I just felt as if I was the only person in the entire world and nobody wanted to know me. It was awful. And they kept doing things like forgetting to bring my meals because I was the only one that … 'oh we didn't know anyone was in there'. So of course there was just floods of tears, 'I'm not even worthy of them bringing me a cup of tea'.
>
> (Felicity)

In the following lengthy account Wendy, who has twin sons following successful IVF treatment, talks of her experiences in hospital and what for her were rational responses to the enormity of becoming a mother.

> I had baby blues in hospital … I stayed in there for a week … Well they told me that I could go home on the Friday. I had them on the Monday and they said I could go home on the Friday. But I said, no I'm staying, and they let me stay and said I could stay for a bit longer if I wanted to. They were saying about this mother and baby place I could go to … because they said we should have been counselled, because they were IVF babies, but we never had anything. Because you just go in and you think, oh my god, I'm having these two babies tomorrow and they're just there and you think, god, what do I do? You just have to know it all. I don't think they've got much time for you up there because I was trying to breastfeed Ben, and I used to ring them to help me to fix him on and that, and it used to take them ten minutes to come along. Fifteen minutes

> and you think, I can't cope with this and I just used to give him a bottle. I had to beg them one night to take them off me for one night and the next night I thought, well I'm not going to ask them again because you just think, do they really want them? It's really bad. They kept saying it was part of postnatal depression, but it wasn't. They sent a psychiatric woman in to see me and she said, do you feel suicidal? and I said no. I was on the seventh floor. I said if I did I'd be jumping out that window by now. We went in on the Sunday and that's all they kept talking about, because I was quite tearful anyway when we went in and she kept saying I've got to tell you about postnatal depression, and I said I haven't got it. I'm just teary because I'm in here and I'm going to give birth in the next 24 hours ... I wasn't the only one up there crying. There was quite a few of us. It was weird though, having these two babies just lying there and thinking, god, what do I do?
>
> (Wendy)

Competing lay and professional perspectives are clearly apparent in this extract. Wendy's perception is that, in retrospect, she had not been properly prepared, 'because they said we should have been counselled, because they were IVF babies, but we never had anything'. Her sense of being unsupported by staff on the ward once the babies were born is also clear: 'well I'm not going to ask them again because you just think, do they really want them?' But Wendy explains that she was not alone in feeling 'teary', '... I wasn't the only one up there crying. There was quite a few of us.' Wendy challenges the diagnosis of postnatal depression and the need for a 'psychiatric woman' (sic); rather she makes sense of her own feelings within the context of the enormity of what she is going through, 'and they're just there and you think, god, what do I do?' Wendy's profound sense of not knowing what to do was echoed across many of the women's accounts. The women were now mothers with responsibilities for their babies, and suddenly an event that had long been awaited and prepared for was not as they had expected.

THE EARLY POSTNATAL PERIOD

Following the birth, women are usually transferred home within one or two days of delivery for postnatal care in the community. Postnatal care in the community is provided initially by midwives and then health visitors. The shift from hospital to home can be a difficult time for women and their families as they come to terms with meeting the needs and developing the skills necessary to care for their child. Whilst women may be socialised from birth into gendered, female roles the experience of becoming a mother may not resonate with their expectations and the tasks of early mothering can seem daunting and the responsibility overwhelming. Yet it is also very difficult to voice what are felt to be problems or 'unnatural' responses at this time, especially if those around you appear to be coping (Miller 2002). The dominance of biomedical discourses in the antenatal period which reinforce particular, morally underpinned ideas about 'good' mothering can be seen to be potentially disempowering. According to Lupton this 'may make it difficult to take back control after the birth, when [a mother] may have no real knowledge of her own feelings, or her baby' (Lupton 1994:148–149). Indeed a sense of not knowing what to do was profoundly felt by some of the women in the study, as the following examples demonstrate.

> I just wanted to go back to hospital actually the whole time … after being home for a couple of days, I thought I just wanted to go back, I want someone else to be in control.
>
> (Philippa)

> [antenatal classes] didn't really prepare you for actually what you'd got to do when you'd got the baby … which wasn't really much use because you just wanted to be told, you know.
>
> (Peggy)

The move from hospital to home marked the beginning of a change in the relationship between the midwives and the new mothers. Whilst the women welcomed – and some depended on – the midwives' visits, the selective basis on which they were made was confusing. Because the visits were selective, some of the new mothers felt they might be labelled as having failed if they requested an additional visit. They still felt they needed expert guidance and someone to share the responsibility and, at times, take control, but this wasn't what they experienced. This new twist in the relationship was confusing and unexpected, as the following extracts show.

> I must admit that one thing I didn't like was that because my emotions were all over the place and I'm a very organised person, I found that it was very difficult for me to get my head round who was supposed to be in charge of me, who I was supposed to ring up and all the rest of it … and I was under the impression that she [midwife] was going to keep coming for ten days, and after the second day she said, you're fine, I won't come anymore. And I have felt a bit abandoned really, and she knew that I was feeling quite emotionally tender, so I think perhaps that could have been dealt with a bit better … and I did feel a bit abandoned … the midwife just dropped me after two days saying that I was fine, the baby was fine and everything was all right … But I didn't feel emotionally all right.
>
> (Rebecca)

> Midwives came for 10 days, well the 10-day period, this is another thing. Because I felt so dreadful I would have liked them to call every day to check sort of my tail end every day, but they assumed that because I was again … I suppose they think this is a fairly nice house, you know you've got everything sorted out, husband was home, they kept saying 'I'll not call tomorrow eh, I'll leave it for a day or two' and I kept … it was almost as if I couldn't say no actually I want you to come back and talk to me tomorrow. So I had to go OK yes, that's fine.
>
> (Felicity)

Others found the relationship more supportive but still felt bewildered by their early mothering experiences. In the following extract Philippa describes the early days at home.

> And I've found the whole way through that they've [midwives] been fairly reactive but then that's OK, once you get used to it. I think I went … I kind of had the attitude … or felt that everything should be a bit more

> black and white than it actually is and that people would actually tell me what to do, and I've found ... I mean even in hospital no-one told me how to sort of bath the baby for example. I had to you know say how do you do ... how do I do this? And they said gosh, hasn't she been bathed for two days you know or whatever? Well no-one's shown me, no-one's given me a bath or whatever, I don't know. And I think emotionally as well I mean they were quite supportive. The occasion when I'd seen the midwife one day and everything was fine and then she said right I won't come tomorrow if that's all right ... have a day off, and I called her and said come round, because we'd had like this sort of 12, I think 12 hours feeding almost continuously right through the night, and I just didn't ... I mean I didn't know what I was doing wrong, whether it was just she wasn't getting enough or whether she just wanted the comfort or whatever. And she was great because she sort of came round and she actually put me to bed and latched the baby on and made me a sandwich ... and I felt quite depressed about you know 'oh my god what have I done' because she [baby] was obviously taking up all my time and all [husband's] time as well and we were both like 'what have we done to our lives?' We quite liked our life before and we were just never going to know ... we just couldn't imagine ever being beyond this kind of 24-hour baby care.
>
> (Philippa)

Becoming a mother, then, usually turns out to be different from what had been anticipated, as expectations are replaced by experiences. Plans that had seemed plausible before the birth have to be rethought. The conflicting, and sometimes overwhelming, feelings of love, guilt, exhaustion, joy and fear are not uncommon experiences in the early weeks and months of becoming a mother but they need to be understood and made sense of and recognised as *normal* reactions to motherhood. For the many women who find that their early experiences are different from what they had expected, the need can appear paramount to provide culturally recognisable accounts of early mothering that show that they are 'good' mothers who *are* coping (Miller 2000b). Women can feel that they must convey an identity of a coping and responsible mother and that difficult or contrary experience must be concealed. This can result in mothers feeling unable to talk to others, including midwives and health visitors, about what they think must be *ab*normal experiences of early mothering, as the following extract demonstrates.

> But I still felt as though it wasn't normal somehow to feel like that ... you know my whole life's falling apart and I can't do anything and they're [other mothers] coping so well.
>
> (Diana)

For midwives providing postnatal care in the community the demands on their professional expertise and time are increasingly challenged. The needs of the mother, her baby and other family members can require different skills and clearly move beyond just identifying physical needs in relation to a return to normal. Different family circumstances may also lead to different needs, as Garcia and Marchant have noted (1996:66): 'midwifery care in the community reaches all types of families, including those who clearly have extra needs and those who do not appear to need help, but may have needs that are not recognised'. However, patterns of care following the birth of a child continue to be largely task-based with an emphasis on routine physical assessments taken to indicate a 'return to normal'. This continued emphasis was recognised in a recent review of literature on the midwife and community-based practice, which concluded that 'there is some evidence that midwives concentrate on the physical aspects of care rather than on the provision of psychosocial support for new mothers' (Dowswell et al 2001:99). Yet given the increasing workload that comes with trying to provide continuity of care and carer and more flexible patterns of practice, this continued focus is perhaps not surprising.

CONCLUDING DISCUSSION: EXPERIENCES AND PRACTICES

So, whilst many women continue to anticipate having at least one child during their lives, studies have shown that women's expectations of motherhood often do not resonate with their experiences and that they come to motherhood with 'quite unrealistic expectations' (Oakley 1993, Richardson 1993, Mauthner 1995, 2002, Barclay et al 1997, Nicolson 1998). New mothers can feel disempowered and de-skilled by their birth and early mothering experiences; after all it is not something they have done before and they may find it difficult to talk about. Mothers and other family members who would at one time have provided practical and emotional support are now more likely to be geographically dispersed and often themselves engaged in paid work outside the home. These changing circumstances clearly have implications for midwifery practice and the ways in which services are organised. In theory the policy shifts that have promoted continuity of care should lead to relationships that are premised on continuity and shared understandings but in practice, as we have seen, this can be difficult to achieve. Whilst having more time to be with women would help to promote a participatory model of care and build partnerships, it does not fit with the current organisation or financing of maternity services. Midwives also have private lives with their own family demands and so cannot always work as flexibly as required if such policy aims are to be fully realised. In reality, then, midwives are constrained in the ways in which they can deliver care because of factors often beyond their control.

In the context of delivering midwifery care this chapter has drawn attention to some of the challenges and difficulties that midwives can encounter in meeting women's different – and similar – needs. Clearly midwives have a key role to play in the development and delivery of future maternity services that can support and meet women's needs and contribute to the Government's wider commitment to improve public health. Recent policy initiatives such as the development of National Service Frameworks lay the foundation for a new public health agenda to be realised, and midwives are well placed to make a significant contribution. The challenge for midwives however will be to continue providing high quality care and support to women whilst at the same time negotiating the contours of medicalisation within often hierarchical working structures. It is to be hoped that the new opportunities offered by these recent shifts in policy will enable midwives to continue to 'be with women' in ways that build upon, and enhance, their unique role.

References

Barclay L, Everitt L, Rogan F, Schmied V, Wyllie A 1997 Becoming a mother – an analysis of women's experience of early motherhood. Journal of Advanced Nursing 23:719–728

Beck U 1992 Risk Society: Towards a New Modernity. Sage, London

Beck U, Beck-Gernsheim E 1995 The Normal Chaos of Love. Polity Press, Cambridge

Chase S E, Rogers M F 2001 Mothers and Children: Feminist Analyses and Personal Narratives. Rutgers University Press, New Brunswick

Davis-Floyd R E, Sargent C 1997 Childbirth and Authoritative Knowledge: Cross-Cultural Perspectives. University of California Press, Berkeley

Department of Health Expert Maternity Group 1993 Changing Childbirth. HMSO, London

Department of Health 2003 Delivering the Best. Online. Available: www.publications.doh.gov.uk/cno/midwives.pdf

Dowswell T, Renfrew M, Hewison J, Gregson B 2001 A review of the literature on the midwife and community based maternity care. Midwifery 17:93–101

Duncan S, Edwards R 1999 Lone Mothers, Paid Work and Gendered Moral Rationalities. Macmillan, Basingstoke

Foster P 1995 Women and the Health Care Industry. Open University Press, Buckingham

Garcia J, Marchant S 1996 The Potential of Postnatal Care. In: Kroll D (ed) Midwifery Care for the Future. Baillière Tindall, London

Garcia Coll C, Surrey J L, Weingarten K 1998 Mothering Against the Odds. Diverse Voices of Contemporary Mothers. Guilford Press, New York

Giddens A 1991 Modernity and Self-Identity. Polity Press, Cambridge

Glenn E N, Chang G, Forcey L R (eds) 1994 Mothering Ideology, Experience and Agency. Routledge, London

Kitzinger S 1988 The Midwife Challenge. Pandora, London

Lupton D 1994 Medicine as Culture. Sage, London

Lupton D 1999 Risk. Routledge, London

McRae S 1999 (ed) Changing Britain: Families and Households in the 1990s. Oxford University Press, Oxford

Mauthner N 1995 Postnatal depression. The significance of social contacts between mothers. Women's Studies International Forum 18:311–323

Mauthner N 2002 The Darkest Days of My Life: Stories of Postpartum Depression. Harvard University Press, Cambridge, MA

Miller T 1995 Shifting boundaries: exploring the influence of cultural traditions and religious beliefs of Bangladeshi women on antenatal interactions. Women's Studies International Forum 18(3):299–309

Miller T 1998 Shifting layers of professional, lay and personal narratives: longitudinal childbirth research. In: Edwards R, Ribbens J (eds) Feminist Dilemmas in Qualitative Research. Sage, London

Miller T 2000a An exploration of first-time motherhood: narratives of transition. Unpublished PhD Thesis, Warwick University

Miller T 2000b Losing the plot: narrative construction and longitudinal childbirth research. Qualitative Health Research 10(3):309–323

Miller T 2002 Adapting to motherhood: care in the postnatal period. Community Practitioner 75(1) January

Murphy E 1999 'Breast is best': infant feeding decisions and maternal deviance. Sociology of Health and Illness 21(2):187–208

National Audit Office 1990 Maternity Services. HMSO, London

National Health Service Management Executive 1994 Woman-Centred Maternity Services. HMSO, London

Nicolson P 1998 Post-Natal Depression. Routledge, London

Oakley A 1980 Women Confined: Towards a Sociology of Childbirth. Martin Robertson, Oxford

Oakley A 1993 Essays on Women, Medicine and Health. Edinburgh University Press, Edinburgh

Office for National Statistics 2001 Social Trends. Office for National Statistics, London

Page L, Sandall J 2000 The third way: A realistic plan to reinvent the profession. British Journal of Midwifery Vol. 8 No.11, November

Richardson D 1993 Women, Motherhood and Childrearing. Macmillan, London

Sikorski J, Clements S, Wilson J et al 1995 A survey of health professionals' views on possible changes in the provision and organisation of midwifery care. Midwifery 11:61–68

Tew M 1990 Safer Childbirth: A Critical History of Maternity Care. Chapman & Hall, London

Treichler P A 1990 Feminism, Medicine and the Meaning of Childbirth. In: Jacobus M, Fox Keller E, Shuttleworth S (eds) Body/Politics. Women and the Discourse of Science. Routledge, London

Winterton Report 1992 Report of the Social Services Select Committee on Maternity Services. HMSO, London

Wrede S, Benoit C, Sandall J 2001 The state and birth/the state of birth. In: De Vries R, Benoit C, van Teijlingen E, Wrede S (eds) Birth by Design. Routledge, London

SECTION 3

The practice reality: public health midwifery

SECTION CONTENTS

Chapter 8

Laying the foundation: the STOMP study

Caroline Homer

CHAPTER CONTENTS

SUMMARY

In 1997, an innovative model of community-based midwifery care was implemented in Australia as a response to numerous state and federal government reports. The St George Outreach Maternity Project (STOMP) provides continuity of care through the antenatal, intrapartum and postpartum period. Hospital salaried midwives and obstetricians provide antenatal care from community-based settings. Community-based antenatal care was unusual in Australian settings at that time. Postnatal care is provided in hospital and in the community.

A randomised controlled trial was conducted to test the efficacy of the new model of care. Women who attended the community-based antenatal clinics perceived that they had a higher 'quality' of antenatal care compared with control group women. Women allocated to STOMP also had a significantly lower caesarean section rate. The model was instituted within the current hospital budget using existing personnel. The mean cost of providing care per woman was lower in the STOMP group compared with the control group.

This endeavour used research as a means to introduce change in an Australian maternity service. The STOMP model was cost-effective, liked by women and had positive clinical outcomes. It is now fully integrated into the hospital system and offered as an option for all women.

INTRODUCTION

Community-based maternity services, particularly those providing antenatal care with midwives, are uncommon in the Australian public health system. This chapter will present the experience of introducing a community-based model of continuity of midwifery care in an Australian public health system. This model is known as the St George Outreach Maternity Program (STOMP). STOMP was implemented in 1997 and was evaluated using a randomised controlled trial. The model continues to operate in much the same manner as it was first designed. The results of the STOMP study have been widely published (Homer 2000, Homer et al 2000a, Homer et al 2001a, b, Homer 2002, Homer et al 2002a, b). Only a summary of the results is presented in this chapter. The chapter will use STOMP to illustrate some of the issues currently facing midwifery and the health system in Australia.

FACTORS INFLUENCING THE DEVELOPMENT OF THE STOMP MODEL

A number of factors influenced the development of the STOMP model. These include recommendations from local, state, national and international policy documents, research evidence and the commitment to improved services that was present at St George Hospital where the study was conducted. A primary health care approach was used to design STOMP. This framework (encompassing equity, access, the provision of services based on need, community participation, collaboration and community-based care) was used as a means to bring about change in a public health system that was generally dedicated to the provision of an acute care model.

Other important determinants that guided the development of the STOMP model included financial considerations, the consultation process within the organisation and the experience of maternity units in the UK, where team midwifery schemes have been discontinued. The evaluation was influenced by the characteristics of the population, the need to address issues of disappointment or measurement bias and the importance of a rigorous appraisal.

POLICY STATEMENTS ADVOCATING CHANGE

A number of state and national government reports in Australia have recommended major changes to the provision of maternity services. Recommendations include providing opportunities for continuity of care, increasing collaboration between midwives, obstetricians and general practitioners (GPs) and moving antenatal care to the community (NSW Health Department 1989, Victorian Department of Health 1990, NHMRC 1996, NSW Health Department 1996, Maternity Services Advisory Committee 1999, Senate Community Affairs References Committee 1999). Essentially these reports recommend moving maternity care from an acute care framework to one which has primary health care as its focus.

Two of the Australian reports were most instrumental in the development of the STOMP model in late 1996. In New South Wales (NSW), the landmark review of maternity services known as the Shearman Report (NSW Health Department 1989) emphasised certain principles in its recommendations. These included: equitable access to quality care; recognition of the needs of women from non-English speaking backgrounds (NESB); maximising each woman's participation in decision-making during pregnancy, childbirth and the postpartum period; and promoting co-operation and collaboration among doctors, midwives and other health professionals. The report recommended that options should be explored to expand and to redefine the role of hospital-employed or salaried midwives, and suggested that these midwives could be located in community health centres to provide care during pregnancy and childbirth for low-risk women. There were also a number of strategies to meet the needs of women from NESB. These included: increased funding for interpreter services; development of new models of care, including midwives' clinics and shared care with bilingual GPs; and the establishment of ethnic obstetric liaison midwives to provide continuity of care and education.

Widespread change in the provision of maternity services and the development of new models of care did not occur in NSW public maternity services as a result of the Shearman Report (NSW Health Department 1989). This dearth of change was one of the driving forces behind the development of STOMP. The Shearman Report provided a valuable framework of recommendations on which to guide the design of the model.

The peak health body in Australia, the National Health and Medical Research Council (NHMRC) released *Options for Effective Care in Childbirth* in 1996 (NHMRC 1996). This report also guided the development of the STOMP model and the evaluation. Recommendations in this report included facilitating continuity of care and carer in the antenatal period and encouraging the development of small teams of midwives and general practitioner obstetricians. The report stated, 'we suggest [a model of joint practice run by midwives and obstetricians providing continuity of care] deserves more attention and appropriate evaluation by both professional and health planners' (1996:26).

Continuity of care and community-based care were important components both in this report and in others conducted in Australia at a similar time (Department of Health Western Australia 1990, Victorian Department of Health 1990). The *Australian National Non-English Speaking Background Women's Health Strategy* (Alcorso & Schofield 1992) also made recommendations which assisted the development of STOMP. For example, the strategy suggested that outreach midwifery schemes offering continuity of care to women from NESB should be introduced in Australian public hospital systems to ensure that care is provided within local communities.

Two reviews of maternity care in the United Kingdom (UK) were also influential in the development of the STOMP model. The Winterton Report (House of Commons 1992) highlighted the need for women to have choice, continuity and control in the birth of their babies. *Changing Childbirth*, also known as the Cumberledge Report (Department of Health Expert Maternity Group 1993), was the English government's response to the Winterton Report. *Changing Childbirth* focused on the provision of maternity services and set specific targets and indicators for the providers of maternity care. The recommendations from the report (1993:18) were based on three fundamental principles of care, which were most relevant in the development of STOMP:

> The woman must be the focus of maternity care. She should be able to feel that she is in control of what is happening to her and be able to make decisions about her care, based on her needs, having discussed matters fully with the professionals involved;
>
> Maternity services must be readily and easily accessible. They should be sensitive to the needs of the local community and based primarily in the community; and
>
> Women should be involved in the monitoring and planning of maternity services to ensure they are responsive to the needs of a changing society. In addition, care should be effective and resources used efficiently.

Despite all these reports and recommendations over a decade, by 1996 it seemed that few public hospital maternity services in Australia had managed to achieve the widespread change necessary to introduce the components of continuity of care and community-based care into the provision of maternity care. The STOMP model was an endeavour to achieve change within a public sector metropolitan hospital in Sydney.

RESEARCH SUGGESTING CHANGE

Previous research into models of care that provide continuity of midwifery care suggested that there were positive benefits for women and health systems. Continuity of midwifery care has been shown to reduce interventions in labour, particularly augmentation of labour, analgesic use and electronic fetal monitoring (Flint et al 1989, Kenny et al 1994, Rowley et al 1995, Waldenström & Nilsson 1993, 1997). A small Canadian trial in 200 women demonstrated a significant reduction in caesarean section rate (Harvey et al 1996) and one of the Australian trials reported a trend towards a reduced elective caesarean section rate in high-risk women (Rowley et al 1995). A retrospective cohort study in California has also shown that supportive nurse-midwifery care in labour was associated with a reduced caesarean section rate (Butler et al 1993).

Continuity of midwifery care has been shown to improve women's experiences with care during pregnancy and childbirth (Flint et al 1989, MacVicar et al 1993, Waldenström & Nilsson 1993, Kenny et al 1994, Rowley et al 1995). In particular, women who have received continuity of care report greater preparedness for birth and early parenting (Flint et al 1989, McCourt et al 1998), increased satisfaction with psychological aspects of care (Waldenström & Nilsson 1993) and higher participation in decision making (Turnbull et al 1996) than women who received standard care.

Continuity of midwifery care has been associated with reduced costs to the health system in two Australian studies (Kenny et al 1994, Rowley et al 1995), although there were deficiencies in both cost analyses, demonstrating the need for more research. Results from these studies were compelling and influential in the development and design of the STOMP model.

LOCAL COMMITMENT TO CHANGE

Another important factor in the development of the STOMP model was the extent of the hospital's commitment to change. The maternity unit at St George Hospital in Sydney had been committed to improving their service over a number of years. This was evident from a series of innovations that had already occurred in the maternity unit. For example, a birth centre was established in 1990 as a result of the Shearman Report (NSW Health Department 1989). The birth centre was one of only three in Sydney at the time. Despite initial difficulties, with opposition from obstetricians and midwives, the birth centre remains a well-established option for women and excellent clinical outcomes have been reported (Homer et al 2000b).

The establishment of a midwives' clinic in 1995 was another example of the maternity unit's commitment to an improved service. The midwives' clinic enables women of low obstetric or medical risk to have continuity of midwife 'carer' throughout the antenatal period. This clinic was established partly as a result of the Shearman Report (NSW Health

Department 1989) but also in response to a customer survey conducted in 1994 (Everitt et al 1995).

This customer survey, known as the Maternity Services Customer Satisfaction Research Project (Everitt et al 1995), was another important factor in the development of STOMP. The survey used a combination of qualitative and quantitative methods to establish customer satisfaction levels and identify problem areas in the service provided by the hospital. A sample of women from English and NESB who were current, recent or potential users of the service were included in the survey. Problems identified included: the lack of continuity of care and carer in the antenatal and postnatal periods; insufficient respect for individual opinions and beliefs; and conflicting advice regarding breastfeeding. Difficulties accessing antenatal care at the hospital (because of a lack of car parking facilities) were also reported. Women from NESB reported difficulties in obtaining culturally appropriate care and accessing adequate information. The survey made 26 recommendations, including the establishment of new models of care that provide continuity of care and carer, and the consideration of community-based antenatal clinics. The STOMP model was developed to target specifically these two recommendations.

THE CONSULTATION PROCESS

The process of implementing the new model of care began during the latter half of 1996 with a series of formal and informal discussions between midwives, obstetricians and managers in the maternity unit. The purpose of these early meetings was to discuss the principles of continuity of care and community-based care and to canvass opinions about the proposed shift to a model of team midwifery. The researcher and others wrote a paper describing the issues around continuity of care and the change to the organisation that would result from the introduction of midwifery teams. This paper was distributed to all midwives, managers and obstetricians. Numerous in-service sessions and frequent informal interactions were conducted with staff members. External consultation also took place. This included discussions with experts in models of midwifery care in Australia (Kenny et al 1994, Rowley et al 1995) and in the United Kingdom through a study tour. A working party, which included midwives, obstetricians, managers and researchers, was established to develop the model initially, and subsequently to guide the implementation and evaluation.

During the consultation and development phase, it was decided that two STOMP teams would be established. Each team would consist of six midwives and provide antenatal, intrapartum and postnatal care for 300 women per year. Establishing two teams of midwives was unusual in Australia. Both previous projects had been based on only one team of midwives (Kenny et al 1994, Rowley et al 1995) which meant that access to the model was limited to fewer than 300 women annually. Other research in the UK and Sweden also involved only one team of midwives (Flint et al 1989, Turnbull et al 1996, Waldenström et al 1997).

FINANCIAL CONSIDERATIONS

The maternity unit at St George Hospital did not have any additional funds to establish new models of care. Therefore, the STOMP model was designed with the understanding that no additional funding would be available for the implementation. The model was aimed at women without private health insurance who were attending a public hospital for maternity care. Charges were not levied on the women receiving care. The STOMP model was implemented by reorganising the current maternity service's existing resources and staff. Internal restructuring provided the midwifery staff for the two STOMP teams by shifting 12 midwives from their existing wards or units, for example antenatal, labour and delivery and postnatal wards, to create the teams.

In many ways, the lack of additional funding was an advantage, rather than a disadvantage. Implementation within an existing budget meant the model was embedded in the organisational structure from the outset. We anticipated that full integration would make the new model less vulnerable to discontinuation in times of budgetary constraint.

Integration of innovation in maternity care has been uncommon in Australia. Pilot programmes have usually been established with the assistance of additional funding either from federal or state government bodies (Kenny et al 1994, Hambly 1997, Thiele & Thorogood 1997). This can mean that programmes are vulnerable to discontinuation when the support ends. It also can mean that the programmes are not seen or managed as a part of the existing or 'mainstream' service.

EXPERIENCE IN THE UK

The 1993 report from the UK, *Mapping Team Midwifery* (Wraight et al 1993), was another important determinant in the development of STOMP. *Mapping Team Midwifery* was a review of team midwifery schemes that had been implemented as a result of *Changing Childbirth* recommendations (Department of Health Expert Maternity Group 1993). Of concern was the finding that more than one quarter of schemes established in 1990 were discontinued by 1991. Discontinuation occurred because of inadequate staffing levels, problems with deployment onto the teams, lack of commitment from midwives and obstetricians, lack of consultation, discontent among midwives, failure to increase continuity of care, and personality clashes within teams. These factors were important in the development of the STOMP model.

SITUATING THE SERVICE

The STOMP model responded to the state and federal government reports that recommended antenatal care be based in the community (NSW Health Department 1989, Victorian Department of Health 1990,

NHMRC 1996). Women in Brisbane, Queensland, have reported choosing community-based care because of availability with appointment times and decreased travel and waiting time (Del Mar et al 1991, Ramsay 1996). Previous models of continuity of midwifery care in Australia have provided antenatal care from hospital-based clinics (Kenny et al 1994, Rowley et al 1995). Community-based antenatal care in Australia is generally only available to women who attend private medical practitioners, either specialist obstetricians or GPs. Midwives have a limited, if any, role in these models.

Community-based antenatal services provided by GPs and midwives have been evaluated in the UK and found to be feasible, satisfactory for the majority of women (Williams et al 1989, Fleissig et al 1996) and offer greater flexibility and choice (Perkins & Unell 1997). The 'One-to-One' midwifery project is an example of a model of continuity of carer in a community setting. 'One-to-One' midwifery (McCourt & Page 1996) was established as a demonstration project in the UK as a result of *Changing Childbirth* (Department of Health Expert Maternity Group 1993). The project provided care for all women regardless of risk group, in both hospital and community settings. The results indicated that women had a strong preference for community-based antenatal care.

Community-based maternity services, other than those provided in the private sector, are uncommon in the general Australian public health system. A review of the literature failed to uncover any reports of a 'mainstream' community-based antenatal program in Australia. A number of small pilot projects have provided community-based antenatal care by midwives (Ramsay 1996, Hambly 1997, Thiele & Thorogood 1997). These projects were small and available to a limited number of predominantly 'low-risk' women. A small number of special community-based antenatal services that have catered for specific disadvantaged groups, for example, adolescent (Brodie 1994) or indigenous women (Bartlett et al 1998) have been reported. These services are unavailable to most women because they only cater for minority groups.

In Australia, the move to community-based care has been interpreted by public health systems as a cost-saving measure. By virtue of the manner in which health services are funded in Australia (Leeder 1999), costs of providing care can be shifted from the state-funded public hospitals to the federally-funded GP in the community. It does not always follow that women receive better care, or indeed more cost-effective care. Problems have been reported in research from Melbourne (Brown et al 1999) including: fragmentation of services and provider; an increase in the number of antenatal visits and costs to women; duplication in investigations; variability in the quality of care; and a lack of co-ordination of care.

Difficulties have been experienced in Australia when midwives have attempted to work in small teams in the community. One of the reasons for this is the system of health care funding in Australia mentioned above. State governments fund public hospitals and their associated services, while the federal government funds GPs through the Medicare system (Leeder 1999). Therefore, there are currently no mechanisms to allow midwives to be contracted to provide antenatal care in GP practices. General practitioners are thus reluctant to employ midwives as they are unable to attract a Medicare rebate for midwifery care. It is unlikely that this current funding system is going to change, at least in the next decade (Senate Community Affairs References Committee 2000).

During the design phase of the STOMP model, it was decided that care during labour and birth would be provided in the delivery suite rather than in a birth centre or at home. Home birth is not a common option in Australia. There has been only one publicly funded home birth service reported in Australia. This was a small pilot project in Western Australia (Thiele & Thorogood 1997). In 1998, only 0.2% of women in NSW chose a home birth (NSW Health 2000), and since this time problems with indemnity insurance for midwives have meant that the rate is even lower. While a publicly funded home birth service is a potential option in the long term, at this stage it would have been unwise to attempt such a radical change in the provision of maternity care.

Birth centres are reasonably well known in Australian maternity care. The philosophy behind birth centre care is to provide care to low-risk women in a less clinical environment with as little intervention as possible in the normal progress of pregnancy and labour. Favourable outcomes have been reported in retrospective reviews of birth centres in Australia (Martins et al 1987, Biro & Lumley 1991, Ryan 1999, Homer et al 2000b) and in a randomised controlled trial conducted in Sweden (Waldenström & Nilsson 1993, Waldenström et al 1997). In a population-based survey of new mothers in Victoria in 1993, women who attended birth centres were significantly more likely to: report having an active say in decisions during labour; have their wishes taken into account; and have known midwives before labour. These are all factors that have been strongly associated with satisfaction with childbirth (Brown & Lumley 1998). Birth centres have a non-interventionist philosophy and are available for women who are expected to have a normal labour and birth. When women develop complications during pregnancy or labour, they are transferred to standard care.

The birth centre at St George Hospital can only cater for 350–400 women per year as it has only two birthing rooms and a staff of five to six midwives. The two teams in the STOMP model would cater for 600 additional women per year. Clearly the resources of the birth centre were inadequate to meet the STOMP model requirements, which meant STOMP care was provided in the delivery suite.

It was also recognised that not all women recruited to STOMP would choose a non-interventionist style of care. We wanted STOMP to be a model of care available to most women, regardless of risk or expectations around birth. We also knew, from retrospective research in the unit, that our delivery suite had similar obstetric outcomes to the birth centre in a matched cohort of women (Homer et al 2000b). This acknowledgement reaffirmed the decision to provide labour care in the delivery suite. The two Australian trials (Kenny et al 1994, Rowley et al 1995) had also provided care in the delivery suite.

CHARACTERISTICS OF THE STOMP MODEL

Each STOMP team consisted of seven full time equivalent (FTE) midwives, which gave a working roster of six midwives per team. The additional FTE position was required to cover the annual leave entitlements within the team. Adequate uptake of annual leave entitlements was seen as an essential component of the STOMP model to ensure that the midwives did not become exhausted and 'burnt out'. Under the current NSW Nurses Award, midwives who work rotating rosters are entitled to 6–7 weeks' annual leave. This meant that there was almost always one of the seven midwives on annual leave.

The caseload of each STOMP team was guided by the Australian research by Kenny et al (1994) and Rowley et al (1995) and informed through our consultation process with others who had expertise in this area. Flint's book *Midwifery: Teams and Caseloads* (1993) was also used, but her recommended personal caseload of 36 women per year was thought to be too low to be financially sustainable in our setting. Each STOMP team was implemented with a caseload of 300 women per year or 50 women per midwife per year.

THE ORGANISATION OF ANTENATAL CARE

Antenatal care was provided in the community with hospital-salaried midwives and obstetricians. It was hypothesised that this would provide greater convenience and access for women. Two different sites were chosen. One clinic was in an early childhood centre (where child and family health services are provided in the community) and the other initially in a family planning centre (this clinic has subsequently moved into an early childhood centre as well). The STOMP clinics became known by their respective localities: Rockdale and Hurstville. The sites were selected as they were easily accessible to women (adequate public transport and car parking options), had appropriate facilities (two rooms for consultation) and were geographically central to the greatest number of the childbearing women in the district. The staff at both the early childhood centre and the family planning centre were very supportive of the project and welcomed the move of antenatal services into community centres.

The STOMP clinics were conducted collaboratively. Two midwives and an obstetrician or obstetric registrar attended each session. This meant that the STOMP model could cater for women with risks. Collaboration also allowed women who requested obstetric care (for reassurance or support) to receive this in a community-based setting. Provision of obstetric antenatal care in conjunction with midwifery care from a community-based setting is unusual in an Australian context. Obstetric staffing was slightly different between the two sites. The staff specialist obstetrician attended the Rockdale clinic but did not routinely see all the women who attended. The midwives requested consultations when necessary. Some of these consultations were scheduled in advance for particular women, and others were on an ad hoc basis. One of two obstetric registrars attended each of the clinics at Hurstville STOMP, with ultimate responsibility provided by the Professor of Obstetrics at the hospital. The decision to staff the Hurstville STOMP clinic with registrars was based on a number of factors, including the need for the hospital to provide adequate training opportunities for medical staff and the clinical demands placed on the department at the time. Obstetric staff reviewed each woman's antenatal record at the first visit to the clinic. Women were assessed only when it was deemed necessary from the record review or as requested by the midwife or the woman. At other times, the obstetric staff contributed to teaching and support of the midwives and attended to other paperwork. Women were also able to have GP shared care. This occurred in the form of alternating visits, that is, every second visit was with the GP. These women all remained in the STOMP group for the analysis.

All women carried an antenatal card, which was a smaller duplicate of the version kept by the hospital. At the time of the study, records held by the women were in the evaluation phase (Homer et al 1999) and not available across the maternity unit. The STOMP teams did not provide antenatal or parenting education classes. Women were offered the regular classes that were provided (at a small cost) by the hospital.

THE ORGANISATION OF CARE DURING LABOUR AND BIRTH IN STOMP

One of the midwives from each STOMP team was always 'available' for women in labour or to answer questions. Women were able to access the STOMP midwife by telephoning the hospital's switchboard and requesting that the respective STOMP midwife be paged. The midwife would then call the woman and discuss her particular situation and plan of care. On occasions, women arrived in the delivery suite unannounced. These women were admitted and cared for by the midwives on duty while the on-call STOMP midwife was contacted.

STOMP midwives worked 12-hour 'available' shifts and most did not come into the hospital unless required to provide labour care for a STOMP woman. The decision to work 12-hour shifts was prompted by a number of factors. Proctor's (1998) research showed that women valued continuity *during* labour and did not want to experience a change of staff when labour was established. Rowley et al's (1995) work has also suggested that having only one caregiver in labour is advantageous. The consultation process at St George Hospital also influenced the decision. Midwives who had only ever worked conventional 8-hour shifts were concerned that a 24-hour period would be too great a change in the initial phase. Once a STOMP midwife's 12-hour shift was complete, she handed over primary responsibility for the woman to the next STOMP midwife. The first midwife was able to remain with the woman if appropriate, for example if she was expected to give birth soon, but the oncoming midwife assumed responsibility. This principle was in place to ensure that an over-tired midwife did not jeopardise the care of the woman. Ideally, women would receive continuity of carer in labour but this did not always occur. As discussed earlier, this compromise was influenced by previous research and was guided by our internal and external consultation process.

In the delivery suite, STOMP midwives received support from the 'core' midwives (that is, midwives who normally worked in the delivery suite and were not in either STOMP team). This support was important for practical reasons: for example, it enabled STOMP midwives to have meal breaks. More importantly, core midwives provided STOMP midwives with advice, guidance and assistance with solving problems. In the event of two women from the same STOMP team being in labour simultaneously, the midwives made a decision based on need and staffing levels. Either the one STOMP midwife provided care for both women with the assistance of the core midwives, or a second STOMP midwife was called. Team work and mutual support were important in making these decisions.

STOMP midwives continued to provide midwifery care in the operating theatre for women who had an elective or an emergency caesarean section. This was usually in the role of preparing the woman and her partner for surgery, and receiving and accompanying the baby and the woman's partner back to the delivery suite or if necessary, the special care nursery (SCN). Midwives at St George Hospital did not 'scrub' or assist in the theatre in any other manner.

THE ORGANISATION OF POSTNATAL CARE

Issues surrounding the provision of postnatal care and support were influential in the development of the STOMP model. It was decided that postnatal care would be provided in the hospital and in women's homes, continuing the cycle back into the community. After the birth, women were transferred to the postnatal ward. Women could either choose to remain in hospital for postnatal care, or be discharged early (4–48 hours) and visited at home by the STOMP midwives.

Ensuring continuity of care and carer in the postnatal period was difficult. A compromise was reached where women were cared for by a STOMP midwife on a morning shift and at other times the core midwives provided care. Every morning shift, a STOMP midwife from each team was rostered for duty on the postnatal ward. This meant that there were two STOMP midwives and two or possibly three core midwives to provide postnatal care for the 24 women on the ward and the STOMP women at home. STOMP midwives worked 8-hour shifts when providing postnatal care. The STOMP midwives predominantly cared for the STOMP women in the ward but also cared for other non-STOMP women if necessary, for example, when there were few STOMP women requiring postnatal care in hospital. STOMP midwives also provided care at home for STOMP women who chose to leave hospital early.

A typical day for a STOMP midwife could include providing care for three STOMP women on the ward and three or four at home. The midwife would come on duty at 7.30 am, review the women on the ward and plan their care for the day. She would discuss the day's workload with the manager of the postnatal ward, the other STOMP team's midwife, and the core midwives. Discussion would include the number of women in hospital and at home, the needs of the ward while the STOMP midwives were in the community, and the use of vehicles. At some stage through the morning the STOMP midwife would visit women at home. While she was out of the ward, the other STOMP midwife or the core midwives and the manager would provide care for the women on the ward. Outside the morning shifts, the core midwives on the postnatal ward cared for STOMP women. The STOMP midwife, in conjunction with the woman, planned the care to be provided on the other shifts. This process ensured that consistent information, care and support were provided for the woman. STOMP midwives usually rostered themselves to the postnatal ward for two to four consecutive days to increase continuity of carer.

THE STOMP MIDWIVES

STOMP midwives were recruited from the existing staff of midwives within the Division of Women's and Children's Health at St George Hospital. As most midwives in the unit routinely rotated through all areas of care, finding midwives with adequate skills in all areas may have been less difficult than in other hospitals where midwives did not move from area to area on a regular basis.

In November 1996, an 'Expression of Interest' for the first team, known as the Rockdale team, was distributed to areas in the maternity unit. This was the culmination of the first series of formal and informal sessions, where the STOMP model and the role of the midwives was described and discussed. Six midwives responded to this advertisement and all were subsequently appointed. These midwives came from different areas within the maternity unit, although most had worked within the hospital for some time. The second team, known as the Hurstville team, was recruited in May 1997. The majority of these midwives had come to St George Hospital recently with the expressed interest of ultimately joining a team providing continuity of midwifery care.

Both teams were made up of midwives with a range of experience and skills. They were not necessarily the most experienced or senior midwives in the unit. Some were newly graduated and others had 10 years of experience. Midwives entering the STOMP teams were required to complete a 'Skills Inventory' which consisted of a self-assessment process aimed at identifying skills that needed 'updating'. This tool was adapted with permission from research in the Midwifery Development Unit in Scotland at Glasgow Royal Maternity Hospital (McGinley et al 1995). Identifying areas of skill deficit gave midwives an opportunity to address these areas prior to commencing on the team and/or during the early days of STOMP. Clinical leadership, teaching and professional support were provided by a midwifery consultant who was attached to the teams for the first year, and by the staff specialist obstetrician. STOMP midwives were also well supported by managers, clinical leaders in midwifery and obstetrics, and by the midwives in the wider maternity unit.

POLICIES AND PROCEDURES

STOMP teams followed the St George Hospital's standard policies and procedures for all aspects of maternity care. This principle was adopted for a number of reasons. Firstly, the research was designed to test the safety, efficiency and cost of the *new* model of care. It was not designed to alter midwifery *practice* but to change the structure and place in which midwifery care was provided. In essence, if procedures were specifically altered, the research findings would have been compromised. It would be impossible to say if the results were due to the effect of the new model or the different procedures. Secondly, the new model was being introduced as a component of the mainstream system, rather than an 'add-on' service. This meant it was important that the service was seen as a whole and the policies as seamless between the community setting and the hospital. Thirdly, a commitment to evidence-based practice was, and continues to be, the philosophy of the maternity unit at St George Hospital. All policies and procedures were grounded in research evidence and therefore were independent of the midwife providing care.

The change in structure aimed to develop the capacity of STOMP midwives to provide individualised care by improving the relationship with the women. It was hoped that this 'relationship' would mean that policies and procedures were applied more appropriately.

LEADERSHIP AND SUPPORT WITHIN THE MATERNITY UNIT

Implementing a new model of care requires fundamental changes at all levels within the organisation as well as a transformed culture (Page et al 1995). In implementing STOMP, we asked midwives, obstetricians and managers to move out of their 'comfort zone' of familiar routines and roles to a new way of providing care that centred on what the women needed rather than what the organisation could provide. The introduction of the STOMP model resulted in considerable disruption to all staff within the maternity unit and resulted in widespread changes to the way people worked and related to one another. This process was facilitated by the commitment and leadership demonstrated by staff within the unit.

STOMP midwives, particularly in the first year, received direct support from a midwife consultant, with additional support from the manager of the delivery suite and the postnatal wards. Fortnightly meetings were held with each team to discuss issues that had arisen, to provide opportunities for solving problems and to ensure consistency of care was maintained. Individual and one-to-one support was also available to the midwives. The meetings provided midwives with time to reflect on their practice and processes for making decisions. Regular social events were also important to assist the midwives to develop cohesive working relationships with one another. Core midwives also required additional support through the transition process. Strategies such as regular ward meetings and newsletters about the research were used. Minutes of STOMP meetings were also circulated and informal communication networks were used to minimise the sense of disruption and alienation that may have occurred. All midwives in the unit attended one of a series of 'team building' days that were provided. These days were designed to help midwives, in their small teams, understand more about the ways in which teams work and develop strategies to help address issues of effective communication and support.

Regular talks were given by members of the working party which guided the development of the model, in a variety of staff forums, to ensure that all midwifery and medical staff were aware of the project and its current status. The research newsletter, which reported on all the research projects being conducted within the maternity unit and was written by the researcher, also provided a source of information for staff. Research support and guidance was also provided through regular meetings.

These processes were extremely important for the successful implementation of the new model of care. The STOMP model required widespread reorganisation of human resources within the maternity unit. Effective communication, shared solving of problems, flexibility and trust were essential components of the organisational processes. The commitment and support provided from managers and senior staff within the maternity unit meant that the model was successfully implemented, evaluated and continues to be an option for women.

SUMMARY

The STOMP model of care was developed to give women increased choice, control, continuity and ease of access to care. Government policy documents, both in Australia and the UK, were used as starting points but previous and ongoing research and experience have also influenced the development of the STOMP model. Compromises were required, as this was a new model of care both for the organisation and the staff. The change needed to be one that was acceptable, sustainable and manageable within the public health system.

STOMP care differs from standard care by its capacity to provide continuity of care and carer, even when women develop complications during pregnancy and labour. Chief differences between STOMP and the standard models of care are presented in Table 8.1.

METHODS

The evaluation investigated whether the STOMP model improved maternal and neonatal clinical outcomes, resulted in a better experience for

Table 8.1 Differences between the STOMP model and standard care at St George Hospital

	STOMP	Standard
Antenatal care provided in community-based settings	Yes	No
Obstetric care available in community-based settings	Yes	No
Same midwives provide antenatal, intrapartum and postpartum care	Yes	No (only birth centre)
Care is collaborative involving midwives and obstetricians	Yes	Yes
Transfer to standard care in event of medical complications	Rarely	Not applicable
Postpartum community midwifery visits	Yes	Yes
Postpartum community midwifery visit from a midwife met in the antenatal period	Yes	No

women and could be implemented within the current resources of this public teaching hospital in Sydney, Australia.

A randomised controlled trial using a Zelen (1979) design was used to compare the STOMP model with standard care. One thousand and eighty-nine women were randomly allocated to either the STOMP model or standard hospital-based care. The Zelen design was used to increase the participation of women from non-English speaking backgrounds and to reduce disappointment bias in women allocated to the control group (Homer 2000, Homer et al 2002b).

Clinical and cost data were collected from medical records once the woman was discharged from the service. Data on the experiences of women were collected using questionnaires administered at 36 weeks' gestation and at 8–10 weeks after the birth, with response rates of 75% and 69% respectively.

RESULTS

The research on the STOMP model of care demonstrated benefits for women and the organisation. The study recruited a diverse range of women, including those from NESB, and did not exclude women who developed complications in pregnancy.

The results showed that the STOMP model of care produced satisfactory clinical outcomes. There was a significant difference in the caesarean section rate between the groups, 13.3% (73/550) in the STOMP group and 17.8% in the control group (96/539). This difference was maintained after controlling for known contributing factors to caesarean section (OR = 0.6, 95% CI 0.4–0.9, P = 0.02). There were no other significant differences in the events during labour and birth.

Eighty (14.5%) neonates from the STOMP group and 102 (18.9%) from the control group were admitted to the special care nursery but this difference was not significant (OR = 0.75, 95% CI 0.5–1.1, P = 0.12). Eight infants died during the perinatal period (four from each group), for an overall perinatal mortality rate of 7.3 per 1000 births.

The mean cost of providing care per woman was lower in the group who had the STOMP model of care compared with standard care. Cost savings associated with new model of care were maintained even after costs associated with admission to special care nursery were excluded. The cost saving was also sustained even when the caesarean section rate in the new model of care increased to beyond that of the standard care group.

In the antenatal period, women in the STOMP group reported waiting significantly less time for antenatal visits, with easier access to care. STOMP group women also reported a higher perceived 'quality' of antenatal care compared with the control group. STOMP group women saw slightly more midwives and fewer doctors than control group women did. STOMP women were significantly more likely to have talked with their midwives and doctors about their personal preferences for childbirth and more likely to report that they knew enough about aspects of labour and birth, particularly induction of labour, pain relief and caesarean section.

Almost 80% of women in the STOMP group experienced continuity of care during labour and birth, that is, one of their team midwives was present. STOMP women reported a significantly higher 'sense of control during labour and birth'. Sixty three per cent of STOMP women reported that they 'knew' the midwife who cared for them during labour, compared with 21% of control women. In a secondary analysis, women who had a midwife during labour who they felt that they knew, had a significantly higher sense of 'control' and a more positive birth experience compared with women who reported an unknown midwife.

Postnatal care elicited the greatest number of negative comments from women in both the STOMP and the control group.

IMPLICATIONS FOR MATERNITY CARE IN AUSTRALIA

The STOMP model was implemented as a strategy to improve clinical outcomes and women's experiences of care, at no additional cost to the maternity unit of a NSW public hospital. While all aspects of the STOMP model may not be appropriate within all contexts, there may be components that can be adapted for particular settings. For example, community-based antenatal care may be possible from other Australian hospitals. It was hoped that the results of the STOMP study could be used by other organisations who wanted to institute change.

The STOMP study showed that maternity units can be reorganised and restructured to enable new models of care to be established within existing budgets. A commitment by the leaders of the service to the process of change is required. Strategies need to be developed to address the difficulties and barriers that will invariably arise. Models of care that are efficient and effective are more likely to be sustainable, that is, continue to exist in the long term.

SUSTAINABILITY

The sustainability of new models of care is dependent on a number of factors, including the satisfaction of the staff who provide the care, and the cost of providing the service. Problems, including industrial award constraints and territorial disputes between obstetricians, GPs and midwives, may contribute to reduced sustainability and a desire to revert to the status quo.

A sustainable model of care for midwives has been related to the avoidance of burnout and the provision of flexible, woman-centred care (Sandall 1997). Sandall (1997) found that having control over the organisation of work, social support at work and home, and being able to develop meaningful relationships with women were important factors associated with the avoidance of burnout. A caseload model gives midwives more control over their workload and an opportunity to 'know' the women better, as there are fewer women to meet. For example, in a caseload model each midwife will be involved in the births of 70 women a year (Leap 1996). In a team model like STOMP, six midwives care for 300 women per year. A midwife in STOMP may provide care during labour for any one of these 300 women. Midwives are usually on-call more often in a caseload model than in a team model. However, as they are on-call for proportionally fewer women they are less likely to be called (Leap 1996).

The STOMP model is by no means the 'ideal' model of maternity care, but it is one that has worked in our context at the St George Hospital. Additional elements could be included and may improve the experience for women. These might include an opportunity to have some antenatal visits in the home and the provision of first stage of labour care at home. Future expansion of the model may also include a home birth option. The inclusion of midwifery students into continuity of care models may educate midwives for whom this way of working is the norm rather than the exception. The 'way of working' refers not only to the system of being available for women in labour, but also a philosophy of women-centred practice. Additional elements would have to be planned and evaluated. The cost and the impact on the clinicians need to be considered in future development of new models of care.

We have found that each team of six midwives should 'book' 35 women per month with the aim of attending the labour and birth of 30 women per month, in order to maximise efficiency and provide a manageable workload. This means that the teams can cater for 720 women a year, which is higher than our original estimations of 600 women a year. From anecdotes, this caseload means that the midwives are efficiently utilised. This caseload and activity level can take some time to achieve. There is an initial 'setting up' phase of 9–12 months as the programme is established, women are booked onto the team, midwives are recruited and any updating of midwifery skills occurs. During this period, considerable flexibility and adaptability of all staff is required.

Flexible systems mean that midwifery resources can be efficiently matched to actual need. For example, when there are no women in labour the staffing levels are low; conversely, when there are more women in labour, additional midwives are available.

Flexibility and a substantial caseload are important factors in ensuring long-term sustainability of models of care. Flexibility is more difficult to achieve when models of care cater for a small proportion of the women at a particular hospital and the new model is not integrated into the wider unit (Audit Commission 1998). The STOMP model now caters for 28% of the women at St George Hospital. The implementation and sustainability of two teams means that STOMP caters for a significant number of women. Implementing the model within existing resources also ensured that it was always part of the maternity service, rather than an 'add-on' model. We believe these factors will be important in assuring long-term sustainability and development.

INTER-DISCIPLINARY COLLABORATION

Inter-disciplinary collaboration was an important factor in the STOMP model and may have contributed to the benefits. Collaboration is an essential part of contemporary maternity care, but there is little written on the topic. Celia Davies (2000) has written that collaboration in health care is 'characterised by the recognition that it is not what people have in common, but their differences, that makes collaborative work powerful' (2000:1021). This observation is highly applicable in provision of maternity care, where both midwives and obstetricians have different but equally valid knowledge, expertise and resources and can combine these to provide a level of care that is highly effective. There are some women who need to see an obstetrician for medical reasons and others who choose to see one for reassurance, for additional information, or because this is their expectation of maternity care. Professional territorial disputes can impede a model of collaborative practice being implemented, often to the detriment of the women who want and need care from both professional groups. Classifying women as 'low' or 'high' risk can contribute to these territorial disputes by creating additional barriers. The assumption can be that high-risk women need doctors and low-risk women need midwives. This supposition denies women choice and means that the inter-disciplinary collaboration is limited. A proportion of low-risk women will want to see an obstetrician (if only for reassurance) and it is likely that many high-risk women benefit from midwifery as well as medical care.

The STOMP model provided care primarily from midwives, with obstetric involvement when indicated (either due to medical reasons or personal choice). It appears that collaboration has been beneficial for women. For example, fewer women had an antenatal hospital admission, thus reducing the costs and the disruption for women. Other benefits, which have not been measured in this study, include those to the midwives and the obstetricians. Midwives have reported an increase in knowledge, skills and personal and professional confidence. Doctors have reported improved communication with midwives and a greater understanding of the role of the midwife. The doctors have also reported that from their perspective, the efficiency of care provided to women was high. For example, midwives ensured that pathology and ultrasound results were acted upon appropriately and efficiently. Results were always available at clinic visits. The level of responsibility and accountability towards the women also appeared to be high in the STOMP model. Both professions described the development of an increased level of trust and support which has improved their clinical practice.

LEADERSHIP AND VISION

Successful implementation of a new model of care requires strong inter-disciplinary leadership from within the organisation. Shifting the organisational culture to one where change is accepted and embraced also requires a clear vision of where the organisation is moving and what might be possible (Page et al 1995). This process requires creativity and imagination, a strong sense of how the vision may be translated into practice, and a capacity to muster support and develop trust and collaborative effort amongst staff. Changing the culture of an organisation is a slow process and one that requires leaders to be determined, savvy and demonstrate political skills. These skills include a capacity to listen to all sides of an argument, to negotiate, persuade and debate as necessary, and to be discerning towards what is important to fight for and what can be left alone (Page et al 1995). Communication and information sharing about the change are also important components of change. It is of little value to drive an organisation towards a vision if no one knows what it is.

Ongoing support from management and inter-disciplinary collaboration are essential elements to ensure sustainability of the new model. It is important that this support is provided for midwives providing care in the new model as well as those who are 'core' midwives (Page et al 2000). Efforts should be made to include all staff in the design and implementation process. Strategies that were used in the STOMP study include: the distribution of a discussion paper to all staff; the establishment of a inter-disciplinary working party with regular meetings; formal and informal education sessions; and constant feedback from senior staff to other staff in the unit. Newsletters, minutes of meetings and use of communication books are other practical measures that have been found to be helpful in ensuring staff are informed and feel a sense of 'ownership' and inclusion in the process.

FURTHER RESEARCH AND DEVELOPMENT

The STOMP model is only one way to provide maternity care, and while there were benefits for women and the organisation, concerns still exist which require further research. The level of intervention in labour, the proportion of neonates admitted to the SCN, postnatal care in general, and the level of information provided to women from NESB are all factors that have been identified as worthy of further research. A new model of care, which addresses the deficits identified in the provision of postnatal care, may need to be developed and evaluated. A caseload model, where groups of two to four midwives provide care to a smaller group of women, may be the next step in the development of new models of maternity care in Australia. Any new model would require evaluation from the perspective of the women, the clinicians and the health care organisation.

The benefits of continuity of care and carer, particularly in labour, continue to be an important question and one that this study has not been able to answer fully. Qualitative methodologies may be the best way to understand continuity of carer in labour because of difficulties understanding the complex nature of values about the topic (Page et al 2000). Qualitative research may lead to the development of a new questionnaire, which can evaluate continuity of carer in labour more effectively.

The provision of continuity of care and carer will undoubtedly impact on the midwives and obstetricians who provide the care. Other research to examine the impact of being 'on call' is important, to understand the long-term effects of continuity of care models.

Many maternity units will not have access to bilingual midwives. Despite this, it is still possible to include women from NESB in randomised controlled trials (Homer 2000). Using interpreter services and translated materials and having a genuine commitment to participation of all women will contribute towards a diverse sample. As translation services are costly, identifying the most common language groups and targeting only these for translation will also facilitate recruitment and reduce costs.

CONCLUSION

The STOMP model of care is associated with benefits for women and for the health care system. Women report positive social and emotional experiences, with a reduced caesarean section rate and reduced use of electronic fetal monitoring. The model is not more expensive for the health care system than standard care, and was implemented within an existing budget and resource base.

Many of the challenges involved in establishing and maintaining the STOMP model revolved around the need to change an inherently inflexible acute care system into one that was flexible and primary health care focused. The systems around the midwives and managers were intrinsically conservative and generally focused on meeting the needs of staff and the system rather than the women. A balance needed to be found, between a model that met the needs of women and one where the conditions of the midwives and the system were paramount and exclusive.

The STOMP model is one way to provide effective and efficient maternity care. It is a model that has been shown to be successful in a culturally diverse teaching hospital. We hope that the STOMP model demonstrates that improvement in maternity care can be achieved even in an

Australian setting which is based on an acute care model. For change to occur, a strong commitment to improving services must come from within the organisation and its staff. Support, collaboration and a clear vision of what is desirable and what might be possible are all required to implement successfully a new model of care. Ensuring that midwives can practise to their full capacity is an important aspect of models which involve continuity of care. Since the study was completed we have been asked by numerous organisations within NSW and throughout Australia for advice and support on how to implement new models of midwifery care. This interest led to the publication of a handbook for midwives and managers which details the 'how to' stages that have been learned from STOMP and other models of midwifery care.

Maternity services in Australia and elsewhere are increasingly recognising that they must change in order to provide women with effective care that is acceptable, cost effective and rewarding for women. In addition, given the current crisis in the number of midwives in Australia and elsewhere, maternity services need to be re-organised so that they are satisfying for midwives as well as for women. Establishing a model of care such as STOMP is one way in which midwives can play a significant role in shifting the balance to a public health, primary health care focus.

References

Alcorso C, Schofield T 1992 The Australian National Non-English Speaking Background Women's Health Strategy. Australian Government Publishing Service, Canberra

Audit Commission 1998 First Class Delivery: A National Survey of Women's Views of Maternity Care. DH, London

Bartlett M, Hecker R, Jan S, Capon A, Conaty S 1998 Evaluation of the Daruk Aboriginal Medical Service antenatal programs. Public Health Association of Australia Inc., Hobart

Biro M A, Lumley J 1991 The safety of team midwifery: the first decade of the Monash Birth Centre. Medical Journal of Australia 155:478–480

Brodie P 1994 Midwifery care for pregnant teenagers: primary health care in action. In: Wass A (ed) Promoting Health: The Primary Health Care Approach. Harcourt Brace, Sydney

Brown S, Lumley J 1998 Changing childbirth: lessons from an Australian survey of 1336 women. British Journal of Obstetrics and Gynaecology 105:143–155

Brown S, Dawson W, Gunn J, McNair R 1999 Review of Shared Obstetric Care: Summary Report. Centre for the Study of Mothers' and Children's Health, La Trobe University, Melbourne

Butler J, Abrams B, Parker J, Roberts J M, Laros R K 1993 Supportive nurse-midwife care is associated with a reduced incidence of caesarean section. American Journal of Obstetrics and Gynaecology 168:1407–1413

Davies C 2000 Getting health professionals to work together [Editorial]. British Medical Journal 320:1021–1022

Del Mar C, Siskind V, Acworth J, Lutz K, Wyatt P 1991 Shared antenatal care in Brisbane. Australian and New Zealand Journal of Obstetrics and Gynaecology 31:305–306

Department of Health Expert Maternity Group 1993 Changing Childbirth. Department of Health/HMSO, London

Department of Health Western Australia 1990 Ministerial task force to review obstetric, gynaecological and neonatal services in Western Australia. Health Department of Western Australia, Perth

Everitt L, Barclay L, Chapman M, Hurst R, Lupi A, Wills J 1995 St George Maternity Services Customer Satisfaction Research Project. St George Hospital and Community Services, Sydney

Fleissig A, Kroll D, McCarthy M 1996 Is community-led maternity care a feasible option for women assessed at low risk and those with complicated pregnancies? Results of a population based study in South Camden, London. Midwifery 12:191–197

Flint C 1993 Midwifery: Teams and Caseloads. Butterworth-Heinemann, Oxford

Flint C, Poulengeris P, Grant A 1989 The 'Know Your Midwife' scheme – a randomised trial of continuity of care by a team of midwives. Midwifery 5:11–16

Hambly M 1997 Community Midwives Pilot Project Evaluation, Alternative Birthing Services in the ACT. ACT Department of Health and Community Care, Canberra

Harvey S, Jarrell J, Brant R, Stainton C, Rach D 1996 A randomised, controlled trial of nurse-midwifery care. Birth: Issues in Perinatal Care and Education 23:128–135

Homer C S E 2000 Incorporating cultural diversity in randomised controlled trials in midwifery. Midwifery 16:252–259

Homer C S E 2002 Using the Zelen design in randomised controlled trials: debates and controversies. Journal of Advanced Nursing 38:200–207

Homer C S E, Davis G K, Everitt L 1999 The introduction of a woman-held record into an antenatal clinic: a randomised controlled trial. Australian and New Zealand Journal of Obstetrics and Gynaecology 39:54–57

Homer C S E, Davis G K, Brodie P 2000a What do women feel about community-based antenatal care? Australian and New Zealand Journal of Public Health 24:590–595

Homer C S E, Davis G K, Petocz P, Barclay L, Matha D, Chapman M G 2000b The obstetric outcomes of low risk women: birth centre versus labour ward. Australian Journal of Advanced Nursing 18:8–12

Homer C S E, Davis G K, Brodie P M, Sheehan A, Barclay L M, Wills J, Chapman M G 2001a Collaboration in maternity care: a randomised controlled trial comparing community-based continuity of care with standard care. British Journal of Obstetrics and Gynaecology 108:16–22

Homer C S E, Matha D, Jordan L G, Wills J, Davis G K 2001b Community-based continuity of midwifery care versus standard hospital care: a cost analysis. Australian Health Review 24:85–93

Homer C S E, Davis G K, Cooke M, Barclay L M 2002a Women's experiences of continuity of midwifery care in Australia: a randomised controlled trial. Midwifery 18:102–112

Homer C S E, Sheehan A, Cooke M 2002b Early infant feeding decision and practices: a comparison of the experiences of women from English, Arabic and Chinese-speaking backgrounds in Australia. Breastfeeding Review 10:27–32

House of Commons 1992 The Health Committee Second Report: Maternity Services Vol. 1. (Chair: N. Winterton). HMSO, London

Kenny P, Brodie P, Eckermann S, Hall J 1994 Westmead Hospital Team Midwifery Project Evaluation: Final Report. Westmead Hospital, Sydney

Leap N 1996 Caseload practice: a recipe for burnout? British Journal of Midwifery 4:329–330

Leeder S R 1999 Healthy Medicine: Challenges facing Australia's Health Services. Allen & Unwin, Sydney

MacVicar J, Dobbie G, Owen-Johnstone L, Jagger C, Hopkins M, Kennedy J 1993 Simulated home delivery in hospital: a randomised controlled trial. British Journal of Obstetrics and Gynaecology 100:316–323

Martins J M, Greenwell J, Linder-Pelz S, Webster M A 1987 Evaluation of outcomes: deliveries at the birth centre and traditional setting at the Royal Hospital for Women, Sydney. NSW Department of Health, Sydney

Maternity Services Advisory Committee 1999 The NSW Framework for Maternity Services. NSW Health, Sydney

McCourt C, Page L 1996 Report on the Evaluation of One-to-One Midwifery. The Hammersmith Hospitals NHS Trust and Thames Valley University, London

McCourt C, Page L, Hewison J 1998 Evaluation of One-to-One Midwifery: Women's responses to care. Birth: Issues in Perinatal Care and Education 25:73–80

McGinley M, Turnbull D, Fyvie H, Johnstone I, MacLennan B 1995 Midwifery development unit at Glasgow Royal Maternity Hospital. British Journal of Midwifery 3:362–371

NHMRC 1996 Options for Effective Care in Childbirth. Australian Government Printing Service, Canberra

NSW Health 2000 New South Wales Mothers and Babies 1998 (State Health Publications No. (EPI) 000029 ed.) NSW Health Department, Sydney

NSW Health Department 1989 Final Report of the Ministerial Task Force on Obstetric Services in NSW: The Shearman Report. (State Health Publication No. (HSU) 89-007 ed.) NSW Health Department, Sydney

NSW Health Department 1996 NSW Midwifery Taskforce Report (State Health Publication No. (NB) 960017 ed.) NSW Health Department, Sydney

Page L A, Bentley R K, Jones B, Marlow D 1995 Transforming the organisation. In: Page L A (ed) Effective Group Practice in Midwifery: Working with Women. Blackwell Science, Oxford, pp 77–95

Page L A, Cooke P, Percival P 2000 Providing one-to-one care and enjoying it. In: Page L A (ed) The New Midwifery: Science and Sensitivity in Practice. Churchill Livingstone, Edinburgh, pp 123–140

Perkins E R, Unell J 1997 Continuity and choice in practice: a study of a community-based team midwifery scheme. In: Kirkham M J, Perkins E R (eds) Reflections on midwifery. Baillière Tindall, London, pp 26–46

Proctor S 1998 What determines quality in maternity care? Comparing the perceptions of childbearing women and midwives. Birth: Issues in Perinatal Care and Education 25:85–93

Ramsay K 1996 Evaluation of the Community Midwifery Service. Mater Misericordiae Mothers Hospital, Brisbane, Queensland

Rowley M J, Hensley M J, Brinsmead M W, Wlodarczyk J H 1995 Continuity of care by a midwife team versus routine care during pregnancy and birth: a randomised trial. Medical Journal of Australia 163(6):289–293

Ryan M 1999 Do clinical outcomes differ between a birth centre and a labour ward? (Abstract). Australian College of Midwives, Hobart

Sandall J 1997 Midwives' burnout and continuity of care. British Journal of Midwifery 5:106–111

Senate Community Affairs References Committee 1999 Rocking the Cradle: A Report into Childbirth Procedures. Commonwealth of Australia, Canberra

Senate Community Affairs References Committee 2000 First Report: Public Hospital Funding and Options for Reform. Commonwealth of Australia, Canberra

Thiele B, Thorogood C 1997 Community Based Midwifery Program in Fremantle WA. Centre for Research for Women (WA) and the Fremantle Community Midwives, Fremantle

Turnbull D, Holmes A, Shields N et al 1996 Randomised, controlled trial of efficacy of midwife-managed care. Lancet 348:213–218

Victorian Department of Health 1990 Having a Baby in Victoria: Ministerial Review of Birthing Services in Victoria. Victorian Department of Health, Melbourne

Waldenström U, Nilsson, C A 1993 Women's satisfaction with birth centre care: a randomised controlled trial. Birth: Issues in Perinatal Care and Education 21:3–13

Waldenström U, Nilsson C A 1997 A randomised controlled study of birth centre care versus standard maternity care: effects on women's health. Birth: Issues in Perinatal Care and Education 24:17–26

Waldenström U, Nilsson C A, Winbladh B 1997 The Stockholm birth centre trial: maternal and infant outcome. British Journal of Obstetrics and Gynaecology 104:410–418

Williams S, Dickson D, Forbes J, McIlwaine G, Rosenberg K 1989 An evaluation of community antenatal care. Midwifery 5:63–68

Wraight A, Ball J, Seccombe I, Stock J 1993 Mapping Team Midwifery. IMS Report 242 to the Department of Health. Institute of Manpower Studies, Brighton

Zelen M 1979 A new design for randomized controlled trials. New England Journal of Medicine 33(22):1242–1245

Chapter 9

Sex education and teenage pregnancy: missed opportunities

Jill Gullidge

CHAPTER CONTENTS

SUMMARY

The high incidence of teenage pregnancy and parenthood in the United Kingdom continues to be a complex issue, and from a midwifery perspective teenage pregnancy is a major challenge because of increased maternal, fetal and infant morbidity and mortality rates.

The main aim of this chapter is to identify whether midwives have a role to play in the teaching of sex and relationship issues to teenagers within schools. This chapter is designed to provide an in-depth analysis of the role of the educator within sex and relationship education. It also looks at the expressed views, opinions and needs of teenagers and professionals concerning sex and relationship education.

One of the main issues identified in this chapter is the unprecedented need to re-organise the teaching of sex and relationship education in light of the high incidence of teenage pregnancies. Within the national curriculum there are certain aspects of sex education that are compulsory, and the remaining element of this subject is left to the discretion of individual schools. The equation for providing effective sex education in the United Kingdom combines not only what is taught, but also the optimum person as the educator.

This work concludes that it is the responsibility of health professionals in conjunction with others to educate the child morally, socially and developmentally within sex and relationship education at school. There is little doubt that the midwife has a part to play in this education, especially as childbearing issues form part of the curriculum recommended by the Department for Education and Employment (2000). However, the midwife cannot work in isolation and professionals all need to work in a collaborative approach to educate teenagers. It also recognises that parents also have to accept the same responsibility towards their children and should also work in partnership with the school and health professionals.

INTRODUCTION

Teenage pregnancy is a major public health problem, and one important solution identified to combat this is improvement within sex and relationship education. The aim of this chapter is to analyse how the role of the midwife could be incorporated in the teaching of sex and relationship education to teenagers. Despite previous massive public health programmes, teenage pregnancy remains a crucial issue affecting our society. Midwives have a clear sense of responsibility in the public health sector in working to reduce inequalities and improve the health and wellbeing of people and communities. The Department for Education and Employment (2000) highlights this point and suggests that part of the curriculum in schools is childbearing issues.

In past decades, teenage pregnancy has been extensively studied and yet in spite of all that is known, our society has yet to gain control of the problem (Porter 1998). The high incidence of teenage pregnancy and parenthood in the United Kingdom continues to be a complex issue and is of increasing concern to society.

From a midwifery perspective, teenage pregnancy is a major challenge because of the increased maternal, fetal and infant morbidity and mortality rates (Sweet 1997). The concerns of teenage pregnancy include the social, psychological and educational health and welfare of the teenager and the subsequent baby (Dignan 2000). Also one cannot ignore the effect on family and society as a whole (Fugelsang 1997).

In 1997 a National Task Group was established to explore issues surrounding teenage pregnancy. In 1998 this task was taken on by the Social Exclusion Unit with the main aim of reviewing and suggesting strategies to decrease the incidence of teenage pregnancy and parenthood. The published report demonstrated the enormity of the problem. It stated that in England alone, there are almost 90,000 teenage pregnancies a year, of which approximately 2200 are to girls under the age of 14 years and 7700 to girls under the age of 16 years (Social Exclusion Unit 1999). This is further discussed in Chapter 11. Whilst the incidence of teenage pregnancy varies between areas of the United Kingdom, it is a problem that affects every part of the country; prevalence is high in affluent areas, but even higher in areas of deprivation and poverty (Smith 1993). International comparisons indicate that the incidence of teenage pregnancy in the United Kingdom is greater than in any other developed country except the United States of America, Canada and New Zealand (National Children's Bureau 1999).

Throughout most of Western Europe, the incidence of teenage pregnancy has steadily declined since 1970. However, by contrast, within the United Kingdom the incidence has increased, so that we now have the highest rate of teenage pregnancies within Western Europe (Social Exclusion Unit 1999). To put this into context, the United Kingdom has teenage birth rates twice as high as Germany, three times higher than France and six times higher than the Netherlands (Social Exclusion Unit 1999).

CURRENT LEGISLATION

Teenage pregnancy has been recognised by the Government as a serious issue that needs addressing and in conjunction with the Social Exclusion Unit (1999) key areas have been identified as part of a national campaign to reduce the rate of teenage pregnancy in the United Kingdom by 50% within the next 10 years. One key issue raised is the present provision of sex and relationship education within schools and its being a possible contributory factor in the high rate of teenage pregnancy.

In response the Education Authority, in conjunction with the National Children's Bureau and the Sex Education Forum, published national guidelines on teaching sex and relationship education. However, these are guidelines only and are open to individual interpretation. At present there is no formal training for the teaching of sex and relationship education and it is left for the school to nominate a member of staff to teach this subject. Whilst the school nurse supports the teacher in this role, she does also have an important role to fulfil in other aspects of child healthcare (Maclean 1997) and therefore limited time is allocated to this support. The expertise of the midwife could be seen as complementary to the role of the school nurse. Yet, part of the strategy from the Social Exclusion Unit (1999) is the review of the content of teacher training courses to ensure sex and relationship education is covered in their initial training. Such training could be seen as unnecessary and a waste of resources when there may be health professionals that could help to provide this type of education. However, the Government has already recognised that the reduction of teenage pregnancy has to be a national effort involving communities, the media, teenagers, parents and many different professionals working together (Social Exclusion Unit 1999).

Sex and relationship education within schools has received increasing attention. In general, teenage sex education is criticised as being inadequate in both content and teaching styles (Jobanputra et al 1999). The focus of such education needs to be for teenagers to have the knowledge required to make informed decisions and avoid negative health outcomes. However, there is still public concern over whether sex education increases promiscuity, despite research demonstrating that ignorance about sex is a risk factor for teenage pregnancy and that good sex education helps to delay rather than accelerate sexual activity (Kirby 1995). Sex education within schools needs to be seen as an opportunity to influence teenage behaviour and appears to represent an important part in reducing the incidence of teenage pregnancies (McEwan et al 1994). Sex and relationship education is lifelong learning about physical, moral and emotional development (Department for Education and Employment 2000). It is a legal requirement for schools to provide some aspects of sex and relationship education (National Children's Bureau 1999). Section 1 (2) of the Education Act (Department for Education 1994) requires all schools to offer a curriculum which:

- Promotes the spiritual, cultural, mental and physical development of pupils at the school and of society
- Prepares such pupils for the opportunities, responsibilities and experiences of adult life.

Whilst there have been no recent changes to the law regarding sex and relationship education, since 1993 there have been a number of national policies that have had an impact on the provision of sex and relationship education within schools. One such policy was the new sex and relationship initiative established as a priority in the 'Teenage Pregnancy Action Plan' launched by the Government and the Social Exclusion Unit in 1999.

In response to the 'Teenage Pregnancy Action Plan' the Department for Education and Employment (2000) proposed that the provision of sex and relationship education within schools be taught from a different perspective. This subject falls into two main categories: firstly sex and relationship education that comes under the science aspect of the national curriculum, which is concerned with anatomy, puberty and biological aspects of sexual reproduction (Box 9.1). The other aspect of sex and relationship education

Box 9.1
National Curriculum for Science (Department for Education and Employment 2000)

Key Stage Three (11–14 years)

- That fertilisation in humans ... is the fusion of a male and female cell
- About the physical and emotional changes that take place during adolescence
- About the human reproductive system, including the menstrual cycle and fertilisation
- How the fetus develops in the uterus
- How the growth and reproduction of bacteria and the replication of viruses can affect health.

Key Stage Four (14–16 years)

- The way in which hormonal control occurs, including the effects of sex hormones
- Some medical uses of hormones, including the control and promotion of fertility
- The defence mechanisms of the body.

comes under the 'Personal, Social and Health Education and Citizenship' framework (Sex Education Forum 1999) (Box 9.2), which aims to support the personal and social development of children and young people.

Whilst the Department for Education and Employment (2000) produced the guidelines listed in Boxes 9.1 and 9.2, the content of sex and relationship education is not clearly defined and is open to different interpretation from schools. Governing bodies of schools are required to ensure that their schools offer a programme of sex education. However, the only criteria for such programmes are that they should include sessions on Human Immunodeficiency Virus (HIV), Auto Immune Deficiency Syndrome and Sexually Transmitted Diseases (Department for Education 1994). Obviously many schools address other aspects of sex and relationship education than just the compulsory elements, but if schools choose not to, it is their choice. Schools can justify these actions providing they keep a written statement of their provision of sex and relationship education.

In the past sex education in schools had a narrow, reproductive focus and was taught only as part of the National Curriculum for science. The publication of *Sex and Relationship Education Guidance* (Department for Education and Employment 2000) now suggests that children of all ages should acquire information, develop skills and form positive beliefs, values and attitudes. This should ensure that young people have the opportunity to receive information, examine their values and learn relationship skills

Box 9.2

Personal, social and health education issues (Department for Education and Employment 2000)

Key Stages Three and Four (11–16 years)

At secondary school level, sex and relationship education should prepare young people for an adult life in which they can:

- Develop positive values and a moral framework that will guide their decisions, judgements and behaviour
- Be aware of their sexuality and understand human sexuality
- Understand the arguments for delaying sexual activity
- Understand the reasons for having protected sex
- Understand the consequences of their actions and behave responsibly within sexual and pastoral relationships
- Have the confidence and self-esteem to value themselves and others and respect for individual conscience and the skills to judge what kind of relationships they want
- Communicate effectively
- Have sufficient information and skills to protect themselves and, where they have one, their partner from unintended/unwanted conceptions, and sexually transmitted infections including HIV
- Avoid being exploited or exploiting others
- Avoid being pressured into unwanted or unprotected sex
- Access confidential sexual health advice, support and if necessary treatment
- Know how the law applies to sexual relationships.

that will enable them to resist becoming sexually active before they are ready, and to prevent unprotected intercourse, enabling young people to become responsible, sexually active adults (Sex Education Forum 1999).

CURRENT EDUCATORS

Sexuality defines our role in society and influences our feelings about relationships (Finan 1997). Walton (1997) suggests that sexuality is concerned with sexual orientation, desires, expressiveness, innate feelings, sexual instincts and identity at every stage of life. The teenager is required to make moral choices, including the choice not to be sexually active. They therefore need to have an understanding of their own sexuality, and yet there is controversy over who teaches these sensitive issues.

There is continual debate and opposition from teachers, parents and health professionals as to what needs to be taught to our teenagers. Perhaps the broader emotional and ethical dimensions of sexual attitudes of different professionals need also to be considered. It may then be possible for health professionals to liaise with teachers and parents to provide a better system. So the equation for providing effective sex education is not only what is taught, but also who teaches this subject (Dolby 1998). As a society we have to take adequate steps to ensure our teenagers are educated, or accept the consequences.

Historically, school governors in conjunction with schoolteachers have decided on the content of sex and relationship education. It has now been suggested by the Sex Education Forum (1999) that such policies should be developed in consultation with parents, young people, teachers, governors and the wider community. There are clear intentions from the Government and the Social Exclusion Unit (1999) in developing specialist sex and relationship education training for teachers. Whilst there is clearly a need for improved teaching in sex and relationship education, it is unclear who the appropriate people are to teach this subject.

Proposals from the Department of Health (1999) include the widening of the midwifery role to inform young people about healthy lifestyles: the midwife may have an effect on the attitudes and values of teenagers. Certainly Bennett and Brown (1999) suggest that a necessary skill of a midwife is the deep perception of the influence of emotions and the effect this can have on an individual's behaviour.

FAMILY INFLUENCE

However, Finan (1997) suggests that the family is the most important source for learning about sexuality issues. Parental attitudes and behaviour definitely have a major impact on the behaviour of teenagers, and this is one issue that has been raised in the teaching of sex and relationship education. Briggs (1998) discusses how parents have a tremendous influence over their children despite the decline of traditional values. A study undertaken by Rosenthal and Feldman (1999) focused on this issue and discussed how parents should play a pivotal role in sex and relationship education of their children, because alongside sexuality come questions of values and morals.

However, the experience of young people is very different today from that of past generations. Fuglesang (1997) suggests the family is noticeably in decline, with the traditional extended multi-generational families giving way to single parent families, and many young people choosing careers over marriage. Whilst this study was performed in Tanzania, it also describes societies in developed countries. Rosenthal and Feldman's study (1999) also highlighted that many parents find the task of teaching sex education to their children difficult, feeling ill-equipped to deal with certain issues. The midwife has an important role to play in family relationships, alongside promoting good physical health and positive emotional health (Page 1999).

THE SCHOOL

Saito (1998) suggests that the first step in teaching sex and relationship education is to recognise the teenager as a sexual being. This may be easier for the health professional who, understandably, views the teenager in a different light from the teacher. There may be difficulties for the teacher and the teenager who are used to a classroom situation. The frequent contact that teachers have with teenagers can itself act as a barrier to sex education (Eisenberg et al 1997). Eisenberg et al also found in their study that teenagers felt uncomfortable receiving information from teachers and recommended using outside health professionals who could ensure more freedom and less embarrassment because of their anonymity compared to teachers. Wight and Scott (1994) also demonstrated this point in their study, showing that a teacher's anxiety often exacerbates pupil embarrassment. They also felt that outside speakers show more expertise, are usually easier to talk to, and can deal with problems that teachers find difficult. Sheridan (1997) discusses how the teacher of sex and relationship education needs to be experienced in the field of health education, and the midwife may be seen as an appropriate professional. This is acknowledged by the Department of Health (1999), recognising the diversity of the role of the midwife and the need for better use of the midwife's knowledge and skills.

A study was also undertaken by Kumar-Bhasin and Aggarwal (1999) to explore the perceptions of schoolteachers and their role in teaching sex education to schoolchildren. This study, whilst undertaken in India where the culture is very different, is significant as the United Kingdom has a multi-cultural society where different social, ethnic, cultural and religious backgrounds need to be taken into account. Within India sexuality is still a 'taboo' subject and is not openly discussed, despite the need to encourage responsible sexual activity in the teenager. India has an estimated 2.5 million people infected with HIV (Kumar-Bhasin & Aggarwal 1999), which indicates that there are many people having unprotected sexual intercourse and could suggest a high rate of unwanted pregnancy. Despite this, 21% of teachers in this study were against sex and relationship education within schools. This was partly due to their culture, but a high percentage of teachers felt that sex education was linked to increased promiscuity. Interestingly, teachers who felt that sex education was appropriate only thought that the anatomy and physiology aspects were suitable. Aggleton (1989) discusses previous research to suggest that unless sex education is properly re-organised in schools it is a missed opportunity to influence the future sexual behaviour of the individual teenager.

There appears to be little doubt that influence within schools can play a major role in shaping the health and lifestyle behaviours of teenagers. Sex education may be more beneficial if centred on teenagers' needs and discussed by health professionals who have an interest in this speciality. Teachers' reluctance to discuss sexuality may be due to a lack of knowledge, or even the fact that they may hold conservative values regarding sexuality. Ruusuvaara (1997) suggests that sex education is also coloured by society's reluctance to accept teenage sexuality.

HEALTH PROFESSIONS' INPUT

Research has demonstrated the value of the professional nurse and patient relationship, particularly when addressing the complex issues of the reproductive health of the teenager (Meisenhelder 1985, Hanna 1993). Donati et al (2000) also raise this issue and suggest that children should be encouraged to question and explore their attitudes and values within sex and relationship education, to develop the ability to exercise independent choice. A small qualitative study undertaken by Lambke and Kavanaugh (1999) highlighted how teenagers need to be empowered in order to make their own decisions and understand the ramifications of their behaviour. This is an interesting concept as midwifery practice is centred on empowerment of the woman.

Donati et al (2000) included in their research both the attitudes and knowledge of teenagers: that is, to provide a quality sex education policy there needs to be collaboration between schools and health professionals. If midwives are not seen as the appropriate professionals to educate teenagers in the UK, perhaps midwives should be concerned with supporting teachers and school nurses in their role as educators of sex and relationship education. The Department for Education and Employment (2000) also raised this issue, and suggested that health professionals have much to offer and should work closely with teachers in supporting sex and relationship education in schools.

THE PEER GROUP AND THE MEDIA

Many societies emphasise sexuality as a problem and would prefer teenagers to postpone sexual activity until they are older (Ruusuvaara 1997). However, surely this leaves teenagers to form attitudes and values from their peers and the media, and as Ruusuvaara (1997) suggests, to form their own social norms. The concern is that these values and beliefs may not always be part of the prevailing value system that they are growing up in.

It needs to be remembered that whoever teaches sex and relationship education within schools, teenagers will form many of their attitudes from sources that are out of the control of parents, teachers or health professionals. There is no doubt that teenagers' values and the media influence attitudes: sex is seen as associated with humour and excitement, and it is only recently that the dangers of unprotected sex have been described (Shelov et al 1995). In research undertaken by Witte (1997), the need for better sex education was universal, together with the need for teenagers to be explicitly informed of the consequences of their actions. Beitz (1998) discusses how a teenager, just watching television in normal hours, is subjected, over the course of their teenage years, to 14,000 sexual references, innuendos and behaviour with very little regard for birth control, abstinence or personal responsibility.

The sexual behaviour of teenage peer groups will also have an influence on the initiation of sexual activity of the teenager. Over the years research has suggested that it is the responsibility of whoever teaches sex education to strongly pursue ways to encourage abstinence in teenagers (Strasburger 1989, Khouzam 1995). This seems a little narrow-minded; if teenagers feel there is some dark secret, it is likely to encourage them to experiment. Beitz (1998) raises the issue that if teenagers in an immediate social group participate in unhealthy sexual behaviour then the other members of the group will act in a similar way. If the teenager receives comprehensive sex and relationship education it may prevent him or her from participating in unhealthy sexual behaviour.

Donovan (1998) discusses how communities could create local advisory committees comprising parents, religious leaders, medical professionals and other community leaders to review and approve sex education curricula within schools. Saito (1998) agrees this point and suggests that all segments of a society should work together. However, one issue that needs consideration is the double moral standards within society that still exist. Male adolescents are often pushed towards the early initiation of their sexual life whilst restrictions are often placed upon the same behaviour in girls. In sex education, relationships and parenthood taught to boys have been overlooked, and the trend often continues into fatherhood (National Children's Bureau 1999).

THE HOLISTIC APPROACH

Health professionals are concerned with the promotion of health and the prevention of illness. However, according to Beitz (1998), health promotion is not just about the early detection and treatment of disease, but is also concerned with the holistic approach of the person. He further suggests that health promotion also includes encouraging healthy lifestyles and involves organisational, economic and political strategies that facilitate environmental and behavioural change. Clearly this is an area where teachers are not trained, and health professionals have an advantage over teachers in teaching sex and relationship education to teenagers. Whilst a part of the role of all health professionals may be to promote health, a large percentage of professionals' role may include prevention following disease or illness. However, the role of the midwife differs in that she is an advisor and a facilitator (Murray 1995).

The content of sex education is questioned throughout the research and is thought to be impersonal and mainly concerned with the biological aspect and not the relationship aspect (Holland et al 1990). Within the study undertaken by Ogden and Harden (1999) it was reported that most teenagers felt that sex education was delivered by facts and information and that the format of their education was too didactic. This particular study was a questionnaire that was sent to almost a thousand teenagers at various schools, of which a high percentage reported a preference for more interactive methods of teaching such as discussions and role-play.

Within the study of 476 teachers undertaken by Kumar-Bhasin and Aggarwal (1999) it was concluded that teachers did not mind teaching anatomy and physiology, menstruation and family planning, but the majority did not want to teach issues surrounding abortion and premarital sex. Interestingly this study also highlighted that over 60% of these teachers felt that the most appropriate person to teach these issues were doctors. This raises the issue as to how non-medical staff actually educate teenagers in the knowledge of reproductive health. This issue was examined by Donati et al (2000), who found that out of 376 students, the majority felt that they would prefer health professionals to discuss sexual issues. This study was undertaken in Italy, where sex education is not included within the school curriculum and yet as a country they have a low incidence of teenage pregnancy in comparison to the United Kingdom. The study was able to demonstrate that teenagers coming from a higher socioeconomic background had higher levels of initial knowledge.

In certain countries such as Sweden the teenage pregnancy rate has decreased and the use of contraception increased, which is thought to be linked to the various campaigns at schools and dissemination of information via teenage health clinics (Persson & Jarlbro 1992, Klanger et al 1993). Within the United States of America however there appears to be little evidence that contraceptive-based sex education programmes have resulted in a decreased incidence of sexual activity in teenagers, a lower incidence of teenage pregnancy, or an increased use of contraception (Stout & Rivara 1989, Genuis & Genuis 1995).

Donovan (1998) suggests that the lack of personal and social skills taught within schools may be due to the reluctance of some teachers to teach sex education which is often exacerbated by a lack of training. She further discusses how some undergraduate teachers now have at least some sexuality education in their training. In the Netherlands many teachers have completed training in 'sexology', but this does not mean they are the most appropriate people to teach sex education (Dolby 1998). This training is surely unnecessary as there are already health professionals who can teach these issues, as was recognised by the Department for Education and Employment (2000). The Department of Health (1999) had already discussed that health professionals are public health workers working with whole communities and individuals.

It has been argued that the timing of sex education is crucial. Within a study from Ogden and Harden (1999) many teenagers expressed concerns over the timing of sex education, suggesting that sex education was 'too little and too late'. This may be clear from the lack of professionals involved in the teaching of sex education. In other countries, such as the Netherlands, children are taught from a much earlier age and this is reflected in their lower teenage pregnancy rate (Ogden & Harden 1999).

A further worrying point highlighted within the research is that not all schools were able to say whether they had a policy for teaching sex and relationship education. This point was demonstrated in a survey of local education authorities in England and Wales in 1991 (McEwan et al 1994). Fewer than 50% of schools were able to state whether their school had a written sex policy. In the same survey it highlighted that school governors were often confused and not sure of their role in sex education.

EMPOWERMENT OF TEENAGERS

There are now many initiatives such as 'Sure Start' (Department for Education and Skills 2003), as discussed in Chapter 10, that recognise the involvement of midwives to minimise health inequalities and to improve the social development of teenagers to reduce the incidence of teenage pregnancy. As a society we have to accept, even if it is not agreed, that teenagers have a choice and the best way to prevent pregnancy is for the teenager to be in possession of all the facts and to be aware of the consequences of his or her actions.

Hiltabiddle (1996) suggests that teenagers may not have accepted their own sexual identity and therefore have problems in complying with contraceptive methods that involve anticipating sexual intercourse. Boyer (1990) argues that this is due to teenage sexual encounters that are often unplanned and infrequent. Perhaps teenagers need to learn life skills to help them cope when faced with a difficult situation. Utilisation of the midwife's skills could influence the development of critical thinking in teenagers.

Donati et al (2000) further state that teenagers need the opportunity to acquire accurate information on sexual health and to develop the skills to evaluate the information in order to make decisions. The midwife has effective listening skills, which could help to support the teenager and build a trusting relationship to assist the individual in making important decisions. The optimal timing for education for healthy pregnancy needs to be before teenagers become sexually active. A study of pregnant teenagers by Witte (1997) took an extremely hard view on how best to prevent teenage pregnancy and recommended that people involved with teenagers need to be more realistic and teach children about birth control and the consequences of unprotected sexual intercourse. In practice, many teenagers continue to have unprotected sexual intercourse and do not become pregnant: this often leads to a teenager wrongly assuming she cannot become pregnant.

Many of the pregnant teenagers in the study by Witte (1997) had a good knowledge base regarding contraception but admitted that they had learnt this from midwives during their pregnancy. It seems inconceivable that as a society we have failed teenagers by only teaching important issues once they are pregnant. This sentiment is echoed by the Report from the Social Exclusion Unit (1999) who stated that a third of teenagers are sexually active by the time they are 16 and yet half of these did not use any form of contraception. These statistics differ from those elsewhere; for example, 80% of girls aged between 16 and 19 years in countries such as the Netherlands and Denmark use contraception (Social Exclusion Unit 1999).

Teenagers in Witte's study expressed a need to have learnt about sexual intercourse from reliable sources such as educators, mothers and physicians, but in reality they received their information from friends and this was often inaccurate. The Department for Education and Employment (2000) have raised this concern and indicated that health professionals need to inform teenagers about the health services that are available to them and help them develop the confidence and skills to use them.

There are now many initiatives, some of which are listed below, which offer teenagers information and advice:

- Sure Start, which aims to improve the health and well-being of families and children before and from birth. Sure Start is a cornerstone of the Government's drive to tackle child poverty and social exclusion. It was anticipated that by 2004 there would be 524 Sure Start programmes helping up to 400,000 children living in disadvantaged areas (www.surestart.gov.uk).
- The Site is produced and managed by Youthnet UK and aims to offer the best guide to life for young adults, believing that all young people have the capacity to make their own decisions and choices, provided they have access to quality, impartial information and an opportunity to get support and empathy from other young people in similar situations (www.thesite.org.uk).
- Teenage Health Freak is a comprehensive website for teenagers including the facility to e-mail questions on a wide range of medical and sexual issues (www.teenagehealthfreak.org).
- There4me is confidential on-line advice for teenagers (www.There4me.com).
- Sexwise is for young people and gives information on contraception, sex and relationships. This site also allows you to search for services anywhere in the United Kingdom (www.ruthinking.co.uk).
- Like it is, a website which provides advice on issues such as contraception, periods, teenage pregnancy, sex and sexuality (www.likeitis.org.uk).
- British Pregnancy Advisory Service provides accurate information on termination of pregnancy and options for dealing with unwanted pregnancy (www.bpas.org.uk).
- LoveLife provides clear, up-to-date information on sexual health issues (now available at www.playingsafely.co.uk).
- No Worries is a major new scheme to help local teenagers in South Gloucestershire to get help and advice on sexual health matters. It was designed with the help of local teenagers and young mothers. The logo No Worries will be displayed in GP surgeries, local pharmacists and young people's sexual health clinics, to show teenagers where they can get help before they enter into a sexual relationship, and they will be directed to a sensitive service designed especially for them (www.noworries.nhs.uk).

However, in practice we are still not supporting teenagers fully. In many areas family planning clinics are inaccessible. Many teenagers report that they cannot go to their medical centre for advice due to the worry of being seen by friends or relatives. Furthermore, to have a clinic appointment during school hours necessitates the need to confide in a teacher.

In a study undertaken by Shelov et al (1995) it was established that approximately 85% of teenagers have sexual intercourse before seeking professional advice regarding the prevention of pregnancy and disease. This may be because teenagers are unaware of how to access professionals that can advise and support them, and could provide an even stronger argument as to why other health professionals, such as midwives, need to be involved in delivering sex education. The Department of Health (1999) discusses how midwives could provide advice and counsel in a range of areas, including with teenagers in the prevention of teenage pregnancy.

In Ogden and Harden's (1999) study of 967 teenagers between the age of 16 and 19 years, 31% thought that sex education was too late, but 4% thought that it was too early. This study also showed a high number of teenagers that would have liked discussions on relationships and family planning or a visit to a family planning clinic. Ogden and Harden conclude that their research supports any previous recommendations to change present sex education as a means to changing behaviour of the teenager in the long term. Donovan (1998) discusses how sex education programmes are seen by professionals as too short, not very comprehensive, and failing to cover important topics, and are thus less effective than they could be. However, Donovan also raises the issue that sex education is often seen by society as immoral.

Interestingly, within the study by Edwards et al (1997) many of the teenagers had an understanding of the importance of preconceptual care. This study demonstrated a need for sex educators to be proactive: when teenagers present themselves to the medical centre already pregnant, it is too late for advice about preconceptual care. The educational role of the midwife within schools could be based around preconceptual care and healthy pregnancy. This issue is evident from the *Midwives' Rules and Code of Practice* (UKCC 1998) which discusses how the work of a midwife involves preparation for parenthood that extends to certain areas of gynaecology, family planning and childcare.

Witte (1997) discusses fear campaigns in relation to sex and relationship education as a common, persuasive strategy. She suggests that they motivate people to act instead of simply offering information and letting teenagers choose whether they want to act. However, surely it is a better approach to make teenagers more aware of all the facts and sure how to deal with situations, rather than being frightened into certain behaviour. This approach does not appear to bode well with teenagers needing to act responsibly and seeking early support if required. Witte (1997) concluded in her study that the feelings of teenagers about pregnancy should be addressed within the constraints of sex education. Many pregnant teenagers do not realise the full impact of pregnancy, such as loss of social life, emotional and physical stresses and the burden of becoming a parent at an early age.

Low levels of knowledge and lack of information among teenagers appears to be a worldwide phenomenon (Donati et al 2000). The task of educating teenagers has to be more than giving information; it also requires receptivity on the part of the listener and mutual understanding and respect of each person. In a qualitative research study undertaken by Eisenberg et al (1997), teenagers expressed concern over the material covered in sex education, which did not address all of their questions and concerns. This point was also raised by a study undertaken by Woodcock et al (1992). Eisenberg et al (1997) also reported that students would like to have a full understanding of their options if they did get pregnant and they all expressed a desire to receive realistic information on parenting as a teenager. In practice, the midwife has experience of dealing with pregnant teenagers and is in a suitable position to discuss the concerns of teenage pregnancy. This may also be a way forward for the midwife to promote the importance of preconceptual care to teenagers, so that if they do get pregnant the incidence of mortality and morbidity may be reduced.

Renker's study (1999) demonstrates the contradictions embedded in the notion of sex education and the denial of the fact that many teenagers are sexually active. She discusses how Sweden is one of the few countries that, through a positive investment into sex education and the setting up of special youth clinics, has effectively reduced the incidence of teenage pregnancy. In Sweden, midwives, nurses, social workers and psychologists work together to teach sex education.

There are some worrying misconceptions within the research that highlight the issue of teenagers not receiving adequate sex and relationship education within schools. In one survey (Health Education Authority 1999) 25% of 14–16 year olds thought that the contraceptive pill gave protection against sexually transmitted diseases. In another study less than one in three 16–24 year olds had heard of chlamydia (Health Education Authority & ONS 1998).

Research by Ford (1991) indicated that approximately 40% of under-15s have had sexual intercourse, 52% at the age of 16 and 67% at the age of 17. International research into teenage pregnancy in developed countries also concluded that access to free, confidential youth advisory centres is a key factor in enabling teenagers to control their fertility (Jones 1985).

COLLABORATIVE APPROACH

Sex education has been criticised for lack of skills training, for example, buying condoms and negotiation of relationships (Ogden & Harden 1999). More than 10 years ago this concern was also raised by Abraham and Sheeran (1993) and yet research shows that this is still not taught in every school. The consequences of such narrow and restrictive sex education are far-reaching and the rate of teenage pregnancy is likely to continue. The Department for Education and Employment (2000) suggests that health professionals could assist teachers by providing up-to-date knowledge about sexual health, well-being and contraception. A part of the midwife's role is to provide sound family planning information and advice (UKCC 1998).

The teenagers in a study by Donati et al (2000) discussed the inaccessibility of family planning clinics. This may be a good reason to provide such a service in school, and yet the publication of information on such clinics and the use of the 'morning after pill' have in the past caused a lot of controversy.

Dolby (1998) discusses how a midwife may be able to provide the necessary link between the skills and information teenagers require for future health, relationships and possible parenthood and the growing awareness of their sexuality. She further suggests that the midwife may be able to liaise with other professionals to enhance the provision and flexibility of services.

In a study by Briggs (1998) in Nigeria, many pregnant teenagers have abortions by unskilled practitioners, leading to all sorts of complications. If as discussed by Witte (1997) fear tactics are used, as a society we may go back to teenagers having illegal abortions. It is interesting to note that abortion is still illegal in Nigeria (Briggs 1998). In this study Briggs noted that 87.8% of parents did not discuss sexual matters with their daughters and that 79.1% of parents did not want their children using contraception as they felt it increased promiscuity.

Donovan (1998) discusses how North Carolina schools are under pressure to eliminate discussion of birth control methods from sex education and instead promote abstinence as a means of preventing pregnancy. Teenagers need to be able to explore all the issues regarding sex and relationships to enable them to make informed choices. Informed consent requires that all methods of contraception should be presented to teenagers, and yet as Lambke and Kavanaugh (1999) discuss, there are contradictions that exist regarding the scope necessary for the empowerment of teenagers: in a qualitative study they discussed with school nurses the barriers to sex education, and found that often the long-term health risks of current behaviour choices for the teenagers are addressed inconsistently, discussed within the context of other information, and often not presented by the same person. The issue of confidentiality was also raised as a barrier to sex education, and led to lack of support for the teenager at crucial times. Certainly the issue of confidentiality is different for teachers, as they are not bound by the same codes of confidentiality as midwives and nurses.

The issue of sex education and sex communication was raised by Warren (1995), and refers to general education as knowledge from expert to novice, and communication involving the viewpoint of both being valued. This may be viewed as a potential problem for teachers in schools discussing sex education, as they may be used to educating teenagers with knowledge from expert to novice, whereas health professionals are more used to a different style of education. This is particularly the case with midwives, who are used to listening and offering choices in people's care. However, it has been argued that an impersonal and objective approach to sex education may be counter-productive (Aggleton 1989).

Young people learn from a range of different sources; sex and relationship education at school prepares teenagers for their 'sexual career' (Thomson 1993). She further suggests that teenagers may see schools as an informal setting which is neither medical nor clinical. The teenager may also feel unable to discuss such an emotive subject at home with the family. It would be interesting to understand the teenager's view of the health professionals. It may be that teenagers mistakenly view the school nurse in association with illness and not in a preventative role, and the midwife as a professional who only deals with pregnancy.

Beitz (1998) believes that teenagers do not always have important sexual health information, and they also often lack the ability to understand the consequences of their actions. Beitz links this inability to chronological age and life experiences. Midwives may be seen as ideal candidates to develop and participate in teaching of sex education because of their clinical expertise and health education focus.

Tucker (1990) found that education directed to mothers of teenage girls is beneficial for promoting healthy behaviour. This obviously raises the issue of whether the nurse/teacher, teenager and parents should be regarded as independent entities. Lambke and Kavanaugh (1999) concluded in their study that more research into interventions to involve parents and support in the community is urgently required. They further suggest that the isolation of teenagers from their communities contributes to their health risks. Page (1999) discusses how the most effective form of midwifery practice has a basis in the primary health care sector, enabling midwives to work in a positive relationship with individual women and their families, integrating family support with physical care and health promotion.

A study undertaken by Jobanputra et al (1999), to determine the feasibility of medical students being involved in sex education to teenagers in schools, found significant benefits to outside speakers. It was found in this study that the age of the medical students was an advantage in building up a rapport with the teenagers, enabling more relaxed discussion in certain aspects of sex education that were felt to be difficult for teachers. Teachers felt that the medical students were able to discuss issues with fewer inhibitions. Teenagers expressed concern over discussing issues with teachers, and found it easier to discuss these issues with medical students. However, some students did express the feeling of difficulty of discussing sexual issues with strangers. This study further suggested that medical students were the ideal people to act as a quasi-peer group in local schools, due to their closeness of age to the target audience, and were generally more approachable than established sex education providers.

Often teachers feel that they have covered topics adequately and yet in the study by Jobanputra et al (1999), 43% of teenagers felt that they did not have, and would have liked, information on pregnancy. Many teenagers in this study worried about the issue of confidentiality and teachers; but 41% worried about this same issue with friends, while few worried when talking to outsiders. This is a disturbing fact when the teenagers normally only talk to teachers and friends.

Jobanputra et al (1999) also found in their study that the sex education providers felt that medical students as a source of knowledge were valuable, but that they required training. This is not surprising: can they really be seen as the most appropriate people to educate teenagers? Their lack of teaching experience may be inappropriate; the midwife however is used to continually teaching her clients.

The Department for Education and Employment (2000) suggests that health professionals can help schools work in partnership with parents and make links between the school and other relevant professionals and services such as local general practitioners, family planning clinics and genito-urinary medicine clinics.

The phenomena of teenage pregnancy and parenting remain complex and multi-faceted, and challenge professionals to search for valid and effective approaches to alleviate the problem of teenage pregnancy (Thompson et al 1995). Teenage pregnancy is one of the most crucial issues affecting our society. Despite rigorous efforts and massive public health programmes, large numbers of teenagers continue to participate in unhealthy lifestyles (Beitz 1998). Every health professional whose sphere of practice teenage pregnancy touches should be concerned (Dignan 2000).

DIVERSITY OF MIDWIVES' ROLE

While there is much debate as to who should teach sex education, it is still not clear where the responsibility lies. Curriculum guidance for sex and relationship education from the Department for Education and Employment (2000) for this age group certainly consists of many child-bearing issues, which poses the question of a midwife's involvement. It could be argued that she is in an ideal position to be involved in teaching sex and relationship education. The definition of the midwife (UKCC 1998) clearly states:

> She has an important task in health counselling and education, not only for women, but also within the family and the community. This work should also involve antenatal education and preparation for parenthood and extends to certain areas of gynaecology, family planning and child-care. She may practise in hospitals, clinics, health units, domiciliary conditions or in any other services.
>
> (UKCC 1998)

May (1992) discusses how pregnant teenagers often delay antenatal care to conceal the pregnancy from their parents. Whilst the teenager may be frightened of the outcome of informing people that she is pregnant, perhaps an important issue to be considered is that if teenagers were aware of the facts, they might decide it is better to receive early antenatal care. If health professionals better supported sex and relationship education, it could result in a decrease in the incidence of teenage pregnancies and also a reduction in the incidence of morbidity and mortality.

The midwife possesses skills and expertise to counsel and advise couples on sexuality (Evans 1992); this role could be extended to teenagers as part of sex and relationship education. Although counselling skills are not included in the midwife's training, it is imperative that she develops these skills to facilitate the most effective communication with her clients. The Department of Health (1999) has raised this issue by stating that:

> Midwives should play a bigger role in public health strategy. For example, working in partnership with school nurses and health visitors, they need to be more involved in helping to ensure young people are well informed about healthy lifestyles. Midwives are especially placed to contribute on issues including contraception, sexual health, relationships and the responsibilities associated with pregnancy and childbirth.

By changing the focus of sex and relationship education to reproductive health, it may be easier for the role of the midwife to be identified and strengthened within this education. The benefits of professionals working together and the sharing of their knowledge and understanding would undoubtedly improve the present sex education system.

CONCLUSION AND IMPLICATIONS FOR FUTURE PRACTICE

Teenage pregnancy is a major area of concern that is not just the responsibility of one segment of professionals, but as Dignan (2000) suggests it is a problem that requires a multi-professional approach.

In the United Kingdom there is still a high incidence of teenage pregnancy that appears to derive from inadequate sex education. However, the controversy over sex education appears to be shifting from whether it should be taught to what should be taught and by whom. Donovan (1998) links this continual controversy with concerns of parents objecting to the content of sex education, and the lack of support for teachers. Forrest and Silverman (1989) discuss how sex education accounts for a small part of teaching responsibilities, less than 10% of their time. Donovan (1998) notes that it is normally Physical Education, Biology or Home Economics teachers who teach sex education. Teachers often limit sex education to safe topics such as anatomy and physiology, and Donovan (1998) attributes this to teachers who would rather play safe and not jeopardise their careers for something that they consider a secondary responsibility.

Within the guidelines for sex and relationship education issued from the Department for Education and Employment (2000), there is a proposal to teach topics that could be construed as childbearing issues. This could justify the argument for the role of the midwife to include the teaching of sex and relationship education.

In the past, several studies have demonstrated that exposure to sex education does not increase the likelihood that teenagers will begin sexual activity earlier and in fact is more likely to delay it (Dawson 1986, Kirby et al 1991). In a study by Renker (1999) it was again demonstrated that sexuality education did not enhance promiscuity, and she reviewed 35 other studies that came up with the same conclusion.

Schools need to be recognised as a powerful resource for the prevention of teenage pregnancies, but there are both disadvantages and advantages to sex education in schools. One major advantage in location is increasing accessibility of health care services to teenagers (Porter 1998) and the teenager's becoming familiar with the staff, and this may help to provide a trusting relationship. Porter (1998) in her study discusses how in an effort to deal with sensitive issues and opposition from parents, schools should have advisory boards that comprise health and educational professionals.

Teenage pregnancy is a major public health programme, and one important solution identified to this is the improvements within sex education (Jobanputra et al 1999) This is an area within schools that is lacking, and as Jobanputra et al (1999) observed, it is also given low priority within school curricula. One of the main strategies highlighted by the Government and the Social Exclusion Unit (1999), in the prevention of teenage pregnancy, was an improved provision of sex and relationship education within schools. It is apparent that many teenage pregnancies result from a considerable level of ignorance and mixed messages regarding sex and its consequences (Social Exclusion Unit 1999). Whilst there are guidelines from the Department for Education and Employment (2000) to teach sex and relationship education, it is apparent from this research that not all schools are using these guidelines. One problem identified in this research may be that the 'Personal, Social and Health Education and Citizenship' framework (Sex Education Forum 1999) is very broad, and it is difficult to determine what should be taught under each section.

Ruusuvaara (1997) notes that countries where sex education has been firmly established and accepted, combined with the use of family planning services and abortion on demand, have the lowest pregnancy and abortion rates in the world. She further suggests that to deliver appropriate sex education, midwives, nurses and doctors need to be aware of all the trends and changes within the young society.

Sex education is often discussed and evaluated in the context of reducing the incidence of teenage pregnancies (Donovan 1998). It is interesting that the Department for Education and Employment merely offers advice on what should be taught within sex education, recognising that each child and young person is different and sex and relationship education should take into account these different requirements.

The teenage years are a time of transition between childhood and adulthood in which behaviour of the individual is a determinant of their present and future health status. Tobias and Ricer (1998) suggest that teenagers are at a crossroads emotionally, physically and socially. There are many health professionals, each of whom has a valuable contribution to make, but lack of communication can lead to duplication. Health professionals can help by advocating improved teacher education, providing resources for educators, and reviewing proposed curricula for accuracy and effectiveness (Tobias & Ricer 1998).

There is an unprecedented need to re-organise the teaching of sex and relationship education in light of the high incidence of teenage pregnancies. We must not be complacent about sex education in the United Kingdom, and must be amenable to new ideas. It may be necessary to search for ways to better prepare the person who is going to teach the subject of sex education. Effective campaigns are desperately needed to combat the problem of teenage pregnancy.

The common theme discussed by most critics of sex education appears to be the violation of children's innocence. We are currently in the midst of a media revolution in which children are constantly surrounded by images of, and references to, sexuality. This has a direct effect on the education of teenagers, especially those who receive inadequate information on sex and relationship education from school.

While still controversial, there has been research for many years to support the idea that teenage pregnancy can be prevented by better sex education (Klein 1978, Kirby 1985). Opposition is based on the belief that sex education can increase promiscuity among teenagers. However, there is strong evidence that providing sex and contraceptive advice to teenagers does not lead to an increase in sexual activity and unwanted pregnancy (Kirby et al 1994, Frost & Forrest 1995, Oakley et al 1995). In fact research has shown that sex education can be effective in reducing sexual risk-taking behaviour (NHS Centre for Reviews and Dissemination 1997).

In conclusion, the provision of sex and relationship education is still a major problem despite initiatives to tackle the problem. This research has highlighted that it is the responsibility of professionals in co-operation, and the community and parents, to educate the child morally, socially and developmentally along with sex and relationship education at school. There is little doubt that the midwife has a part to play in this education, especially as some of the issues that are recommended to be taught by the Department for Education and Employment (2000) are childbearing issues.

Midwives have a clear sense of responsibility in the public health sector in working to reduce inequalities and improve the health and well-being of people and communities (Page 1999). The midwife is in the unique position to highlight areas of concern such as social deprivation and poor housing. McCrea (1993) discusses how the midwife has already mastered the 'chameleon effect' by being able to integrate herself into the woman's environment without prejudice for her lifestyle, race, religion or personal idiosyncrasies. This appears to be an essential quality when dealing with teenagers.

It would be foolish to compare the status of professionals, as the midwife cannot work in isolation and there needs to be a cohesive approach between all professionals. Parents have to accept the same responsibility towards their children, and should work in partnership with the school and health professionals. As professionals we also need to listen to the needs of the teenager to provide a better service. After all, who at present is benefiting from the current sex education offered in schools? Certainly not teenagers, as is proven by the high incidence of teenage pregnancy.

References

Abraham C, Sheeran P 1993 In search of a psychology of safer sex promotion: beyond beliefs and text. Health Education Research: Theory and Practice 8:245–254

Aggleton P 1989 HIV/AIDS education in schools: constraints and possibilities. Health Education Journal 48:167–171

Beitz J 1998 Sexual health promotion in adolescents and young adults: primary prevention strategies. Holistic Nursing Practice 12(2):27–37

Bennett R, Brown L 1999 The midwife. In: Bennett R, Brown L, Uprichard M (eds) Myles Textbook of Midwifery, 13th edn. Churchill Livingstone, London, pp 2–11

Boyer C 1990 Pyschosocial, behavioural and educational factors in preventing sexually transmitted diseases. Adolescent Medicine 1:597–613

Briggs L 1998 Parents' viewpoint on reproductive health and contraceptive practice among sexually active adolescents in the Port Harcourt Local Government Areas of River State, Nigeria. Journal of Advanced Nursing 27:261–266

Dawson D 1986 The effects of sex education on adolescent behaviour. Family Planning Perspective 18(4):162–170

Department for Education 1994 Education Act 1993: Sex Education in Schools. Circular 5/94. Department for Education, London

Department for Education and Employment 2000 Sex and Relationship Education Guidance. DfEE Publications, Nottingham

Department for Education and Skills/Department for Work and Pensions 2003 Sure Start. DfES Publications, London. Website: www.surestart.gov.uk

Department of Health 1999 Making a Difference: Strengthening the Nursing, Midwifery and Health Visiting Contribution to Health and Health Care. TSO, London

Dignan K 2000 Teenage pregnancy. In: Kerr J (ed) Community Health Promotion. Baillière Tindall, London, pp 83–99

Dolby L 1998 Is sex education in the Netherlands better organized than in Britain? British Journal of Midwifery 6(2):96–100

Donati S, Medda E, Spinelli A, Grandolfo M 2000 Sex education in secondary schools: an Italian experience. Journal of Adolescent Health 26:303–308

Donovan P 1998 School-based sexuality education: the issues and challenges. Family Planning Perspectives 30(4):188–193

Edwards G, Stanisstreet M, Boyes E 1997 Adolescents' ideas about the health of the fetus. Midwifery 13:17–23

Eisenberg M, Wagenaar V, Neumark-Sztainer D 1997 Viewpoints of Minnesota students on school-based sexuality education. Journal of School Health 67(8):322–326

Evans K 1992 Getting back to nature. Modern Midwife 2(1):14–17

Finan S 1997 Promoting healthy sexuality: guidelines for the school-age child and adolescent. Nurse Practitioner 22(11):62–72

Ford N 1991 Regional overview of socio-sexual lifestyles of young people in the South West of England. Institute of Population Studies, University of Exeter, Exeter

Forrest J, Silverman J 1989 What public schools teachers teach about preventing pregnancy, AIDS and sexually transmitted diseases. Family Planning Perspectives 21(2):65–72

Frost J, Forrest J 1995 Understanding the impact of effective teenage pregnancy prevention programs. Family Planning Perspective 27:188–195

Fuglesang M 1997 Lessons for life – past and present modes of sexuality education in Tanzanian society. Social Science and Medicine 44(8):1245–1254

Genuis J, Genuis S 1995 Adolescent sexual involvement: time for primary prevention. Lancet 345:240–241

Hanna K 1993 Effect of nurse–client transaction on female adolescents' oral contraception adherence. Journal of Nursing Scholarship 25(4):285–289

Health Education Authority 1999 Young People and Health: Health Behaviour in School-Aged Children (1997). Health Education Authority, London

Health Education Authority and Office for National Statistics 1998 Omnibus Survey of 1,602 Adults Aged 16 and Over Living in Great Britain Conducted in Home Using Face to Face Questionnaire. Office for National Statistics, London

Hiltabiddle S 1996 Adolescent condom use, the health belief model and the prevention of sexually transmitted disease. Journal of Obstetric, Gynecologic, and Neonatal Nursing 25(1):61–66

Holland J, Ramazanoglu C, Scott S 1990 Managing risk and experiencing danger: tensions between government AIDS health education policy and young women's sexuality. Gender and Education 2:125–146

Jobanputra J, Clack A, Cheeseman G, Glasier A, Riley S 1999 A feasibility study of adolescent sex education: medical students as peer educators in Edinburgh schools. British Journal of Obstetrics and Gynaecology 106:887–891

Jones E 1985 Teenage pregnancy in developed countries: determinants and policy implications. Family Planning Perspectives 17(2):53–62

Khouzam H 1995 Promotion of sexual abstinence: reducing adolescent sexual activity and pregnancies. Southern Medical Journal 88(7):709–711

Kirby D 1985 Sexuality education: a more realistic view of its effects. Journal of School Health 55:421–424

Kirby D 1995 Sex and HIV education in schools. British Medical Journal 311:403

Kirby D, Barth R, Leland N 1991 Reducing the risk: impact of a new curriculum on sexual risk taking. Family Planning Perspective 23(6):253–263

Kirby D, Short L, Collins J 1994 School based programs to reduce sexual risk behaviours: a review of effectiveness. Public Health Report 109(3):339–360

Klanger B, Tyden T, Ruusuvaara L 1993 Sexual behaviour among adolescents in Uppsala, Sweden. Journal of Adolescent Health 14:468–474

Klein L 1978 Antecedents of teenage pregnancy. Clinical Obstetrics and Gynaecology 21:1151–1159

Kumar-Bhasin S, Aggarwal O 1999 Perceptions of teachers regarding sex education in National Capital Territory of Delhi. Indian Journal of Pediatrics 66:527–531

Lambke M, Kavanaugh K 1999 Nurses' description and evaluation of reproductive health counselling for adolescent females. Health Care for Women International 20:147–162

Maclean G 1997 Community health and the social services. In: Sweet B (ed) Mayes' Midwifery, 12th edn. Baillière Tindall, London, pp 956–975

May K 1992 Social networks and help-seeking experiences of pregnant teens. Journal of Obstetric, Gynecologic, and Neonatal Nursing 21(6):497–502

McCrea H 1993 Valuing the midwife's role in the midwife/client relationship. Journal of Clinical Nursing 2:47–52

McEwan R, Bhopal R, Atkinson A 1994 AIDS and sex education in Newcastle schools: policy, priority and obstacles. Health Education Journal 53:15–27

Meisenhelder J 1985 Self-esteem: a closer look at clinical interventions. Journal of Nursing Studies 22(2):127–135

Murray G 1995 A Midwife – The Definitions. New Zealand College of Midwives, Christchurch. April 23–24

National Children's Bureau 1999 Sex Education. National Children's Bureau, London

NHS Centre for Reviews and Dissemination 1997 Effective Health Care Bulletin 3: Prevention and reducing the adverse effects of unintended teenage pregnancies. University of York, York

Oakley A, Fullerton D, Holland J 1995 Sexual health education intervention for young people: a methodological review. British Medical Journal 310:158–162

Ogden J, Harden A 1999 The timing, format and content of school based sex education: an experience with a lasting effect? The British Journal of Family Planning 25:115–118

Page L 1999 Midwives make a difference. British Journal of Midwifery 7(8):490

Persson E, Jarlbro G 1992 Sexual behaviour among youth clinic visitors in Sweden: knowledge and experiences in an HIV perspective. Genitourinary Medicine 168:26–31

Porter L 1998 Reducing teenage and unintended pregnancies through client-centred and family-focused school-based family planning programs. Journal of Pediatric Nursing 13(3):158–163

Renker P 1999 Physical abuse, social support, self-care and pregnancy outcomes of older adolescents. Journal of Obstetric, Gynecologic and Neonatal Nursing 28(4):377–388

Rosenthal D, Feldman S 1999 The importance of importance: adolescents' perceptions of parental communication about sexuality. Journal of Adolescence 22:835–851

Ruusuvaara L 1997 Adolescent sexuality: an educational and counselling challenge. Annals of the New York Academy of Sciences 816:411–413

Saito M 1998 Sex education in school: preventing unwanted pregnancy in adolescents. International Journal of Gynaecology and Obstetrics 63:157–160

Sex Education Forum 1999 The Framework for Sex and Relationships Education. Sex Education Forum, London

Shelov, S, Baron M, Beard L 1995 Sexuality, contraception and the media. Pediatrics 95:298–300

Sheridan V 1997 Health promotion and education. In: Sweet B (ed) Mayes' Midwifery, 12th edn. Baillière Tindall, London, pp 285–304

Smith T 1993 Influence of socio-economic factors on attaining targets for reducing teenage pregnancies. British Medical Journal 306:1232–1235

Social Exclusion Unit 1999 Teenage Pregnancy. TSO, London

Stout J, Rivara F 1989 Schools and sex education: does it work? Pediatrics 83:375–379

Strasburger V 1989 Adolescent sexuality and the media. Pediatric Clinics of North America 36(3):747–770

Sweet B 1997 Antenatal care. In: Sweet B (ed) Mayes' Midwifery, 12th edn. Baillière Tindall, London, pp 208–239

Thompson P, Powell J, Patterson R, Ellerbee S 1995 Adolescent parenting: outcomes and maternal perception. Journal of Obstetric, Gynecologic and Neonatal Nursing 24(8):713–718

Thomson R 1993 Sex education starts at school. Primary Health Care 3:8–11

Tobias B, Ricer R 1998 Counselling adults about sexuality. Adolescent Medicine 25(1):49–70

Tucker S 1990 Adolescent patterns of communication about the menstrual cycle, sex and contraception. Journal of Pediatric Nursing 5(6):393–399

United Kingdom Central Council for Nursing, Midwifery and Health Visiting 1998 Midwives Rules and Code of Practice. UKCC, London

Walton I 1997 Sexuality and childbearing. In: Sweet B (ed) Mayes' Midwifery, 12th edn. Baillière Tindall, London, pp 741–747

Warren C 1995 Parent–child communication about sex. In: Socha T, Stamp G (eds) Parents, Children and Communication: Frontiers of Theory and Research. Erlbaum, Englewood Cliffs, NJ, pp 26–43

Wight D, Scott S 1994 Mandates and Constraints on Sex Education in the East of Scotland (Preliminary study for a sex education initiative). Medical Research Council, London

Witte K 1997 Preventing teen pregnancy through persuasive communications: realities, myths and the hard-fact truths. Journal of Community Health 22(2):137–154

Woodcock A, Stenner K, Ingham R 1992 'All these contraceptives, videos and that …' Young people talking about sex education. Health Education Research 7(4):517–531

Chapter **10**

Midwives playing their part: Sure Start

Eileen Stringer and Carole Butterfield

CHAPTER CONTENTS

SUMMARY

Whilst we know that many recent government documents emphasise that midwives are 'well placed' to pass on health messages due to the unique relationship we have with women (DH 1999), many of us are also in a dilemma about how to introduce a core theme of public health into our everyday work. This chapter provides a personal overview of some of the practical aspects and challenges of working in this way. It describes how we have to use the opportunities presented to us to build a maternity service that fits the public health paradigm. It demonstrates to the reader some of the approaches used on a day-to-day basis that help us to promote good health. We discuss our experiences of working with Sure Start programmes and the need to address mainstreaming issues. The chapter also contains examples of how to tackle some key health targets with reference to practical planning and monitoring tools. Finally, we have tried to incorporate some of the learning that took place along the way and take a look at the future.

WIDENING OUR PERSPECTIVE

The new public health model embraces a much wider perspective than many of us were taught as students. There is now a greater understanding of why people make the choices they do, and simply informing them that certain behaviour carries risk is not always enough to produce change. However, trying to work with this approach in mind has not always been highly valued by colleagues or managers in the past, and the time limitations placed upon individual clinicians and services in general are a major factor in this. In a study published by the ENB 'Research Highlights' series, the authors acknowledge that public health work is seen as difficult to define and not 'core' activity by nurses. The study demonstrated that public health work tended to take second place to that which is more concretely measurable, and these findings are echoed within the experience of many midwives (ENB 2000). Nevertheless, the shift in emphasis towards a population approach to health and ill health means that we need a wider and more innovative approach. That is, we need to work within and with communities to influence changes in policy and environment. This philosophy is at the very heart of the Sure Start programme and even where the opportunity to work within such a programme does not exist, there are still lessons to be learned and transferred over to a mainstream setting.

SURE START LOCAL PROGRAMMES

We have been fortunate as a medium sized maternity unit to have worked with Sure Start since the first trailblazer programmes were being planned in 1998. We took the view early on that Sure Start would give us the opportunity to work differently and we have worked tirelessly and continue to do so in order to reach our goal. It took a little while to grasp, but not too long after we started working with local programmes, we realised our main aim was not to enhance the skills and achievements of any one individual midwife or local programme. Rather, the aim was for all midwives to have a working knowledge of Sure Start and public health and incorporate this into their daily working lives, regardless of whether they were in a Sure Start area or not.

From the beginning, with the first trailblazer programme, we identified that we as midwives were able to deliver services that were key to achieving the targets of the programme, as set out in Box 10.1.

Box 10.1
Sure Start objectives

Objective 1 – Improving social and emotional development (e.g. identifying and supporting mothers with postnatal depression).

- Contact 100% of families within the first 2 months of birth

Objective 2 – Improving health

- Achieving a 6% point reduction in the proportion of mothers who continue to smoke during pregnancy by 2005–6
- Providing parenting support and antenatal information
- Providing support and guidance on breastfeeding, hygiene and safety.

Objective 3 – Improving learning

- Achieve by 2005–6 an increase in the proportion of children having normal levels of communication, language and literacy
- Increase the proportion of young children with satisfactory speech and language development at age 2 years (e.g. this might include joint visits with midwife/speech therapist or inclusion of speech and language development in antenatal classes).

Objective 4 – Strengthening families and communities

- To achieve by 2005–6 a 12% reduction in the proportion of young children (aged 0–4) living in households where no one is working (e.g. this might include development of breastfeeding peer counsellors from the local community).

(DfES 2003)

In addition to these targets, each programme will identify specific targets that are of concern to their particular community, for example, a high incidence of domestic violence.

We submitted a bid to the first programme that demonstrated how our services could make a positive contribution to health, and as a result were successful in securing funding for a midwife to join the programme.

Within the next 3 years, the number of programmes established or about to commence within our catchment area had swelled to seven, with funding for midwifery activity built into each one. Each programme had a different lead body and we found ourselves working with many different agencies for the first time, including Early Years and Play services, Education, Primary Care Trusts (PCTs) and Family Support Services. While we welcomed the chance to concentrate extra resources in those areas of greatest need, we had to consider two points. The first was that with so many bedfellows there was a danger of each 'Sure Start' midwife going off at a tangent, developing albeit much-needed services within the remit of the local programme area, but in isolation from the core midwifery service itself. The second was the need to ensure that we didn't view these initiatives as a 'one-off' event; rather we would use them as a catalyst to transform core midwifery services in order to take on a Sure

Start/public health approach. We knew the funding for the local programmes, although finite, would probably last for up to 10 years. The challenge lay in fitting our plans into this time-frame and across several programmes. We needed to deliver on targets agreed through the service level agreements for each programme, but take a wider view of what we were trying to introduce as a whole service. With this in mind, we undertook a brief review of each programme, identifying the specific traits and targets and how they translated into midwifery services that needed to be established in each area. The review demonstrated that we required strong co-ordination from a midwifery perspective, in order to identify areas of best practice across the programmes, particularly giving direction to the fledgling programmes. The review also demonstrated that some of our existing practice, for example our adapted caseload midwifery model of care, might be a good vehicle for taking some of the Sure Start/public health philosophy forward.

MAINSTREAMING

Tackling Health Inequalities (DH 2003b) specifically looks at the recommendations of the Acheson Report (DH 1998), how we are progressing and how we plan to achieve the recommendations by 2010. One of the key messages contained within the Report is the importance of integrating public health interventions into the mainstream of service delivery with a focus on disadvantaged areas and groups. The document specifically mentions 'mainstreaming Sure Start'.

Fortunately, as we arrived at the conclusion of our Sure Start local programme review, the Department for Education and Skills invited bids to pilot ways of addressing some of the mainstreaming issues that would inevitably arise from the local programmes, particularly as funding is withdrawn. We were invited by colleagues from Early Years and Play, on behalf of Manchester City Council with whom we had worked closely in Sure Start, to contribute to a larger joint bid. Our part of the bid included funding for a midwifery 'mainstreaming' co-ordinator and the pump-priming extension of our adapted caseload midwifery service to become a vehicle for delivering midwifery care with a public health/Sure Start philosophy. In January 2002 we learned our bid had been successful.

THE ROLE OF THE MAINSTREAMING CO-ORDINATOR

The remit of the Midwifery Mainstreaming Co-ordinator has been to work closely with Sure Start in order for the midwifery work within the local programmes to be co-ordinated, best practice and effective interventions to be identified and then carried over to other programmes and non-Sure Start areas. The role also included providing midwifery representation on each local programme board, which in turn helped to identify and resolve potential or existing problems. Other aspects of the role include raising awareness of Sure Start and public health issues for midwives;

identifying ways of mainstreaming some of the lessons learned in the local programmes, for example improving multi-agency working; liaison with the La Leche League Peer Counsellor Training team; organisation of this training and supporting the midwives in different areas until their initiatives became established; establishing a data collection system, promoting multi-agency partnerships and helping all midwives to have high-quality information and contacts for available local services.

In order to establish some of the best practice and new ways of working, it was necessary for the Co-ordinator also to secure funding from non-Sure Start sources for those areas that do not have a local programme.

INTEGRATED APPROACH

Extending the adapted caseload midwifery model was the second part of our mainstreaming bid. It was already established in two of our local catchment areas. This model of care helps midwives to provide care in the antenatal and postnatal period and some intrapartum care (30%) to women within their caseload. The model consists of a small group of midwives working together in a defined area. The group approach to care has allowed midwives to support each other in developing extra services for women in their locality, for example parent education. We felt that if we could extend this model to three other areas, the group midwifery approach would allow us to include public health interventions in each area, including breastfeeding support groups, parent education and improved smoking cessation services.

A key element in utilising the adapted caseload model was the consideration of how midwives funded by Sure Start could remain close to the provision of the core service, while at the same time helping existing midwives in the area to be exposed to the Sure Start way of working. We made a decision that where an adapted caseload group was established in a Sure Start local programme area, the midwife funded by the programme could be integrated into the midwifery group. This integrated approach had been tried in the first local programme, an area with traditional midwifery. The existing community midwife and the midwife funded by Sure Start worked in close partnership, with a great deal of success. Extending this integrated approach to the adapted caseload meant that a greater number of core midwives would have the opportunity to work with a Sure Start programme. They would do this by sharing a collective responsibility to reach the local programme targets whilst continuing to provide clinical care. Their colleague funded by Sure Start working within the group would assist them. The long-term aim is that eventually there will be little difference in the way core and Sure Start midwives work. This will enhance the possibility of the roles being absorbed into the mainstream and remaining where they have greatest effect. Other benefits of this approach include being able to continue the input into the local programme in times of absence of the Sure Start funded midwife. The funded midwife is still the official 'link' to the programme and she retains responsibility for monitoring.

COLLABORATION

We realised we cannot change from a management perspective alone, and those at grass roots level cannot change without management support. Regular communication and a shared vision are crucial to this. Our learning is that this doesn't happen overnight. One cannot assume a vision is shared or accepted in one or two presentations, discussions or debates. It is an ongoing process and is often achieved incrementally over a long period of time. Small areas of conflict need to be resolved, or at least articulated. When a vision or aim conflicts, it is important to articulate both parties' opinions. Agreement is a welcome outcome, but we should recognise that this is not always the case. People may still have different views, but what is important is that they have been able to articulate their concerns and from doing this, they each come to understand and respect one another's position. Acknowledgement and acceptance is often enough for people to agree to move on and to try to work differently. Much of the success of the changes is down to the core midwives being flexible and willing to become involved in Sure Start and share the work with their colleagues. However, we have found that not all midwives like to work in this way. This issue has to be addressed and individuals need to be supported.

SUCCESSFUL TRANSITION

Mainstreaming to us meant a successful transition from 'Sure Start initiative' to core service component. It would have been impossible to recreate the work of Sure Start in its entirety, so we agreed that we would initially identify a small number of alternative practices that had worked well in the local programmes and set about breaking them down into key components. We would then be able to transfer these over to other areas with support until the practice became well established. Some of the key areas that we felt could be developed and taken into mainstream services in the long term were:

- Breastfeeding peer support
- Smoking cessation
- Perinatal depression
- Multi-agency working.

The evidence for focusing on these is well established (DH 1998, 2003a, Protheroe et al 2003) and applying this evidence to our practice means working in a more creative manner in order to improve health outcomes. We have had varying degrees of success, not surprisingly those where we have spent the most time and effort being the most successful.

BREASTFEEDING SUPPORT

One such initiative is the roll-out of the La Leche League (LLL) Breastfeeding Peer Counsellor Programme. It is recognised that increasing the number of women who choose to breastfeed and encouraging them to breastfeed for longer is an important public health issue. Within the Sure Start programme, giving guidance on breastfeeding is part of a larger health target that includes reducing the number of infants admitted to hospital with gastro-enteritis and respiratory infection. There is evidence to suggest that by increasing breastfeeding rates, the incidence of these infections will fall (Howie et al 1990, Kramer et al 2001, La Leche League 2003).

This approach to encouraging breastfeeding was ideal for our core service as it is also a health target for the PCTs and is highlighted within the 'Priorities and Planning Framework' 2003–2006 targets (DH 2002).

As we began to look at this area, our first reaction was that we had always encouraged women to breastfeed – Sure Start wasn't telling us anything 'new'. However, Sure Start required baseline statistics at a local, rather than unit, level. This exercise demonstrated how ineffective we had been in certain areas. Many of the rates were well below 10% and some areas had no reliable methods of data collection at all.

It is clearly documented that breastfeeding rates tend to be well below the national average within disadvantaged communities (Dunkerley 2000, Jamieson & Long 2001, Protheroe et al 2003). In order to change a culture within a community it is important to empower those living there to make healthier choices in their lives (Dunkerley 2000). Training local women to become breastfeeding peer counsellors is one way of trying to change the culture around breastfeeding and empower local women. Evidence within the recent HDA report (HDA 2003) suggests that women are more likely to choose to breastfeed if they see other women breastfeeding, rather than reading or talking about it, and that peer support for breastfeeding is the way forward in increasing rates within deprived areas (Protheroe et al 2003). There are different organisations that provide training programmes for local women to become breastfeeding peer counsellors and these include the Breast Feeding Network, the National Childbirth Trust and the La Leche League, which is an international organization. There are also some well-established individual Trust-based training workshops.

Having met with and been inspired by some of the LLL trainers and women who were working as peer counsellors at a conference in London 2001, we decided to implement the LLL programme within one local area if we could manage to meet the not inconsiderable £6,000 cost. Fortunately, the area was one of the Sure Start trailblazers with a breastfeeding rate of 20% and we successfully secured funding to try this innovative approach.

WHAT DOES THE TRAINING ENTAIL?

The LLL training package has a two-pronged cascade approach, training 10 'workers' (not necessarily health professionals) who then train 10 local women. We decided to make this training multi-agency and included senior crèche workers, health visitors, midwives, the Sure Start centre manager and the special care community midwife. This was to ensure

Box 10.2
The LLL Training Package (La Leche League 2003)

The curriculum covers the following topics:

- The barriers to breastfeeding
- The benefits of breastfeeding
- The anatomy of the breast and the hormones of lactation
- The composition of human milk
- Management of breastfeeding, including correct positioning, etc.
- Getting ready for baby – ideas to make breastfeeding work in day-to-day living
- Breastfeeding in different situations
- Understanding baby's needs from infancy to toddlerhood
- Communication skills and examining our attitudes towards other people.

that there was a cross-section of workers within each area that would be giving a consistent message to local women about breastfeeding. The training (Box 10.2) consisted of 5 full days split over 3 weeks for the 'workers' and 10 weekly 2-hour sessions for the mothers.

The training for the 10 local women uses the same curriculum format. The topics are delivered in 2-hourly sessions over 10 weeks with crèche facilities available. It is important to try to have a cross-section of women who are breastfeeding at different stages. For example, newly delivered mothers, mothers with older babies and even toddlers. It is also important to have a lead professional, preferably two, for example a midwife and a health visitor, who will oversee the training and be able to offer support to the peer counsellors. This also gives a message to the women that midwives and health visitors work together to provide a seamless service in supporting women to breastfeed.

When the training is complete, the women graduate with a certificate. This has had a major impact on some of the women taking part in the training programme in ways not originally anticipated. For example, this is often the first time that some of them will have achieved a certificate in any subject, and it has been empowering. It is interesting to see the changes that take place within the women as they grow in confidence and self-esteem, including the confidence to exercise choice. For example, two of the peer support counsellors became pregnant and both decided to have a home birth. They acknowledged that whilst considering this option in previous pregnancies, they had not had the confidence either to make the decision or to articulate their wishes, before becoming a peer counsellor. Some of the women have been able to go on to further education and paid employment. Others have trained as intermediate smoking cessation advisors, and offer support with smoking cessation as well as breastfeeding. One mother within the area where we first introduced the peer counsellor programme became pregnant with her fourth child. She had formula-fed her first three children but decided to breastfeed her fourth child after spending time with the peer counsellors during her pregnancy. This was due to the fact that the midwife within the area runs a drop-in clinic for pregnant

Table 10.1 Effects of peer support on breastfeeding rates

Area	Breastfeeding rate (%)		Comments
	Before April 2002	End of March 2004	
Area 1 support established	22	41	Peer support in place
Area 2 support established	20	32	Peer support in place
Area 3 support established	27	40	Peer support in place
Area 4 support established	10	37.2	Peer support in place
Area 5	30	34	Training programme commenced, not yet complete

women; the waiting area is the room where the peer counsellors hold their support group. This means that pregnant women are exposed to other mothers breastfeeding. This mother successfully breastfed her fourth child and is now trained as a peer counsellor herself. Empowering women in this way also meets other Sure Start objectives, including the target for strengthening families and communities. In September 2003, the peer counsellors in the initial area were awarded the Sylvia Pankhurst award for outstanding services to women within a local community.

We have since been able to roll out the LLL programme throughout our areas, and at the end of 2004 there were six breastfeeding peer support groups, including non-Sure Start areas. This has been an excellent opportunity to promote close working with local women and has seen an increase in the breastfeeding rates where this support has been implemented (see Table 10.1).

The LLL training complements the Baby Friendly Initiative that is being implemented in some of the local maternity hospitals. We have been encouraged and supported by the Sure Start local programme managers and the Manchester Joint Health Unit in order to progress this objective. Once training is undertaken, the midwives in different areas are offered support with their groups until they become established. It has been an excellent example of how the midwifery mainstreaming co-ordinator role can have a positive and wide-reaching impact.

One of our main learning points in implementing peer support within the communities is that we should never underestimate the knowledge, power and enthusiasm that women have to be good mothers and to help others to succeed. On reflection, we have perhaps in the past been paternalistic in our views on what is right for women and their families, and have not listened to them as well as we might have done.

SMOKING CESSATION

Another area identified for mainstreaming via the co-ordinating role has been the improvement in the smoking cessation Quit rates within the past 18 months. We recognised that our existing approach to smoking cessation required a rethink. Again, looking across the local programmes and non-Sure Start areas, we realised midwives needed better skills in order to have a positive impact on Quit rates. The co-ordinator established links with the citywide smoking cessation team to develop a strategy that allowed midwives to become more involved with smoking cessation in a manner that would have a positive impact on reducing the number of women who smoke during pregnancy. Again, we approached it in both Sure Start and non-Sure Start areas and used a collaborative approach with other agencies. Reducing the number of women who smoke during pregnancy is not only a Sure Start target but is a major goal within the NHS Plan (DH 2000) and other government drivers.

The midwifery co-ordinator arranged for the majority of midwives working in the community to be trained as intermediate level advisors in smoking cessation. This level is the next step up from the basic information and awareness training that some midwives had previously had. Midwives are able to offer information and advice and facilitate women setting Quit dates with the use of nicotine replacement therapy (NRT) if needed. The midwives have taken on board this extra dimension to their role and have been able to work more closely with others in the community and with the smoking cessation team. Some areas have been more successful than others. Time constraints can be a factor in how far we can progress this – it is difficult to offer this in-depth service to pregnant women by midwives with busy caseloads. However, some midwives with the busiest of workloads acknowledge that they have success because they have used their newly developed skills opportunistically, being able to offer more in-depth help and advice at the moment when the mother is most determined to quit. Other midwives observe that their enhanced relationship with women has also helped women to take the message on board.

Some GPs have been reluctant to prescribe NRT for pregnant women, and this has caused some delay in women setting Quit dates. However, a major success for us is that we have recently received agreement from our Trust Drugs and Therapeutics Committee to introduce a Group Directive for the prescribing of NRT. This will provide a great deal more flexibility when trying to offer smoking cessation advice and support.

As a result of the extra smoking cessation training, 96 pregnant women set Quit dates with midwives between April 2003 and March 2004, when in the previous year this was zero. A modest start but definitely heading in the right direction, as one particularly deprived area prior to March 2003 had a smoking in pregnancy rate of nearly 70%. This has now decreased to 38.3%.

PERINATAL DEPRESSION (PND)

In response to the Sure Start target of improving social and emotional development with an emphasis on supporting women with postnatal depression, we needed to review our current service provision. This review highlighted three issues:

- The need for a specific care pathway to be developed for women who may develop or have existing depression in either the antenatal or postnatal period, i.e. perinatal depression (PND)
- The need of training for midwives around PND
- The need to introduce or adopt an assessment tool that can be used in the antenatal period.

We established a steering group to develop a more cohesive service for women suffering from PND. Initially, after reviewing several existing tools, it was decided to try to introduce the use of the Edinburgh Postnatal Depression Scale (EPNDS) by midwives in the antenatal period. We took advice from health visitor colleagues who had been working on this subject area for 6 years and had developed in-depth knowledge. We wanted to collaborate in order to ensure that the tool would be used by midwives and health visitors alike as necessary, and that it should complement and build upon each other's work. In order to achieve this, we agreed to develop joint training.

However, our plans have been delayed, due to the recent publication of both NICE and National Screening Committee guidance that does not support the use of the EPNDS in the antenatal period (NICE 2003, NSC 2003). Neither recommendation addresses the needs of women with existing or developing depression in the antenatal period, and this is a concern for us. Further work needs to be done, and links have been made with a citywide steering group chaired by a senior member of the Manchester Mental Health Joint Commissioning Executive. We are hopeful that with further collaboration and work we will be able to find a suitable approach, deliver the appropriate training and extend it to other areas.

In the interim, we facilitated a small, basic awareness-raising study day for midwives and health visitors in a local setting. The session looked at the latest legislation and different assessment tools. A small number of midwives and health visitors from various areas attended the training session. The evaluation of the training by the participants was very positive, supporting the notion that there is a need for practitioners to be trained in this sensitive area.

The learning from this piece of work centres on the fact that however well intentioned we are, we do not work in isolation, and outside agencies may influence our approach more than we originally realised. We learned that the messages we receive from government or other professional bodies might be conflicting, and this makes it very difficult for clinicians to establish new practices (CEMD 2002, DH 2003a, NICE 2003, NSC 2003).

MULTI-AGENCY WORKING

In terms of multi-agency working, there is an improvement in communication between agencies. We established quarterly meetings with the

Director of Nursing Services and the lead public health professionals within the local PCTs, and value the relationships we have developed. In other areas, we are working with other agencies on the developments for the future Sure Start Children's Centres. However, some staff, both from midwifery and other professions/agencies, find multi-agency working difficult. We have learned that there is a considerable amount of work to be undertaken in order to dissolve inter-agency and professional boundaries. If we are to take one of the major successes of Sure Start, that is, true multi-agency working, and integrate that into our mainstream service, then we need to consider working within the same defined communities as health visitors, other members of the primary health care team and even other agencies. We need to deliver cohesive services that have meaning to a family, a joint approach to tackling health inequalities rather than the fragmented approach that exists in some areas, with health professionals only discussing care issues depending on which GP a woman or her family belongs to. The same professionals may experience difficulty linking into the housing or other social networks for a community – usually because they cover conflicting boundaries and historically, these are not seen as a 'health' problem. Some PCTs have addressed this by reorganising their services into Community Health Teams. These teams are based on Wards and cut across Health Visiting, District Nursing, etc. and we may in the future include midwives in these teams. There is a considerable way to go before this may be possible, not least because of concerns about removing midwives from being GP-attached. There are fears that women based with a particular GP but living in another Ward/postcode area may not be seen by the same Primary Health Team members other than the GP. There can also be a lack of understanding about who employs midwives, that is, the Acute Trusts and not the PCTs in the majority of cases.

We have learned that some of the work we have been doing around multi-agency working is actually very time-consuming, and it will take much longer than first anticipated to implement a change in practice that will have the correct impact for women and their families. We are positive that, given time, we will overcome the current obstacles and will establish a valuable service.

TOOLS FOR CHANGE

During this process of change, we have invented or adapted simple tools that help us to create and share a clear vision of what we are trying to achieve with midwives. Some of these, for example the workplans, are useful on a practical, day-to-day level and can be incorporated into Personal Development Plans. Others, such as the '4 Rs', are useful when trying to plan a more strategic approach to changing a service as a whole. Although we realise there may be many other, more sophisticated systems and tools, we have shared them in the hope that some of you may find them helpful.

WORKPLANS

This concept originally started with the co-ordinator role. Once in post, it became clear that such a large and hitherto unexplored role would need to be broken down into desirable and achievable targets/objectives/outcomes. A half-day session was set up to discuss the work ahead. Each objective merited discussion, with suggestions as to how it might be achieved. Each step identified led to a subsequent step, with the overall aim being achieved when the last steps/objectives were completed. Against each of these a timescale was applied. At the end of the session our thoughts, originally written on flip charts during the session, were transferred to paper and we were left with a developed workplan (Table 10.2). The workplan provides a clear plan of action that we can evaluate our progress against, and a quick guide to the work required over the coming year. Although a basic tool, it has proved to be successful and gives a clear direction. We decided to roll this out to each programme, and included all midwives working in the area as well as the Sure Start midwife. Programme managers are also invited to the session, which usually takes half a day. The key is in the discussion and formulation of the workplan, as this provides an opportunity to get the whole team

Table 10.2 Example of a workplan – part 1: Aims, Objectives and Evaluation (one for each aim)

Aim: To establish effective data collection and monitoring systems

Objective	**Action by**	**Timescale**
Collect baseline data	CB/SC	December 02
Improve existing data collection: update existing Sure Start database, including:	MK/CB	Feb 03
Number of teenage pregnancies		
Number of smoking cessation		
Low birthweight		
Breastfeeding estab. cont. on discharge		
Partner support		
Postnatal visiting		
Asylum seekers		
Parent education		
Diet		
Support score postnatal and antenatal		
Employment		
Collect case studies	All	Jun 03
All midwives to complete Sure Start monitoring forms	All	1/4ly from Mar 03
SS link to liaise with other midwives/training	CB	Jan 03
Submit to SS Office	CB	1/4ly
Evaluation		
IT systems updated		Jan 03
Review database – accurate data retrieved		Mar 03
Sure Start monitoring forms – complete and submitted		Mar 03
Case studies available		Jun 03

Table 10.2 Part 2: Annual plan

ACTION	Dec	Jan	Feb	Mar	Apr	May	Jun	Jul	Aug	Sep	Oct	Nov
Contact LLL/Collect baseline data	X											
Commence A/N info card/contact IT	X											
Identify named M/Ws and H/Vs for LLL		X										
CB to liaise with Monitoring Officer and MWs		X										
Training on monitoring forms		X										
Involve AR and H/Vs in S.C. Plans			X									
Update IT system			X									
Make links with FSU and parents' forum				X								
Commence training for workers – LLL					X							
Identify venue for parent ed./Rota						X						
Case study each							X					
Identify nurse and GP prescriber/use of PGD								X				
Set up drop-in with H/Vs								X				
Advertise drop-in/parent ed.									X			
Commence training for PSW										X		
Research A/N information and healthy eating in pregnancy. Link with dietician											X	
Set up PSW group												X
Ongoing data collection	X	X	X	X	X	X	X	X	X	X	X	X
Reports/Update/data			X			X			X			X

together and take ownership of how the work will develop. We identify the needs and targets of each programme, and all the midwives indicate particular areas that they wish to lead on or develop. Again, timescales are attached, each workplan spanning approximately 1 year. The workplans feed into and are shaped by the milestones from each local Sure Start programme.

THE FOUR Rs

Other tools were gradually created, such as the '4 Rs' (Table 10.3). The concept of the '4 Rs' was developed early on as we struggled to put our thoughts into context. Particularly, how would our plans fit into a bigger strategy on different levels? We felt that the changes we were trying to make would fit into four different stages. They are Review, Relinquish,

Table 10.3 Example of how the 4 Rs might be used to put plans into context

The 4 Rs	Individual midwife	Managerial	Organisation	National
Review (Where are we now?)	Review own practice Audit own activity Survey patient satisfaction Identify gaps	Do we have support at the top? How is our work organised?	Are we developing links to external initiatives? Are we securing external funding?	Are we using current research, government documents/papers as evidence for change?
Relinquish (How do we give ourselves time to do this?)	Identify what you don't need to do any more – i.e. that which has no positive impact on health	Dropping historical working patterns and practices that obstruct – e.g. skill mix review	Is there an opportunity to relinquish systems that obstruct development, e.g. traditional controls over budgets?	Do we understand that purchasing power has been relinquished from a central point to PCTs, and are we using that knowledge?
Reorganise (Change the way we do things – a step at a time)	What can I change on a daily basis?	Is there a system for effective change management?	Are we developing our aims into a strategy? Do we have Executive support for changing the service?	How do we tap into the National Agenda for Leadership in Midwifery?
Reshape (What we want our service to look like?)	Working in a different way	New Service	Joint budgets with other agencies High level of leadership Reaching Targets	New Service is in line with the targets in the Local Delivery Plans for PCTs

Reorganise and Reshape. As we have progressed, we put our thoughts down on paper and realised that the different stages can also relate to different levels within the organisation and even at a National level. This can be useful when trying to establish if the changes you are making fit into a wider strategy and will therefore be supported.

TRANSFORMING SERVICES AND THE CHANGE PROCESS

We feel we have achieved some excellent progress against our goal although we recognise we are only a third of the way through our long-term programme and there is still much to learn. The support throughout from the midwifery managers and Associate Director of Nursing has been essential to the success of our mainstreaming pilot and the ongoing mainstreaming work, and we feel this is a key factor in trying to transform any service.

Time and how it unfolds, often in a painfully slow way during change, is a fact that must be acknowledged and accepted in order to successfully traverse the change process. Changing people's paradigm nearly always takes longer than first anticipated, as different people will change at different paces. Many of the initiatives have been very well received by the practitioners, and some less so. In many areas we are still at the 'freezing' stage in the management of change and still have some way to go (Cross 1996).

We have learned that creating models of care on a small scale can often be highly successful, not least because the midwives chosen or applying for these new ways of working are already subscribing to that particular philosophy. However, when we start to extend the model, members of staff who may not have necessarily volunteered, but have had to participate, can impose negative influences: but these can be overcome. There are times when it feels as if no progress has been made, and it is then worthwhile to reflect on the previous 12 months. Invariably, the reflection demonstrates that there has in fact been movement and this can be immensely reassuring.

We have learned that we cannot change or develop in isolation and that however great our desire to implement new services and ways of working, we are sometimes tempered by a greater strategy. Nevertheless we are proud of some of our achievements to date. Box 10.3 sets out some of the main topics we have learned.

In many areas within our catchment, by the end of 2004 we had:

- Parent education classes in suitable, accessible venues
- A breastfeeding peer support group
- Smoking cessation advisors and referral services
- Drop-in clinics to access a midwife without an appointment
- Discussion with all pregnant women about healthy eating, including 'five-a-day'
- Improved methods of collecting data
- Aqua-natal sessions provided in two locations, with transport provided.

Box 10.3
Summary of main learning points

- Managing change can be difficult and usually takes longer than planned
- Events and strategies outside the control of those working in an innovative scheme can have a great influence on its success/development
- Working together in a group setting in midwifery provides a greater opportunity to integrate a Sure Start and public health approach into the core service
- We can deliver services differently to local women and their families
- We have learned how to collaborate better with local women and their families on delivery of care
- Support at a senior and executive level for change is essential to its success.

RESOURCES

One of the biggest threats to change is if the resources to sustain it are not in place or are withdrawn. Developing a service that will become a community-based model of care will inevitably mean moving a higher percentage of the workforce out into the community. However, it is important to ensure that in doing this we do not jeopardise other vital areas of the service, for example Delivery suite, and therefore the movement of the workforce has to be managed carefully.

Other initiatives involving a shift of emphasis away from the hospital unit have experienced negative perceptions of staff 'being taken away' from the service, especially when it is busy (McCourt & Page 1996). We have experienced similar perceptions, largely unfounded. It is therefore important that continued good communication between hospital and community staff is established in order to avoid such perceptions.

We have recently merged with other local units to become one large Trust with links to 16 local Sure Start programmes. It has also widened our catchment area considerably. We hope that this will provide us with the opportunity and resources to extend our work into many new areas.

We are aware that the resources for the La Leche League training can be an obvious stumbling block for those trying to implement a similar approach. It is difficult to find such funding from within Acute Health services, but our experience has demonstrated that if a case can be presented on the benefits of such a programme to those with a public health commitment to the local population, there is usually a positive response and funding can be secured. Another approach would be to submit a bid to several PCTs/Sure Start programmes/local governing body within a particular area and each could contribute a small amount to one training programme across the area.

THE FUTURE

The experience of Sure Start local programmes has informed and influenced the government's decision to introduce further developments, in particular the Children's Centres initiative. The Sure Start way of working will be continued through these Centres, putting the focus on the child, finding out through consultation with families what services are needed, and planning how to deliver these locally in a co-ordinated way. Another core theme that is intended to continue is how neighbourhood-based Sure Start Centres deliver services locally in a defined community, including health, early learning, child care, etc., via a multi-agency team committed to working in partnership.

Other points that could positively influence service delivery for children and families in the future include:

- Improved multi-agency working/training
- Recognition of the need to allow sufficient time to develop and establish initiatives. Replacing short-term funding with longer-term financial commitment
- Built-in evaluation that will assist us to determine the value of initiatives, e.g. local IT facilities to collect data and to help us to inform future service delivery
- Recognition that some of this work needs to be measured by qualitative evidence, and that the emphasis on statistics does not always determine value.

If we are to make a difference, it means looking differently at how we deliver care. We have got to make best use of our time. The evidence is there to show us how to do that. In addition, care should be based on need, not the routine, and involving consumer groups for regular feedback is essential if we are to achieve this.

CONCLUSION

Taking a long-term preventative perspective means recognising that family well-being is important to the health of mothers, which, in turn, is strongly related to the health of unborn babies (DH 1998). Seizing the opportunity to work within Sure Start and learn from it has given us a greater opportunity than ever before to provide the type of care we want to for women and families. Working in this way has brought benefits to the communities we work with in ways that we had not originally anticipated. It has demonstrated that the agenda we have all been working to, that is to improve the lives of children and families, can be achieved with investment, time, energy and commitment.

Reflection on practice

- How do you think you can implement a local breastfeeding peer support group within your area?
- How can you implement Sure Start/public health principles within your area within the resources that you have?
- How can you find champions within your organisation or amongst your colleagues to change practice and incorporate the principles of Sure Start and public health into mainstream working?

References

Confidential Enquiries into Maternal Deaths in the United Kingdom 2002 Why Mothers Die 1997–1999. Royal College of Obstetricians and Gynaecologists, London

Crafter H 2001 Health Promotion in Midwifery. Principles and Practice. Arnold, London

Cross R E 1996 Midwives and Management. A Handbook. Books for Midwives, London

Department for Education and Skills and Department for Work and Pensions 2003 SureStart. DfES Publications, London

Department of Health 1998 Independent Inquiry into Inequalities in Health (the Acheson Report). TSO, London

Department of Health 1999 Making a Difference: Strengthening the Nursing, Midwifery and Health Visiting Contribution to Health and Healthcare. TSO, London

Department of Health 2000 The NHS Plan. TSO, London

Department of Health 2002 Improvement, Expansion and Reform: the next 3 years. Priorities and Planning Framework 2003–2006. DH, London

Department of Health 2003a Women's Mental Health: Into the Mainstream. Strategic Development of Mental Health Care for Women. DH, London

Department of Health 2003b Tackling Health Inequalities: A Programme for Action. DH, London

Dunkerley J 2000 Health Promotion in Midwifery Practice: A Resource for Health Professionals. Baillière Tindall, London

English National Board 2000 Research Highlights: Evaluation of the Developing Specialist Practitioner Role in the Context of Public Health. ENB Publications, London

Health Development Agency 2003 The Effectiveness of Public Health Interventions to Promote the Initiation of Breastfeeding. HDA, London

Howie P W, Forsyth J S, Ogston S et al 1990 Protective effect of breastfeeding against infection. British Medical Journal 300:11–16

Jamieson L, Long L M 2001 Part 3: Practice of health promotion. In: Crafter H (ed) Health Promotion in Midwifery: Principles and Practice. Arnold, London

Kramer M, Chalmers B, Hodnett H et al 2001 Promotion of Breastfeeding Intervention Trial (PROBIT). Journal of the American Medical Association 285:413–420

La Leche League 2003 Breast Feeding Peer Counsellor Programme. La Leche League, Great Britain

McCourt C, Page L (eds) 1996 Report on the Evaluation of One-to-One Midwifery. Thames Valley University, London

National Institute for Clinical Excellence 2003 Antenatal Care: Routine Care for the Healthy Pregnant Woman. NICE, London

National Screening Committee 2003 Screening in England: Programme Director's Report Period Summer 2002–2003. NSC, Oxford. Online. Available: www.nelh.nhs.uk/screening

Protheroe L, Dyson L, Renfrew M J et al 2003 The Effectiveness of Public Health Intervention to Promote the Initiation of Breastfeeding. Evidence Briefing. Health Development Agency, London

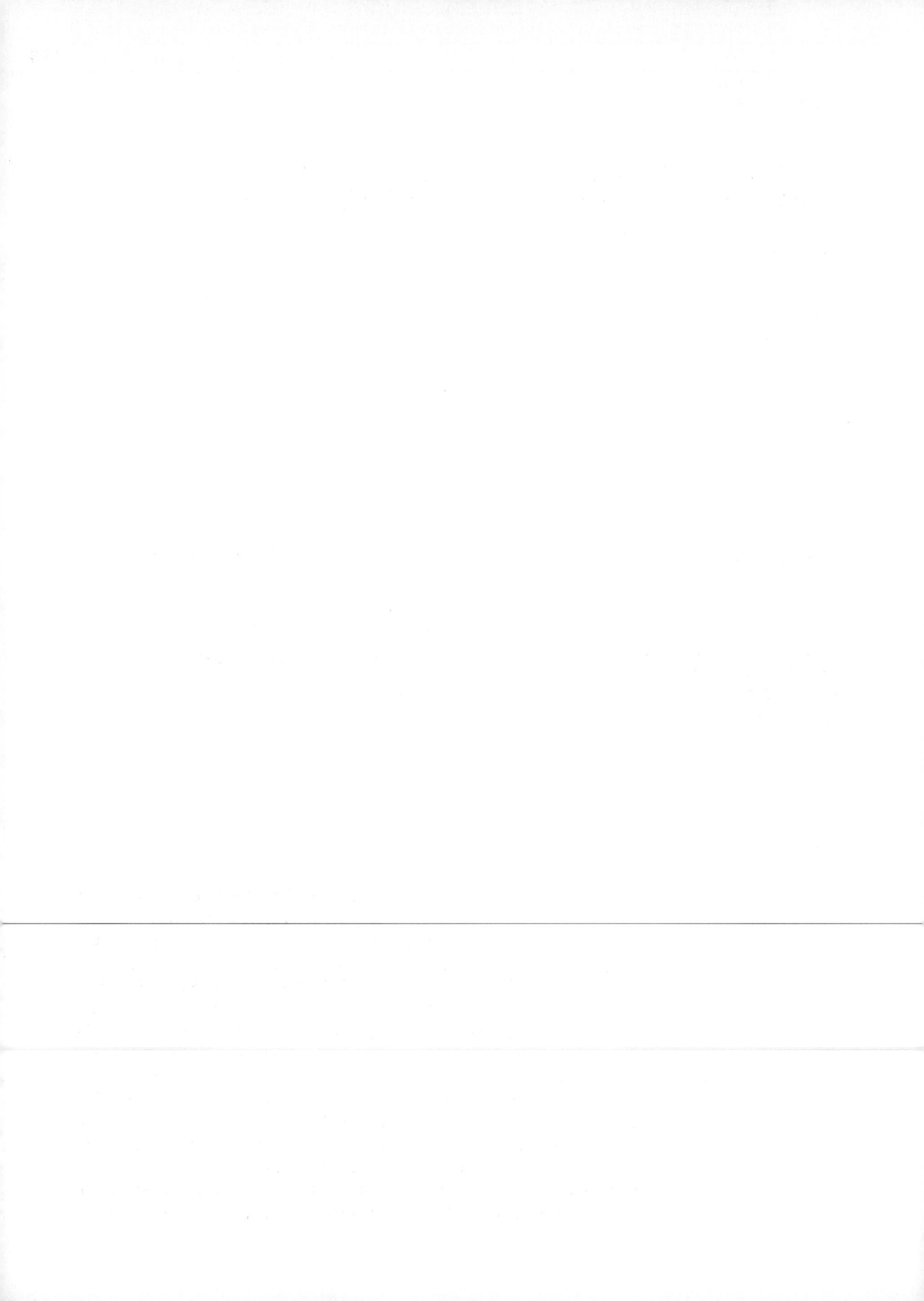

Chapter **11**

Postnatal care: meeting the public health challenge

Debra Bick

CHAPTER CONTENTS

SUMMARY

This chapter examines the past, present and future potential of midwifery practice during the postnatal period. The historical factors which led to the instigation of the statutory provision of midwifery postnatal care, as well as the proscriptive content of care, are described. The recent evidence on specific public health outcomes which midwives could contribute to directly or indirectly is critiqued and presented in sections on teenage mothers, smoking, breastfeeding, and psychological morbidity. Each section describes the outcomes of specific postnatal interventions that may have been undertaken to improve health behaviour or well-being, and where appropriate, antenatal interventions that included impact on postnatal outcomes. Ways in which midwifery postnatal care could be enhanced to incorporate successful interventions are outlined. Referral to national and international policy initiatives in each topic area provides the context for why change in practice may be appropriate, and will enable readers to access the full documents for further information. The importance of providing midwifery postnatal care which is flexible and tailored to needs of women, their babies and their families, is emphasised throughout the chapter.

INTRODUCTION

Midwives have always provided care to promote the public health of women, their infants and their families. For much of the first half of the last century, the majority of midwifery care was provided in women's homes, with medical consultation only sought if deemed appropriate. During the latter half of the century hospital was assumed to be the safest place for women to give birth, and consequently the home birth rate declined steadily. This decline increased the focus of community midwifery on the provision of antenatal and postnatal care.

Midwives continue to play a vital role in enhancing the short- and long-term well-being of women and their families during and after pregnancy, despite the move of maternity care into the acute sector. This chapter describes the background to the provision of midwifery postnatal care, the content and organisation of current care, and how this could be tailored to meet public health needs of women and their families and achieve specific health targets. The chapter concludes with a series of recommendations for practice and further research to enhance the contribution of postnatal care to public health.

POSTNATAL CARE PROVISION BY MIDWIVES

HISTORICAL PERSPECTIVE

When the first Midwives Act was passed by Parliament in 1902, it was one of a range of initiatives aimed at improving public health. The Act led to the subsequent establishment in 1905 of the Central Midwives Board, which published the first Midwives Rules and Regulations, which clearly defined the roles and responsibilities of midwives. In relation to postnatal care, the rules and regulations were very proscriptive, probably as a consequence of the major public health concerns of the time.

At the turn of the twentieth century maternal mortality was extremely high, with one in every two hundred women dying as a consequence of childbirth, the main causes of death being puerperal sepsis and haemorrhage. The impact of pregnancy and childbirth on the lives and health of working women is beautifully illustrated in letters first published in 1915, many written by women prevented from seeking advice or assistance because of prevailing views of modesty and the expected behaviour of 'respectable' women (Llewelyn Davies 1977). The maternal mortality rate continued to be high, despite a fall in death rates from all diseases in the general population from around 1870 onwards. This dramatic reduction was not solely a consequence of improvements in medicine, but resulted from improvements in social and sanitary conditions that led to fewer people dying from infectious disease. Ironically, maternal mortality was often higher amongst middle-class women, whose families were most likely to pay for medical rather than the less expensive midwifery care.

Despite concerns over maternal mortality, midwifery care was not freely available to all women until 1936. This was a period during which there was increased professional rivalry between general practitioners and midwives, with the British Medical Association opposing the report of the Joint Committee of Midwives that there should be free access to midwifery care. Despite the opposition, the incentive to pass legislation to integrate midwives in private practice within public maternity services culminated in the passing of the 1936 Midwives Act. Changes to social services, welfare benefits and the health service during and after the Second World War contributed to a sudden and dramatic decline in maternal mortality, alongside advances in antibiotic therapy, drugs to control haemorrhage, increased availability of blood transfusion services and the establishment of obstetric flying squads. In 1943, the death rate fell to 2.3 deaths per 1,000 registered births. The most recent triennial Confidential Enquiry into Maternal Death which covered all deaths occurring between 1997 and 1999 found a maternal mortality rate of 11.4 deaths per 100,000 maternities, including both *direct* and *indirect* deaths (Lewis & Drife 2001).

Since the passing of the first Midwives Act, there have been few changes to the rules and regulations governing what midwives should do when they visit postnatal women and how often they should be visited. In 1905 the Central Midwives Board established the minimum duration after delivery during which women should receive midwifery care at 10 days. During this time, the woman was expected to take strict bed rest and receive daily visits from the midwife, the focus of the visits being the identification and prevention of infection. The rules stated that a woman was to be visited twice a day for the first 3 days following her delivery, and then to receive daily visits until day 10.

The content of each postnatal visit followed a ritualistic pattern, with set timings for the completion of each observation and examination and strict protocols for hand washing (Leap & Hunter 1993), such was the great fear of infection. Midwives were expected to undertake daily observations of a woman's temperature, pulse, blood pressure and assess uterine involution (to ensure the uterus is returning to a pelvic organ) and vaginal blood loss (the lochia). The woman's legs were also to be examined for the possible occurrence of deep vein thrombosis (DVT), although confining women to bed for 10 days probably increased the risk of DVT.

Although intrapartum care gradually transferred from the home to the hospital, community-based postnatal care has continued to adhere to a very traditional pattern in both content and duration. The only changes include reduced in-patient stay after delivery and the dropping in 1986 of the specification that a midwife had to make twice daily home visits for the first 3 days, followed by daily visits until day 10, in favour of a policy of 'selective' home visiting (UKCC 1992). The policy of selective visiting was introduced with no evidence to support or facilitate the alteration to practice, and no guidance on how to determine the number and frequency of visits appropriate to meet individual postnatal needs.

Thus, postnatal care provision has remained largely unaltered during the century since its inception, with no guidance on how care could be tailored to meet need and, until recently, little evidence of whether the provision of care benefited women's physical and psychological health (Marchant & Garcia 1995, MacArthur et al 2002). The most recently issued Nursing and Midwifery Council rules state only that midwives should 'care for and monitor the progress of the mother in the postnatal period and give all necessary advice to the mother on infant care to enable her to ensure the optimum progress of the new-born infant'. In relation to the duration of postnatal care provision by midwives, the NMC defines the postnatal period as a 'period of not less than 10 and not more than 28 days after the end of labour, during which the continued attendance of a midwife on the mother is requisite'. There are currently no plans to revise the rules with regard to postnatal care.

The midwifery contribution to the public health agenda during the postnatal period can include support for nationally and/or locally agreed priorities to reduce health inequalities. For example, smoking cessation and reduction in teenage pregnancy were two areas highlighted in the first national health inequalities targets (DH 2001). Postnatal care can also address other areas known to enhance short- and long-term health of the public, such as promotion and support for breastfeeding, advice on infant immunisation, nutrition, health promotion, and provision of information on screening. Midwives can also contribute to government programmes to assist women and their families in targeted areas of deprivation, for example through Sure Start projects and involvement with local health needs assessment initiatives. These are all important public health initiatives, but ways in which appropriate and timely care can be targeted to those with the greatest need have to be considered against the need to provide a statutory midwifery service to all women after childbirth.

POSTNATAL CARE AND PUBLIC HEALTH PRIORITIES

The following sections focus on four public health topics that can be addressed within the current organisation and content of midwifery care during the postnatal period. These are teenage mothers; smoking; breastfeeding; and psychological morbidity. Reference will be made to how the content and organisation of midwifery postnatal care can address health needs in these areas. It is acknowledged that other postnatal health topics also fall within the public health agenda, such as puerperal infection and postpartum haemorrhage. However, topics have been included which are priorities from a national perspective and commonly encountered by midwives providing postnatal care. Evidence in relation to public health practice (for example, the provision of an intervention) and public health science (for example, demonstrating evidence of benefit) are described, which are not mutually exclusive and should be viewed as a continuum. The importance of midwives being able to identify and manage some commonly experienced health problems after childbirth, which may impact on a woman's short- and long-term physical and psychological well-being, will also be highlighted.

TEENAGE MOTHERS

> In the world's rich nations, more than three quarters of a million teenagers will become mothers in the next twelve months.
>
> (United Nations Children's Fund 2001)

Until recently, becoming pregnant during the teenage years was viewed as normal and even desirable; physiologically, giving birth at 18 or 19 may be better than commencing childbearing later in life, which is the current trend in the UK and other developed countries. Concerns from a public health perspective relate in the main to the inequalities in health and socio-economic status faced by teenage women and their infants. Teenage pregnancy is almost ten times higher for a woman whose family is in social class V than those in social class I, and infant mortality for babies of teenage mothers is 60% higher than for infants born to older women. There is debate as to whether a higher frequency of adverse perinatal outcome among first teenage pregnancies is an independent association, or explained by confounding factors such as socio-economic class and maternal smoking (Berenson et al 1997, Olausson et al 1999). A recent retrospective cohort study from Scotland found that second births to non-smoking teenage mothers aged 15–19 were associated with an almost threefold risk of pre-term delivery and stillbirth (Smith & Pell 2001).

The achievement of a reduction in the teenage pregnancy rate in the UK, as described in Chapter 9, will clearly involve contributions from a range of health, education and social support agencies. The postnatal role of the midwife caring for a teenage mother can be targeted across a range of activities within this remit, as well as in relation to other areas, to enhance maternal and infant health. For example, midwives should advise on infant care and support for breastfeeding (described later in this chapter), facilitate access to social support, and identify and manage postnatal morbidity. Care provision could also include advice on sexual health problems, including protection against future unwanted pregnancy and sexually transmitted diseases (STDs).

Traditionally, midwifery postnatal care has included provision of advice on contraception, although guidance for midwives is limited and there is a dearth of information on the benefit of any advice thus given and optimal timing of it. Nevertheless, midwives should ensure teenage women they care for are asked about their contraceptive needs as soon as appropriate after the birth, especially as it is now apparent that over a third of women may have resumed intercourse within 6 weeks of giving birth (Sleep et al 1984, Klein et al 1994, Barrett et al 2000). It has been well documented that use of contraception by young people is inconsistent (Ingham et al 2001), and improvement of access to contraceptive services is seen as key to the government's strategy to reduce the rate of conceptions among the under-18s (DH 2000a). The Teenage Pregnancy Unit, which is based in the Department of Health and co-ordinates implementation of the Teenage Pregnancy Strategy in England, has issued Best Practice Guidance on the provision of effective contraception and advice services for young people (DH 2000a). These include the need to involve young people in the planning of services, ensuring confidentiality is maintained and any advice is non-judgemental. Teenagers who do not wish to have another pregnancy in the near future should be advised of the need to recommence contraception within at least 21 days of the birth, when ovulation may recommence. Referral to the GP or Family Planning Clinic should be made for those who may wish to commence oral contraception, or if they wish to discuss other options for contraception. Consideration when providing advice on a request for contraception made by someone under 16 has to be given within the current legal framework, and midwives should ensure they are familiar with this. If midwives require advice on action to co-ordinate the Teenage Pregnancy Strategy in their locality, each local authority has a teenage pregnancy co-ordinator. Twenty Sure Start Plus pilot projects are also underway, which provide support for pregnant teenagers and teenage parents on a variety of health, social and childcare issues.

A recent Australian trial aimed to ascertain if a postnatal home visiting service for teenagers under 18, the content of which was structured to particular needs of this group, could reduce the frequency of adverse neonatal outcomes and improve knowledge of contraception, infant vaccination schedules and breastfeeding (Quinlivan et al 2003). Of the young women who attended a teenage pregnancy clinic, 139 were entered into the trial antenatally and 136 allocated immediately after delivery to receive either five structured postnatal home visits by nurse-midwives in addition to routine postnatal care (n = 71), or usual care (n = 65). Three women were withdrawn before randomisation because of late fetal loss. All teenagers were asked to complete an antenatal questionnaire designed to assess their knowledge of the health areas described above. The questionnaires were completed with the assistance of a midwife, their unprompted answers being recorded verbatim. Level of knowledge was scored later by a member of the research team who was unaware of the teenager's identity or group allocation. For contraception the total score achievable was 9; for infant vaccination it was 10; and for benefits of breastfeeding the maximum available overall score was 11. Those in the intervention group received structured home visits at 1 week, 2 weeks, 1 month, 2 and 4 months after the birth, with visits lasting for 1–4 hours. Each visit was to include advice related to a specific health area for the teenager and her infant, appropriate to expected recovery and development and relevant to service provision at that point in time, as well as ensuring screening and other social issues were addressed. Information to support why five postnatal visits were provided was not presented. The primary trial outcomes were knowledge in the health areas of interest and incidence of predefined adverse neonatal outcome. At 6 months post partum, a postnatal assessment visit was undertaken during which a questionnaire identical to that administered antenatally was completed and scored. In addition, the teenagers were asked about use of contraception, compliance with infant vaccination schedules and duration of breastfeeding.

The results showed that the addition of the structured home visits resulted in a reduction in adverse neonatal outcomes, and increased knowledge and use of contraception. There was a small non-significant increase in knowledge of infant immunisation schedules in the intervention group, but the proportion of women whose babies had been vaccinated at 6 months did not differ between the groups and there was no increase in knowledge of benefits of breastfeeding or the median duration of breastfeeding.

Contraception and sexual health should not be discussed in isolation from resumption of intercourse. Research into women's experiences of sexual health problems after delivery is limited, with information on prevalence arising from observational studies and trials of perineal management. Data that are available are therefore only applicable to groups of particular parity or mode of delivery. Brown and Lumley (1998) contacted 1336 women 6–7 months post partum in a cross-sectional study of all deliveries occurring over a 2-week period in one region in Australia, and found 26% had experienced a 'sexual problem' some time since their delivery. No information on the specification or duration of the problem was elicited. Barrett et al (2000) conducted a cross-sectional study of all primiparous women who delivered at one maternity unit in London, to enquire about a range of sexual health problems. Postal questionnaires were sent at 6 months post partum to 796 primiparae, asking about sexual health problems since the birth and prior to pregnancy; 484 (61%) women replied. Women were asked to recall when they had first resumed intercourse; by 6 weeks 32% had resumed intercourse, 62% had done so by 8 weeks and 81% by 3 months. The researchers asked women about experiences of dyspareunia, which they described as including painful penetration and/or pain during intercourse or orgasm. This was reported by 62% of women at some time during the first 3 months after the birth, and still experienced by 31% at 6 months post partum. Other sexual health problems included loss of sexual desire, reported by 53% in the first 3 months and 37% at 6 months. Several other problems were also reported at 6 months, including vaginal tightness (20%), vaginal looseness or lack of muscle tone (12%) and lack of vaginal lubrication (26%). Although only two thirds of women returned a questionnaire, these data do highlight that sexual health problems after childbirth are common and persistent.

The importance of the midwife asking teenage mothers about sexual health problems is highlighted as they may have one or more risk factors for dyspareunia. These have been identified as mode of delivery, perineal trauma and primiparity, which are all highly interrelated and likely to be variables that include higher proportions of younger women. Higher rates of perineal pain have been reported after instrumental delivery. Glazener et al (1995), in a representative sample of all deliveries over a defined period, found 42% reported perineal pain when questioned in hospital, 22% reported experiencing this between then and 8 weeks post partum; and when questioned again at 12–18 months post partum, 9.8% had experienced perineal pain at some time between 8 weeks and 12–18 months. Differences in perineal pain were clearly related to mode of delivery. Prevalence of pain whilst still in hospital was 84% after instrumental delivery, 42% after a spontaneous vaginal delivery and 5% after caesarean section. Barrett et al (2000) in the study described earlier found that dyspareunia occurring some time during the 3 months after delivery was reported by 62% of women following spontaneous vaginal delivery, 78% after instrumental delivery (forceps or ventouse), 41% after an emergency caesarean section and 47% following elective caesarean section. Logistic regression showed that the difference for instrumental relative to spontaneous vaginal delivery remained significant (OR 2.41, 95% CI 1.24–4.69), but differences for both types of caesarean section did not.

Evidence to support the most effective interventions to relieve dyspareunia is limited, as many studies have only examined experience of pain. One Cochrane Review of the use of therapeutic ultrasound to treat acute and persistent perineal pain and dyspareunia following childbirth, which included four trials involving 659 women, concluded that there was insufficient evidence to evaluate benefit (Hay-Smith 2004). One way midwives could help is to advise women who have had perineal trauma that resumption of intercourse may be painful, which may provide some reassurance, and ensure that referral is made to their GP if pain persists.

Many teenage mothers will have specific health and social support needs, as well as needs which are as relevant for all new mothers. There is limited guidance on optimal organisation and content of services in the UK for teenage parents, including specific interventions to reduce future unplanned pregnancies (DH 2000a), and although the trial by Quinlivan and colleagues (2003) suggests tailored interventions to very young mothers may increase awareness of contraception and improve outcomes for their babies, it would have to be replicated in a UK population. It is important that midwives discuss contraception and sexual health, and ensure teenage mothers have every opportunity to state what they want from postnatal care, rather than providing care based on their own perceptions of the needs of the teenager. Other public health initiatives relevant to the health and well-being of teenage mothers and their infants, such as smoking cessation and uptake and prevention of early cessation of breastfeeding, are discussed later in this chapter.

SMOKING

There is a strong association between smoking and socio-economic status, with higher proportions of regular smokers found amongst people in lower socio-economic groups. It is the biggest cause of preventable death in the western world, killing more than 120,000 people in the UK each year (Health Development Agency 2003). Over half (54%) of babies and young children from lower socio-economic backgrounds are exposed to 'passive smoking' or environmental tobacco smoke (ETS), compared to 18% of those from higher socio-economic backgrounds (Health Development Agency 2003). The current Government's national target is a reduction from 23% to 15% in the proportion of women who smoke during pregnancy by 2010 (DH 2001).

Smoking during pregnancy can contribute to potentially adverse effects on the health of the woman and the fetus. It is one of the few potentially preventable factors associated with low infant birth weight (<2.5 kg), premature birth and perinatal death (Lumley et al 2004).

Smoking has also been strongly associated with elevated risk of placenta praevia, abruptio placentae, ectopic pregnancy and premature rupture of the membranes (Castles et al 1999). Infant exposure to ETS has been associated with development of other adverse events including serious respiratory illness and asthma attacks, sudden infant death syndrome (SIDS) and middle ear disease (Blair et al 1996).

Despite a plethora of general population studies investigating a range of interventions to encourage people to stop or reduce smoking, there has been little change in prevalence in recent decades. Because of their more frequent contact with the health services during and after pregnancy, many studies have developed, implemented and evaluated interventions specifically targeted at pregnant women. Outcomes were mostly related to reduction of smoking at specific points during the pregnancy, but some studies included outcomes on smoking prevalence in the immediate postnatal period. No studies were identified during the preparation of this chapter that examined specific *postnatal* interventions to reduce smoking prevalence. Findings in relation to smoking cessation interventions during pregnancy, some of which included postpartum outcomes, and studies that investigated specific postnatal effects, are therefore described.

A Cochrane Library review of interventions for promoting smoking cessation in pregnancy (Lumley et al 2004) aimed to assess the effects of smoking cessation programmes implemented during pregnancy on the health of the fetus and infant, the woman and the family. A total of 44 trials were identified and included in the review, comprising data on over 17,000 women. Only seven studies were from the UK. Based on pooled data from 34 randomised controlled trials (reasons for excluding trials from the pooled analyses included, for example, lack of adjustment to take account of the effects of clustering in cluster randomised trials), there was a significant reduction in smoking in the intervention groups (OR 0.53, 95% CI 0.47–0.60), an absolute difference of 6.4% women continuing to smoke. Eight trials which used a validated smoking intervention package had high-quality study methodology and high-intensity interventions, with an absolute difference in quit rates of 8.1%. The studies used a diverse range of interventions, intervention duration times and personnel to deliver the intervention. The difficulties of implementing an intervention developed for a previous study using a sample drawn from a different population setting, and variation in replication of findings, suggest that smoking cessation interventions have to be culturally appropriate for the intended target population. The reviewers recommended that although effect sizes were small, given the findings that programmes increased smoking cessation, increased mean birth weight and reduced low birth weight, they should be implemented in all maternity care settings. The most appropriate intervention to use remains unclear.

One recent cluster randomised controlled trial from the UK, not included in the above review, designed to evaluate the effectiveness of a self-help approach to smoking cessation in pregnancy using booklets, found this was ineffective when implemented as part of routine antenatal care (Moore et al 2002). The study took place across three NHS trusts in England and recruited 1527 women who smoked at the start of their pregnancy (724 intervention, 803 control). Women who could speak English and who smoked before becoming pregnant were eligible for recruitment, after giving written consent to participate in the trial. Community midwives (128) were randomised to provide the intervention or current care. Those providing the intervention were instructed to spend at least 5 minutes introducing the first of five booklets to the pregnant women they provided care for, in addition to providing routine care. The booklets were developed specifically for pregnancy and designed to enable the women to use the smoking cessation programme flexibly and in a way that suited them individually. The remaining four booklets were mailed to the woman at weekly intervals. The primary outcome measure was validated smoking cessation at the end of the second trimester of pregnancy, with other outcomes reported, including smoking status and cigarette consumption. All participants who stated they had not smoked for at least 7 days in a self complete postal questionnaire sent at 26 weeks' gestation were visited by a research midwife who collected a urine sample for cotinine assay.

There were no significant differences between intervention and control groups and validated smoking cessation rate (18.8% and 20.7% respectively, 95% CI −3.5 to 7.3) and no differences in self reported smoking status or self reported mean daily cigarette consumption. Qualitative data collected on the delivery of the intervention showed this was variable; some midwives reported spending longer than 5 minutes introducing the first booklet, whilst others reported spending less time. The intervention midwives reported that they found the booklets prompted them to give consistent and coherent smoking cessation advice in a non-judgemental and positive way, but none of the women who received the intervention said the booklets helped them to quit. The researchers postulated that in view of increased evidence showing that behaviour does not change as a consequence of receiving written materials alone, the lack of verbal reinforcement from the midwife may have attenuated the potential effect of the intervention.

Some of the effects of smoking in pregnancy have been assessed in relation to specific postnatal health factors, including determinants of breastfeeding duration within 3 months of the birth (Horta et al 2001). Horta and colleagues (2001) undertook a systematic review and meta-analysis of studies that had observed a shorter duration of lactation among women who smoked. The authors identified 28 papers, 13 of which provided sufficient data to enable a meta-analysis to be performed. Studies were excluded if they included infants who had never been breastfed. The results showed that even after taking account of possible confounding factors, such as age and socio-economic status, in smoking compared with non-smoking women, the random effects pooled odds ratio for weaning before 3 months was 1.93 (95% CI 1.55–1.93). Women who smoked during and after pregnancy and who commenced breastfeeding, increased their risk of early weaning.

In addition to smoking cessation programmes that rely on educational, cognitive behavioural and other self help interventions, pharmacological interventions are now available, but these are contraindicated for pregnant women and some groups of postnatal women. Nicotine replacement therapy (NRT) and bupropion were recently recommended by the National Institute for Clinical Excellence (NICE), which provides guidance for NHS care in England and Wales, including medications available on NHS prescription. The treatments can be prescribed for smokers who want to quit, but only if they have made a commitment to stop smoking on or before a specific date (NICE 2002). Smokers under 18, who are pregnant or breastfeeding, or have unstable cardiovascular disorders, are recommended to discuss use of NRT with a relevant health care professional before use, whilst bupropion is not recommended for women who are pregnant or breastfeeding.

It would now seem appropriate for midwives providing postnatal care to routinely ask women at their first postnatal home visit if they smoke and if they would like help and support to stop smoking, as opposed to restricting this question to their antenatal booking visit. This is particularly important given the high relapse rate for women who have stopped smoking during pregnancy (Walsh et al 2001). Although the type of support most appropriate for postnatal women has not been identified, it is likely that some form of high quality smoking cessation intervention used in antenatal or general populations would be appropriate, but this would have to be tailored to needs after childbirth. Although midwives have an important role in identifying postnatal women who want support to continue to reduce or to stop smoking, conclusive evidence that they are the most appropriate health professionals to implement the intervention is not yet available. Whatever cessation programme is implemented, it is imperative that it is undertaken within a strategy for smoking cessation adopted by the whole primary health care team. Further research in this area is required in relation to postnatal care.

BREASTFEEDING

One of the most important contributions to public health that can be directly supported by midwives after the birth, is increased uptake and reduced early cessation of breastfeeding. Several health benefits have been associated with breastfeeding, including protection of the infant from gastro-enteritis, respiratory infection, otitis media, urinary tract infections and diabetes mellitus (Howie et al 1990). Health benefits for the woman include protection against pre-menopausal breast cancer, ovarian and endometrial cancers (DH 1994) and a possibility of protection against hip fractures in older age (DH 1998).

Despite evidence of benefits for the woman and her infant, successive 5-year surveys of infant feeding undertaken by the Office of National Statistics show breastfeeding rates in the UK have, until recently, remained static. In 1980, 65% of women in England and Wales commenced breastfeeding and in 1990, 63% of women commenced breastfeeding. There have since been small increases, with 68% of women in England and Wales in the 1995 survey commencing breastfeeding (Foster et al 1997) and 71% in 2000, which presented results from the sixth national survey (Hamlyn et al 2002). It is important to note, however, that the composition in the profile of the sample used in the 2000 survey differed from the previous sample, in that there were more mothers aged

30 or over, and more who had continued in education beyond 19 years of age. Both of these factors are strongly associated with breastfeeding uptake. Hence, overall rates would have increased simply as a consequence of changes in the composition of the sample, even if the rates for different groups remained constant.

Department of Health guidance on breastfeeding published in 1994 estimated that the NHS could save £35 million pounds each year in treatment for gastro-enteritis alone if all babies were breastfed, representing a saving of £300,000 for the average health district (DH 1994). Savings at current costs are likely to be much higher. Policies to increase the prevalence of breastfeeding have been recommended to reduce health inequalities. The Infant Feeding Initiative was launched in 1999 as part of the Government's commitment to reduce health inequalities by increasing the incidence and duration of breastfeeding amongst groups in the population with the lowest breastfeeding rates. The initiative also aims to assist all women make an informed choice about how they feed their infant.

Initiation of breastfeeding

Uptake of breastfeeding in the UK is strongly associated with social class, with 90% of women in social class I commencing breastfeeding in 1995 compared with only 50% of women in social class V (Foster et al 1997). In the 2000 survey (Hamlyn et al 2002), socio-economic classification was based on the mother's as opposed to her partner's occupation, and the system of classification was based on the new Office of National Statistics (ONS) classification – the National Statistics Socio-Economic Classification (NS-SEC) introduced in 2001. Although a different classification system was used, mothers in the UK classified into higher occupations were more likely to commence breastfeeding; 85% of women classed to higher occupations, compared with 73% in intermediate and 59% in lower occupations. When social class data using information on the husband's or partner's occupation were used to examine changes in breastfeeding incidence over time, a significant increase was observed between 1995 and 2000 in social class group IIINM in England and Wales. In Scotland significant increases were observed in non-manual social class groups I and II, manual group IV and no partner, whilst in Northern Ireland, significant increases were found in social class groups II, IIINM, IIIM and IV. Women from ethnic minority groups included in the 2000 survey were considerably more likely to commence breastfeeding than white women; comparative data on ethnicity from 1995 were not available (Hamlyn et al 2002).

The majority of women will have decided during the antenatal period which method of infant feeding they will commence. White et al (1992), reporting on the national infant feeding survey for 1990, found 93% of women had made this decision during their pregnancy. A recent systematic review evaluated the effectiveness of interventions to promote the initiation of breastfeeding (NHS Centre for Reviews and Dissemination 2000). Interventions were classified into five categories: health education; health sector initiatives; peer support programmes; media campaigns; and multifaceted interventions. Many of the studies identified were implemented and evaluated in the USA, where health care funding and organisation are very different from the UK; nevertheless a number of recommendations for policy and practice were made by the reviewers. These included the need to consider a revision of local and national policy to reflect an evidence-based approach to the promotion of breastfeeding, with emphasis placed on reduction of health inequalities in line with The NHS Plan (Department of Health 2000b). The reviewers found limited evidence on the cost effectiveness of interventions to promote breastfeeding initiation and the acceptability of these interventions to the women.

One of the most significant variables that appear to affect a woman's decision to breastfeed (and when she should stop – see below) is the support of her partner; a partner's indifference to breastfeeding is associated with much higher rates of formula feeding (Bick et al 1998). When midwives are advising women antenatally about benefits of breastfeeding, involvement of their partner and other supportive family members would appear to be of benefit. It would also appear to be important to involve a woman's partner and/or her relatives when discussing the commencement of breastfeeding.

There may be some cases where an infant is not ready to commence breastfeeding. Infants have been shown to exhibit a wide range of feeding behaviour following a normal vaginal birth (Henschel & Inch 1996), and taking longer time to first feed has been reported following particular obstetric intervention such as induction of labour, use of pethidine and caesarean section (Rajan 1994). In the 2000 Infant Feeding survey, there was a difference in incidence of breastfeeding according to type of analgesia women received during their labour. Only 62% of women who had a general anaesthetic breastfed, compared with 71% who had an epidural and 72% who had no analgesia (Hamlyn et al 2002). The survey also found that women who first held their infants within an hour of birth were more likely to start breastfeeding than those who did not hold their infants within this hour, although this was only in evidence for Scotland and Northern Ireland, and not England and Wales.

Support to continue breastfeeding

The majority of women who wish to breastfeed will commence this whilst on the postnatal ward, although lactation is unlikely to start until after discharge home, highlighting the importance of the role of the midwife working in the community to support women who choose to breastfeed. It is apparent, however, that many women who commence breastfeeding will stop within a few weeks of delivery (Foster et al 1997, Hamlyn et al 2002). Almost half of women stop within 6 weeks of the birth (Bick et al 1998), well below the recommended minimum duration of 6 months (WHO 2002). In 2000, 15% of women who commenced breastfeeding in England and Wales gave up within a week of delivery, some of whom may still have been on a postnatal ward. One of the most frequent complaints about postnatal care is the provision of advice from health professionals that is inconsistent, especially on breastfeeding (Rajan 1993, Audit Commission 1997). As it is likely that the majority of breastfeeding problems could be prevented if women are able to feed their infants effectively and efficiently from the first breastfeed (Inch 1999), the importance of providing correct, consistent and timely advice is highlighted. The Baby Friendly Initiative, a worldwide programme established by the World

Health Organization (WHO) and UNICEF, includes among its ten steps to successful breastfeeding that all staff are trained in the skills required to implement the policy (WHO/UNICEF 1989).

Despite national initiatives to increase breastfeeding uptake and duration, women continue to report a range of problems experienced on the postnatal ward and at home, which in some cases will inform a decision to change to bottle feeding. Of women questioned for the Infant Feeding Survey 2000, 32% who breastfed reported they experienced problems in hospital, more commonly that the infant would not latch on or would not suck; sore or cracked nipples; that the infant appeared to be hungry or they had insufficient milk (Hamlyn et al 2002). Of women still breastfeeding when discharged home, 35% reported breastfeeding problems within the first few weeks. More commonly reported at this stage were sore nipples (40%) and the infant appearing to be hungry (32%); 24% still reported having problems when trying to get the infant to latch on to the breast. Women who gave up within a week of the birth were more likely to report different problems from women who gave up within a second week of the birth, findings which have implications for the type of support that should be offered. Women who gave up within a week were more likely to report that this was because their baby did not suck or rejected the breast, whereas those who gave up in the second week reported insufficiency of milk, painful breasts and breastfeeding taking too much time.

As referred to earlier, relatives and friends can exert a strong influence on a woman's decision to breastfeed; they can also influence when a woman decides to stop breastfeeding. In the 2000 Infant Feeding Survey, breastfeeding mothers who were themselves entirely bottle-fed were more likely to stop breastfeeding within 2 weeks of the birth (Hamlyn et al 2002). In consequence, women who had been entirely breastfed were more likely to be still breastfeeding at 4 weeks (77%) than those who had been bottle-fed (63%). The importance of the influence of a woman's family and friends as to whether she will breastfeed at all, and whether she will continue to do so beyond 2 weeks of the birth, were highlighted by the authors of the survey. As studies that have examined factors affecting breastfeeding duration have usually been based on quantitative methods, subtle social and cultural influences that may affect decisions to choose and continue to breastfeed have not been identified, and research using appropriate methodology to identify these is required.

There remains uncertainty as to the most effective way of providing support to women who choose to breastfeed (Sikorski et al 2003). A Cochrane Review to assess the effects of breastfeeding support which identified 20 trials involving over 23,000 mother–infant pairs found a beneficial effect on the duration of any breastfeeding in a meta-analysis of *all* forms of additional support, the effect being greater for exclusive breastfeeding (Sikorski et al 2003). Extra professional support (which included medical, nursing, midwifery and allied health professionals) appeared beneficial for any breastfeeding (RR 0.89, 95% CI 0.81–0.97) and for exclusive breastfeeding, although the effect did not achieve full statistical significance (RR 0.90, 95% CI 0.81–1.01). Lay support was effective in reducing the cessation of exclusive breastfeeding (RR 0.66, 95% CI 0.49–0.89), but its effect on any breastfeeding did not achieve statistical significance (RR 0.84, 95% CI 0.69–1.02). The reviewers concluded that consideration should be given to the provision of supplementary breastfeeding support as part of routine health service provision, but further evidence was required to assess the clinical and cost effectiveness of both lay and professional support in different health care settings.

Midwives were the health professional group women were most likely to turn to for advice on breastfeeding issues in the 2000 Infant Feeding Survey (Hamlyn et al 2002). Thus in addition to knowing how to support women to commence effective and pain-free breastfeeding, midwives also need to know how to identify and manage breastfeeding problems if they do occur and support women to resolve these, particularly in light of the findings of the review described above. All advice offered should be consistent and reflect best practice. Evidence-based guidelines are available to inform practice in relation to a series of problems such as painful breasts and engorgement (Bick et al 2002), as well as the management of women who may require additional breastfeeding support, for example, multiple birth or babies who develop physiological jaundice. It is also appropriate to refer women to voluntary organisations such as La Leche League and the National Childbirth Trust, which can provide additional breastfeeding support.

PSYCHOLOGICAL MORBIDITY

Psychological morbidity after childbirth is a major public health problem, with prevalence rates for depression ranging from 10% to 15% depending on assessment times and diagnostic criteria. Recent studies have found long-lasting consequences of psychological morbidity for the woman and her child, with increasing evidence of an association between maternal depression and the child's behavioural and cognitive development (Sharp et al 1995, Hay et al 2001). Studies have examined the impact of a range of interventions implemented during the antenatal and postnatal periods to reduce adverse health outcomes, including postpartum psychological morbidity.

Antenatal interventions

One antenatal intervention examined the effect of additional support from midwives for women at high risk of delivering a low birth-weight baby (<2.5 kg) and also assessed the impact on maternal physical and psychological morbidity (Oakley et al 1990). Women who had previously delivered a low birth-weight baby were invited to participate in the trial; 243 were randomised to the intervention group and 234 to the control. The intervention comprised a programme of three antenatal home visits, two further brief visits or a telephone consultation, and access to a 24-hour helpline provided by midwives. The primary study outcome was infant birth weight, with effects on psychological well-being of the mother and other aspects of postnatal health included as secondary outcomes. At 6 weeks postpartum, analysis of the secondary outcomes showed that women in the intervention group were less likely to have reported feeling depressed (40 vs 47%), to have reported a feeling of having no/low control over their lives (28 vs 37%), or to have consulted their GP (27 vs 32%). These effects persisted when the study population was followed up at

1 and 7 years later (Oakley 1992, Oakley et al 1996). Larger studies with maternal psychological and physical well-being as primary outcome measures are now required, to assess if these findings can be replicated.

Educational and psycho-social interventions, some provided by midwives, have also been evaluated in several studies to assess impact on prevention of postnatal depression. Stamp et al (1995) in a randomised controlled trial from Australia, asked women at 24 weeks' gestation to complete a Modified Antenatal Screening Questionnaire to identify those more likely to develop postnatal depression. The study hypothesis was that women identified as vulnerable to develop depression who attended two antenatal and one postnatal group session provided by a midwife educator would be less likely to develop the symptom. Of the 249 women screened, 144 (58%) were identified as more vulnerable and were randomly allocated to the intervention (n = 73) or control (n = 71) groups. There were no differences between the groups when measured using the Edinburgh Postnatal Depression Scale at 6 weeks, 3 months and 6 months after the delivery. However, overall attendance at the classes was very low at only 31%. As postulated by the researchers, this may have been because the classes were held separately from the usual antenatal classes offered.

Sikorski and colleagues (1996) compared clinical and psycho-social effectiveness of the traditional antenatal visit schedule (13 visits) with a reduced schedule of visits for low-risk women (7 for primiparous and 6 for multiparous women). Antenatal consultations were undertaken by the midwife or the GP. Of the 2794 women randomised to the trial groups, 1416 had the traditional and 1378 the new model of care. Main study outcomes were fetal and maternal morbidity, health service use and psycho-social health, data on which were obtained at 34 weeks' gestation and 6 weeks post partum. There were no differences in psychological outcomes at either time point, although women who received the new model of care were significantly more likely to be concerned about fetal well-being and had more negative attitudes to their baby during and after their pregnancy. The study findings should be interpreted with caution, as there was divergence in the visit schedule, with women in the traditional care arm receiving 1.65 fewer visits than planned and women in the new model group receiving 2.60 more visits. As the unit of randomisation was the individual and not the GP practice, it is possible that contamination occurred between the groups, as women receiving one form of care may have talked about this to women receiving the other form of care.

The impact of midwifery-led care has also been evaluated in relation to women's psychological health (Turnbull et al 1996, Shields et al 1997). A Midwifery Development Unit (MDU) was established at Glasgow Royal Maternity Hospital to provide care to women classed antenatally as having low obstetric risk; of 1299 women thus identified, 648 were randomised to receive care from the MDU and 651 to receive usual care (Turnbull et al 1996). The primary trial outcome was obstetric intervention; however, secondary outcomes for assessment at 7 months post partum included a woman's EPDS score (excluding one of 10 items which asks if women have considered thoughts of harming themselves within the previous 7 days); infant feeding; ratings of postnatal care and preparation for parenthood. There was a significant difference in questionnaire return rate at 7 months, with 72% of women in the intervention group returning a questionnaire compared with 63% in the control (Shields et al 1997). The mean EPDS score for women who received MDU care was significantly lower (8.1) compared with women in the control (9.0), a lower score indicating 'better' mental health. However, the EPDS has not been validated as a nine-item scale. Other aspects of care were also rated more highly by women in the MDU group. The findings of this study should also be interpreted with caution, given the differential in the questionnaire return rate and that MDU midwives had volunteered to work on the unit and may have had characteristics that differed from the general midwifery population.

The most recent UK Confidential Enquiries into Maternal Deaths which covered the triennium 1997–1999 recommended women should be screened at antenatal booking for previous psychiatric history, recording severity of depression, care received and clinical presentation, to enable prompt and appropriate management of any recurrence during the maternity episode (Lewis & Drife 2001). Midwives undoubtedly have an important role in ensuring this recommendation is complied with, but evaluation of training needs and implications for health service provision are required before implementation of the recommendation.

Postnatal interventions

The provision of midwifery-led debriefing to prevent postnatal depression has been evaluated in two recent trials from the UK and Australia. Lavender and Walkinshaw (1998) carried out a small randomised controlled trial at a regional teaching hospital in the north-west of England to examine if postnatal debriefing by midwives reduced psychological morbidity after childbirth. Primiparous women who had a normal vaginal delivery of a term infant were allocated to the intervention (n = 56) or routine care (n = 58): total 114. The intervention comprised an interview with the research midwife (who had not been present at the delivery), which included questions on the woman's labour and her feelings about this. The interviews, which took place on the postnatal ward, lasted for between 30 and 120 minutes. Women were then sent a questionnaire at 3 weeks after the delivery which included the main outcome measure, the Hospital Anxiety and Depression Scale (HAD). A score for the sub-scales of anxiety and depression of more than 10 was taken as an indication that the woman 'probably' had depression and should receive a clinical consultation to confirm the diagnosis.

The women in the control group were more likely to have a high HAD anxiety score or HAD depression score, but as this scale has not been validated for use after childbirth and the definition of a high score used in the analysis (≥10) differed from that used to calculate the sample size (≥7), interpretation of the study findings should be undertaken with care. It is also possible that the intervention was affected by 'the blues', a transient state of postpartum dysphoria, rather than postnatal depression.

Small and colleagues (2000) also assessed the effectiveness of midwife-led debriefing during the in-patient postnatal period in a well-designed RCT from Australia. Women were included if they had undergone an operative or instrumental delivery. The main outcome measures were depression at 6 months post partum based on an EPDS score of ⩾13, which indicates a higher risk of developing depression, and overall health status as assessed using the SF36. Of the 1041 women randomised to the trial, 624 had a caesarean section, 353 a forceps delivery and 64 a ventouse delivery. The intervention group (n = 520) had time with a research midwife who had not been involved with their care, to discuss their labour, birth and postnatal experiences.

At 6 months, 917 women responded to a postal questionnaire: 467 (90%) of the 520 intervention women and 450 (86%) of 521 women in the control group. Analysis showed that the odds of depression in the intervention group at 6 months after the birth were raised, but this difference was not statistically significant (OR 1.24, 95% CI 0.87–1.77), and mean EPDS scores did not differ between the groups. The authors postulated that their findings raised the possibility that provision of the intervention may have contributed to an experience of poorer psychological health.

There are ongoing discussions as to appropriateness and need for debriefing after childbirth, given the dearth of evidence to support provision of this intervention. A recent systematic review included in the Cochrane Library, based on 11 trials of debriefing for preventing post-traumatic stress disorder (PTSD), including the two postnatal trials, concluded that there was no evidence that this was a useful treatment to prevent PTSD and compulsory debriefing of victims of trauma should cease (Rose et al 2003). With respect to postnatal care, there is an urgent need to define what debriefing entails for women, as this may not be the correct term to describe what is offered, the optimal time for provision of such an intervention, and who should be providing it.

One recent cluster randomised controlled trial of midwifery-led care in the postnatal period did find a difference in women's psychological well-being. MacArthur and colleagues (2002) developed, implemented and evaluated a new model of midwifery-led postnatal care, which focused on the identification and management of commonly experienced maternal health problems. The intervention comprised a package of care implemented by community midwives that incorporated the use of symptom checklists and the EPDS to screen for physical and psychological health problems and evidence-based guidelines to manage any problems thus identified. GP contact was to be based on need, and not routine. Midwifery care was extended from 10 to 28 days for all women, and included an additional visit at 3 months, at which point the woman was discharged from the maternity services. The visit at 3 months replaced the routine 6–8 week consultation with the GP. Women's physical and psychological health and well-being at 4 and 12 months were the primary study outcomes, which were assessed using the EPDS and the physical and mental health components of the SF36. All outcome data were collected using a postal questionnaire.

A total of 2064 women were recruited from 36 general practice clusters (17 intervention and 19 control), 1087 of whom were randomised to the intervention and 977 to the control, with care in the clusters provided by a total of 80 midwives. Totals of 77% of the intervention group and 76%

of the control returned a questionnaire at 4 months. Analysis was performed using multi-level modelling to take account of possible cluster effect. Women who received the intervention had significantly better mental health and a lowered risk of depression. Physical health scores did not differ between the groups. When further multi-level models were performed, including maternal and cluster characteristics which may have been potential confounders, the effect sizes for mental health increased a little. Twelve-month data and data on cost effectiveness will be published in the near future.

One explanation for the difference in mental health may be that women who were identified as having physical health problems had these promptly managed by the midwife, which could have had a positive influence on their psychological well-being. The relationship between women's postnatal physical and psychological well-being is not well documented or researched. Bick and MacArthur (1995) reported the extent, severity and effect of long-term health problems after childbirth, and for the first time documented the effect of health problems on women's lives. In this retrospective study, women who delivered at one maternity unit in the West Midlands were contacted 6–7 months after the birth and asked to complete a postal questionnaire which asked about their experience of nine commonly experienced postnatal health problems; 1278 (80%) of 1667 women returned a questionnaire. Symptoms were included in the analysis if they occurred within the first 3 months of delivery and lasted for over 6 weeks; they did not have to be new symptoms. Backache, urinary stress incontinence and fatigue were the three most commonly experienced problems. Of these, fatigue was more likely to be rated by the women as severe, in contrast to backache and stress incontinence which were generally rated as less severe (although 47% of the women with stress incontinence reported that they had to wear pads to protect against leakage of urine). Symptoms affected various aspects of their lives. Backache resulted in difficulties carrying baby equipment or older children, or it restricted movement. Women who had stress incontinence reported an effect on participation in sporting activities such as aerobics. In contrast, fatigue appeared to have a much more pervasive effect on women's physical and psychological well-being. Women reported reluctance to socialise, inability to concentrate and increased irritability, although it did not appear to affect their ability to care for their baby.

Brown and Lumley (2000), in a study from Australia, examined the relationship between physical health and depression. Data were collected from a postal questionnaire sent 6–7 months after delivery to 2138 women and a telephone interview with a random selection of those who had a higher or lower EPDS score. A total of 1336 (63%) women returned a questionnaire, 255 of whom had a high EPDS score (classed as a score of ⩾13). Several health problems were associated with greater odds of a higher score, including fatigue, backache, urinary incontinence, and relationship problems. Telephone interviews were conducted with three groups of women at 7–9 months post partum, categorised according to their earlier EPDS score (⩽9, 9–11 and ⩾13), conducted by a researcher blind to the scores. A group of 204 women were interviewed in total (66, 72 and 66 respectively) and again a high EPDS score was associated with a range of health problems, including urinary incontinence, fatigue and relationship difficulties. Physical and psychological morbidity should not be considered as separate entities.

OTHER MATERNAL AND INFANT HEALTH NEEDS

There is increasing evidence that many women experience health problems after childbirth which are chronic and not currently identified or managed by members of the health team responsible for the routine provision of postnatal care (MacArthur et al 1991, Bick & MacArthur 1995). Reference has been made thus far to specific areas that are high on the public health agenda, but it is important to note that other health problems may also be experienced, including urinary and/or faecal incontinence, headache, and perineal pain, which may impact on well-being as described earlier. Midwives providing postnatal care should ensure all women are asked about their experience of health problems, in order that appropriate and timely management can be instigated, if necessary by referral to the most appropriate health professional. Midwives should also ensure that women who may be more vulnerable, because of their particular social circumstances or because they are unsupported, receive care tailored to their needs, again ensuring where appropriate that reference to other health professionals or social agencies is made.

In addition to the identification and management of maternal health problems, the midwife should advise the woman of the infant immunisation programme, and the need to make an appointment with her GP to commence the programme. If a woman requires advice or further information on this, she should be referred to her health visitor or GP.

CONCLUSION

During the course of the last century, midwifery postnatal care made a significant contribution to improving the health of women and their infants. The shifting of the maternity services to the acute sector during the latter half of the century reduced the midwifery profile in public health, but within the last decade the importance of the midwifery contribution has once again been emphasised (DH 2000b). Whilst it is important to work towards achieving targets to reduce health inequalities, midwives providing postnatal care must continue to ensure that the physical and psychological health needs of all women are met. Factors affecting public health are complex and often interrelated; nevertheless, ensuring that postnatal services are reviewed and revised to enable care that is flexible and tailored to meet individual need, midwives will continue to promote the public health of women, their families and ultimately the communities they live in.

RECOMMENDATIONS FOR PRACTICE

- The organisation and content of postnatal care should be flexible and tailored, and based on the best available evidence to meet the needs of individual women and their infants.
- Women should be routinely asked about their physical and psychological well-being during the postnatal period.
- Maternity service providers should work together to challenge and overcome barriers which impact upon health behaviour following childbirth, acknowledging the contribution each makes to the public health agenda.
- Postnatal care provision has to be 'seamless'. Good communication between the woman, her family and all relevant care providers is essential.

RECOMMENDATIONS FOR FUTURE RESEARCH

- New models of care which reflect the multi-disciplinary, multi-agency contribution to public health should be developed, implemented and evaluated.
- Joint training programmes which focus on public health initiatives should be developed for health and social care professionals and voluntary sector agencies who work with women and their families after childbirth.

References

Audit Commission 1997 First Class Delivery: Improving Maternity Services in England and Wales. Audit Commission Publications, Abingdon

Barrett G, Pendry E, Peacock J et al 2000 Women's sexual health after childbirth. British Journal of Obstetrics and Gynaecology 107(2):186–195

Berenson A B, Wiemann C M, McCombs S L 1997 Adverse perinatal outcomes in young adolescents. Journal of Reproductive Medicine 42:559–564

Bick D E, MacArthur C 1995 The extent, severity and effect of health problems after childbirth. British Journal of Midwifery 3:27–31

Bick D E, MacArthur C, Lancashire R 1998 What influences the uptake and early cessation of breast feeding? Midwifery 14:242–247

Bick D, MacArthur C, Knowles H, Winter H 2002 Postnatal Care. Evidence and Guidelines for Management. Churchill Livingstone, London

Blair P S, Fleming P J, Bensley D et al 1996 Smoking and sudden infant death syndrome: results of 1993–1995 case-control study for confidential inquiry into stillbirths and deaths in infancy. British Medical Journal 313:195–198

Brown S, Lumley J 1998 Changing childbirth: lessons from an Australian survey of 1336 women. British Journal of Obstetrics and Gynaecology 105(2):143–155

Brown S, Lumley J 2000 Physical health after childbirth and maternal depression at six to seven months postpartum. British Journal of Obstetrics and Gynaecology 107:194–201

Castles A, Adams A, Melvin C et al 1999 Effects of smoking during pregnancy. Five meta-analyses. American Journal of Preventive Medicine 16:208–215

Department of Health 1994 Weaning and the weaning diet. TSO, London

Department of Health 1998 Department of Health, Nutrition and Bone Health COMA Expert Group. Report on health and social subjects 49. TSO, London

Department of Health 2000a Teenage Pregnancy Unit. Best Practice Guidance on the Provision of Effective Contraception and Advice Services for Young People. Online. Available: www.teenagepregnancyunit.gov.uk

Department of Health 2000b The NHS Plan. A plan for investment. A plan for reform. TSO, London

Department of Health 2001 Tackling Health Inequalities: Consultation on a Plan for Delivery. TSO, London

Foster K, Lader D, Cheesbrough S 1997 Infant feeding 1995. TSO, London

Glazener C M A, Abdalla M I, Stoud P et al 1995 Postnatal maternal morbidity: extent, causes, prevention and treatment. British Journal of Obstetrics and Gynaecology 102:282–287

Hamlyn B, Brooker S, Oleinikova K, Wands S 2002 Infant Feeding 2000. TSO, London

Hay D F, Pawlby S, Sharp D et al 2001 Intellectual problems shown by 11-year-old children whose mothers had postnatal depression. Journal of Child Psychology and Psychiatry 42:871–889

Hay-Smith E J C 2004 Therapeutic ultrasound for postpartum perineal pain and dyspareunia (Cochrane Review). In: The Cochrane Library, Issue 1, 2004. John Wiley, Chichester

Health Development Agency 2003 Research and Evidence. Online. Available: www.hda.nhs.uk/research/evidencebase.html

Henschel D, Inch S 1996 Breastfeeding: A Guide for Midwives. Books for Midwives Press, Hale, Cheshire

Horta B L, Kramer M D, Platt R W 2001 Maternal smoking and the risk of early weaning: a meta-analysis. American Journal of Public Health 91(2):304–307

Howie P W, Forsyth J S, Ogston S A et al 1990 Protective effect of breastfeeding against infection. British Medical Journal 300:11–16

Inch S 1999 Breast feeding update. In: Alexander J, Roth C, Levy V (eds) Midwifery Practice. Core Topics 3. Macmillan, Basingstoke

Ingham R, Clements S, Gillibrand R 2001 Factors affecting changes in rates of teenage conception. Teenage Pregnancy Unit, London. Online. Available: www.teenagepregnancyunit.gov.uk

Klein M C, Gauthier R J, Robbins J M et al 1994 Relationship of episiotomy to perineal trauma and morbidity, sexual dysfunction and pelvic floor relaxation. American Journal of Obstetrics and Gynecology 171(3):591–598

Lavender T, Walkinshaw S 1998 Can midwives reduce postpartum psychological morbidity? A randomised trial. Birth 25:215–219

Leap N, Hunter B 1993 The Midwife's Tale. An Oral History from Handywoman to Professional Midwife. Scarlet Press, London

Lewis G, Drife J 2001 Why Mothers Die 1997–1999. The Confidential Enquiries into Maternal Deaths in the United Kingdom. RCOG Press, London

Llewelyn Davies M (ed) 1977 Life as We Have Known It – by Co-operative Working Women. Virago, London

Lumley J, Oliver S, Waters E 2004 Interventions for promoting smoking cessation in pregnancy (Cochrane Review). In: The Cochrane Library, Issue 1, 2004. John Wiley, Chichester

MacArthur C, Knox E G, Lewis M 1991 Health After Childbirth. TSO, London

MacArthur C, Winter H R, Bick D E et al 2002 The effects of re-designed community postnatal care on women's health four months after birth: a cluster randomised controlled trial. Lancet 359:378–384

Marchant S, Garcia J 1995 What are we doing in the postnatal check? British Journal of Midwifery 3:34–38

Moore L, Campbell R, Whelan A et al 2002 Self-help smoking cessation in pregnancy: cluster randomised controlled trial. British Medical Journal 325:1383–1387

National Institute for Clinical Excellence 2002 Guidance on the use of nicotine replacement therapy (NRT) and bupropion for smoking cessation. Online. Available: www.nice.org.uk

NHS Centre for Reviews and Dissemination 2000 Promoting the initiation of breast feeding. Effective Health Care 6:1–12

Oakley A 1992 Measuring the effectiveness of psychosocial interventions in pregnancy. International Journal of Technology Assessment in Health Care 8(1):129–138

Oakley A, Rajan L, Grant A 1990 Social support and pregnancy outcome. British Journal of Obstetrics and Gynaecology 97:155–162

Oakley A, Hickey D, Rajan L et al 1996 Social support in pregnancy: does it have long-term effects? Journal of Reproductive and Infant Psychology 14:7–22

Olaussson P O, Cnattingius S, Haglund B 1999 Teenage pregnancies and risk of late fetal death and infant mortality. British Journal of Obstetrics and Gynaecology 106:116–121

Quinlivan J A, Box H, Evans S F 2003 Postnatal home visits in teenage mothers: a randomised controlled trial. Lancet 361:891–900

Rajan L 1993 The contribution of professional support, information and consistent advice to successful breast feeding. Midwifery 9:197–209

Rajan L 1994 The impact of obstetric procedures and analgesia/anaesthesia during labour and delivery on breastfeeding. Midwifery 10:87–103

Rose S, Bisson J, Wessely S 2003 Psychological debriefing for preventing post traumatic stress disorder (PTSD) (Cochrane Review). In: The Cochrane Library, Issue 1, 2004. John Wiley, Chichester

Sharp D, Hay D, Pawlby S et al 1995 The impact of postnatal depression on boys' intellectual development. Journal of Child Psychology and Psychiatry 36:1315–1337

Shields N, Reid M, Cheyne H et al 1997 Impact of midwife-managed care in the postnatal period: an exploration of psycho-social outcomes. Journal of Reproductive and Infant Psychology 15:91–108

Sikorski J, Wilson J, Clement S et al 1996 A randomised controlled trial comparing two schedules of antenatal visits: the antenatal care project. British Medical Journal 312:546–553

Sikorski J, Renfrew M J, Pindoria S, Wade A 2003 Support for breastfeeding mothers: a systematic review. Paediatric and Perinatal Epidemiology 17(4):407–417

Sleep J, Grant A, Garcia J et al 1984 West Berkshire perineal management trial. British Medical Journal 289:587–590

Small R, Lumley J, Donohue L et al 2000 Randomised controlled trial of midwife-led debriefing to reduce maternal depression after operative childbirth. British Medical Journal 321:1043–1047

Smith G C S, Pell J P 2001 Teenage pregnancy and risk of adverse perinatal outcomes associated with first and second births: population-based retrospective cohort study. British Medical Journal 323:1–5

Stamp G E, Williams A S, Crowther C A 1995 Evaluation of antenatal and postnatal support to overcome postnatal depression: a randomized controlled trial. Birth 22(3):138–143

Turnbull D, Holmes A, Shields N et al 1996 Randomised controlled trial of efficacy of midwife-managed care. Lancet 348:213–218

UKCC 1992 Registrar's Letter No. 11. United Kingdom Central Council for Nursing, Midwifery and Health Visiting, London

United Nations Children's Fund 2001 Innocenti Report Card. Issue No. 3, July 2001

Walsh R A, Lowe J B, Hopkins P J 2001 Quitting smoking in pregnancy. Medical Directory of Australia 175:320–323

White A, Freeth S, O'Brien M 1992 Infant Feeding 1990. OPCS Social Survey Division. TSO, London

WHO 2002 Infant and Young Child Nutrition. Global Strategy on Infant and Young Child Feeding. WHO, Geneva

WHO/UNICEF 1989 UK Baby Friendly Initiative Self Help Appraisal Tool. UK Baby Friendly Initiative, London

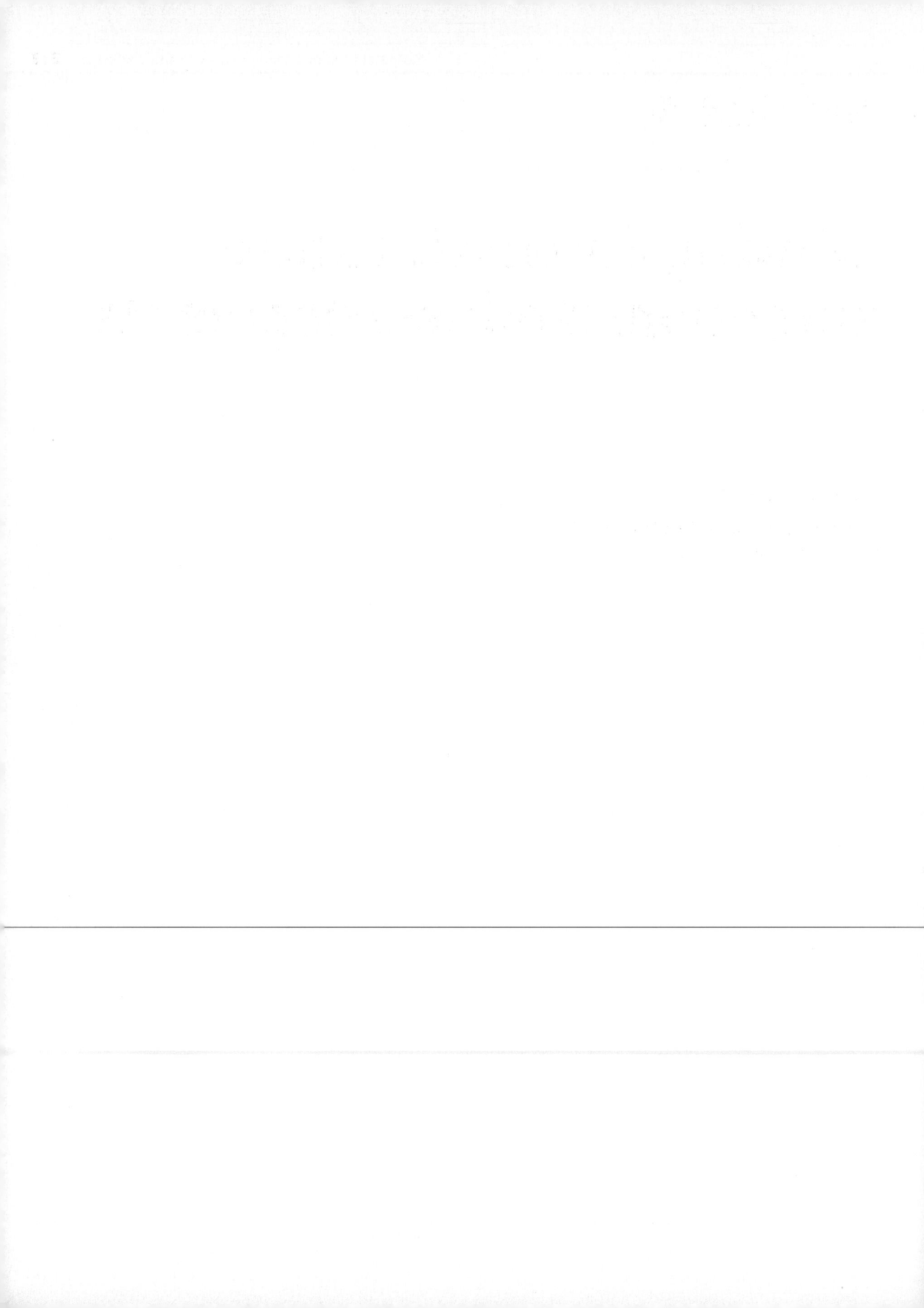

SECTION 4

Moving forward: future directions and developments

SECTION CONTENTS

Chapter 12

Next steps: public health in midwifery practice

Maralyn Foureur

CHAPTER CONTENTS

SUMMARY

This chapter provides a closing critique of the public health agenda for midwives, and presents a case for a major focus on keeping birth normal as the key contribution that midwives can make to public health. It provides insight into some of the evidence of the potential short- and long-term consequences of intervention in childbirth with serious public health implications, and argues that an understanding of the importance of keeping birth normal appears to have been largely overlooked in the setting of the public health agenda. Recent research exploring midwives' perspectives on their preparedness for a public health approach to midwifery is discussed, and recommendations made for a new focus in midwifery education and research.

INTRODUCTION

The preceding chapters have provided insights into how the health agenda of governments in many developed countries has changed. The past focus on preventative health care and individual education for appropriate lifestyle choices has been recognised as limited and largely ineffectual in addressing the poor health of certain population groups. Governments have now embraced a broader understanding of the complex interactions and contribution to health outcomes of not only individual behaviour but also socio-economic inequalities. This has led to a new public health agenda that seeks to engage communities, in concert with a range of health providers including midwives, to improve the health status of those who are currently disadvantaged.

This chapter will add to the previous discussions by exploring three further issues. The first considers midwifery philosophy and the shape of clinical practice. It explores the compelling evidence available to support a focus on keeping birth normal as the primary public health focus for midwives. The second outlines the notion of an enhanced role for midwives and will explore the debate that has begun within the midwifery profession around the issue. It explores the place of the midwife in the multi-disciplinary team, and reveals some of what has been written about educating midwives to fulfil enhanced roles. The final pages focus on the future and discuss the potential barriers to be overcome if we are to fulfil our public health potential.

MIDWIVES' CONTRIBUTION TO PUBLIC HEALTH

The title of this chapter might suggest to you that putting public health into midwifery practice is part of a new agenda for midwives. Undertaking a review of the many government documents cited in the preceding chapters might lead you to the same conclusion. Midwives are on notice. Authoritative figures in numbers of developed countries have discovered the enormous potential that exists within the midwifery workforce and in midwives' unique role in relation to practically every child-bearing woman and her family. We need to rejoice because at last, our full potential may be realised.

An increased awareness of the health inequalities experienced by women who endure socio-economic disadvantage has now placed new demands on service providers and challenged current midwifery roles. Midwives are being asked to take on a greater role in community development to improve social capital and reduce health inequalities, as well as providing core maternity services. Governments have suggested many additional services that midwives could provide, and the preceding chapters have examined some of these in detail. Many midwives will regard such lists of 'additional' services as integral to their primary health role and something they have been actively pursuing already (Henderson 2002a). Others will see such lists as an unattainable radical change to current maternity services, particularly where new services are called for such as comprehensive sex and relationship education in schools, pre-conceptual care, assessing dental health and assisting with the engineering of community-based social and cultural renewal. What this chapter will argue is that most of the calls for a new public health focus for midwives, no matter how comprehensive, fail to recognise the core role that midwives have in ensuring the health of current and future generations by simply keeping birth normal.

INFLUENCING HEALTH IN LATER LIFE

Every midwife no doubt will be familiar with what has come to be called the Barker hypothesis (Barker 1998, 2003). The story of the epidemiological investigation triggered by the discovery of the meticulous birth records of the people of Hertfordshire makes compelling reading from both a midwifery and a public health perspective. By matching the birth records of 15,000 Hertfordshire men and women born between 1911 and 1930 with the National Health Service Registry, Barker and his colleagues were able to identify a large population cohort and gain their co-operation to provide a range of health data for analysis. This enabled Barker to determine that coronary heart disease (CHD) (and other diseases of later life) has its origin in specific patterns of disproportionate fetal growth that result from fetal under-nutrition in middle to late gestation. When failure to breastfeed, early weaning, and smoking are added to an inadequate maternal diet and low birth-weight, the risk of CHD later in life is increased substantially. Many other studies have found similar associations, thus adding weight to the hypothesis that the prenatal, perinatal and early childhood environment can have a long-term effect on many health outcomes (Howden-Chapman & Cram 1998, Dorling et al 2000, Huffman et al 2001, Robinson 2001, Hypponen et al 2003).

Reflection on practice

- Prenatal, perinatal and early childhood experiences can have a long-term effect on many health outcomes.
- CHD and other diseases of later life originate in specific patterns of disproportionate fetal growth.
- What does this mean for the women in my care?

The UK government has recognised the potential for intervention to change this pattern of disease through programmes such as Sure Start, as described in Chapter 10. This programme aims to reduce the incidence of low birth-weight babies by 5%, by targeting women in particularly high-risk areas where there is a high rate of teenage pregnancies, high incidence of domestic violence, high youth unemployment and the highest number of child referrals to health services (Garrod 2002, Hutchings &

Henty 2002). It is a significant step to have midwives employed to deliver the maternity component of Sure Start, since this acknowledges the preventative health role midwives can play in not only improving maternal nutrition and birth-weight of infants but also in increasing rates and length of breastfeeding. However, there is also an inherent challenge for midwives working in this way, to keep birth normal.

KEEPING BIRTH NORMAL

Midwives are, and always have been, primary health care providers with a public health agenda. Unfortunately the last 100 years of midwifery practice has seen our focus diverted from our primary role by the move to a hospital-centred, medicalised approach to childbirth. Midwives' ability to assist women to give birth naturally, which is our primary task, has been gradually eroded until some estimates suggest fewer than 25% of women will give birth without some form of medical intervention (Downe 2001). The rhetoric has been that the increase in scientific medicine and subsequent rising intervention rates in childbirth are to make childbirth safe. However, far from being pleased, women's sense of well-being has deteriorated to the point where most women are fearful of childbirth and are afraid of the pain of labour and of losing control. Childbirth is seen as risky and fraught with complications, and some women are shocked and emotionally scarred by the experience (Walsh 2002). The idea that birth is only normal in retrospect has been finally assimilated into the body and mind of society (Bates 1999) as the medicalisation of childbirth has gone too far (Johanson et al 2002). This situation is the first challenge that individual midwives and the midwifery profession must address if we are to realise our potential contribution to public health.

There are compelling reasons why we need to keep birth normal. There are numerous unintentional and serious consequences of unnecessary intervention in childbirth that have public health implications. There are short- and long-term effects in both mother and baby, revealed in studies ranging from basic science research in individuals (animals and humans) to large epidemiological investigations of population groups. An examination of two of the most common events which childbearing women experience will provide insights into this proposition.

LABOURING UNDISTURBED

The potential public health effects of perinatal environmental disturbance were investigated over 30 years ago by psychologist Niles Newton. In a series of elegant experiments conducted with mice, Newton established that supporting the mother to labour undisturbed is crucial not only for ensuring labour progresses normally but also for the health of the infant (Newton et al 1966, 1968). Placing the labouring mother in a hostile environment, or simply moving her from one place to another during labour, resulted in both a significant slowing of labour and the death of some of the pups.

While we assume that human behaviour is much more complex than that of animals, it is reasonable to extrapolate from studies of parturient animals. Comparative obstetrics has demonstrated that '... different species have made specific adaptations to the ecology of which they form a part ... and ... common mechanisms which have a fundamental value, are observed in all mammals. This is just as true for the behavioural as for the physiological, endocrinological, anatomical (and many other) aspects of parturition' (Naagteboren 1989:796). Therefore while the results of research in mammals is not directly transferable, it does need to be given due attention. Newton asked (1990:37), '... are mammals with more highly developed nervous systems than the mouse equally sensitive to perinatal environmental disturbance... what effect if any do variations between home and hospital environments have on the course of labour and on perinatal mortality?'

How often are women disturbed during the course of their labour in your unit? Why should we be surprised that the two main reasons for all operative intervention in childbirth are uterine inertia and fetal distress? Where is the call for labouring undisturbed placed on the public health agenda?

Reflection on practice

- Keeping birth normal is our primary public health task – ensuring well women remain well.
- Labouring undisturbed is crucial for labour to progress normally.
- Is labouring undisturbed a priority of the public health agenda?

LABOUR ANALGESIA: SHORT- AND LONG-TERM HEALTH IMPACT

A growing body of evidence is available to describe how early breastfeeding behaviour is disturbed by labour analgesia, but few policy documents have made links between labour analgesia, breastfeeding and the public health implications of failure to breastfeed (Ransjo-Arvidson et al 2001, Righard 2001, Stafford 2002, Torrance et al 2003). Many resources are currently being allocated to the Baby Friendly Hospital Initiative in order to change the behaviour of health care professionals and clients to increase the uptake and success of breastfeeding (UNICEF 2003). However, fewer resources have been invested in enabling midwives to provide continuity of care, which has been demonstrated in numerous evaluations to be associated with both less use of analgesia and higher rates of successful breastfeeding. In so doing we are arguably focusing on a downstream effect modifier, rather than a potentially more positive preventative health intervention (Fowler 2000).

Labour analgesia administered to the mother has also been implicated in increased susceptibility to drugs in later life for her offspring, due to an imprinting process when the neonate is exposed to drugs in utero (Nyberg et al 1992). Research by Kerstin Uvnas-Moberg and her colleagues has revealed the crucial role that oxytocin plays in human attachment and relationship behaviour and how this can be blocked or inhibited, by epidural analgesia in particular (Uvnas-Moberg 1997, 1998). Further studies by Swedish researchers also found the mother's labour analgesia and other obstetric procedures were implicated in an increased risk of suicidal tendencies and anti-social behaviour for their offspring (Jacobson et al 1987, 1990, Jacobson & Bygdeman 1998). How can we ignore the public health implications of these findings?

Reflection on practice

- Breastfeeding behaviour is disturbed by labour analgesia.
- What are the public health implications of failure to breastfeed?
- What are the potential long-term health implications of labour analgesia?

Ensuring that well women remain well is the first priority of midwifery practice and maternity care. We must continue to address this issue, at the same time as focusing on disadvantaged groups of women in our communities. Midwives' perspective is long term and preventative, and the foundation of our philosophical approach is that childbirth is a normal (albeit stressful and life-changing) event in women's lives. Supporting and encouraging women in holistic and respectful ways in order to keep birth normal must be our primary function. We have much work to do in order to fulfil just that key component of our role.

CONTINUITY OF CARE: A MEANS TO AN END, NOT AN END IN ITSELF

The potential health gains from midwifery care, especially that provided in a continuity of care model, are well established, having been explored in 19 randomised controlled trials, 15 prospective non-randomised comparative studies, 21 retrospective studies and 4 descriptive studies in the UK, Scotland, Canada, North and South America, Sweden, Hong Kong and New Zealand (Biro 2003). More than 20,000 women have participated in the randomised controlled trials alone, which indicates the level of interest women have in how their care is delivered. Almost all of the trials have found decreased rates of all interventions in childbirth. In Chapter 6, Caroline Homer provides details of one of the studies conducted in Australia which found significant differences in the rate of caesarean section for women receiving continuity of care provided by a small team of midwives located in the community (Homer et al 2001). Not only are well women kept well; their babies are well, women are more satisfied with the process and feel valued and listened to, but costs to the health system and therefore to society are lower. This is surely one of the most significant contributions we can make to public health. Or is it? What is becoming more apparent, as we examine and reflect on models of continuity of care, is that while it is a model that women prefer, it may not provide the health gains we anticipate.

Over 10 years ago I conducted a randomised controlled trial of continuity of care provided by a team of midwives in an Australian maternity unit (Rowley et al 1995). Although there were significantly lower rates of interventions between team and routine care groups, I was somewhat dismayed to discover that only one third of women receiving continuity of care had given birth with no intervention at all. As observed by Johanson and colleagues in a recent publication which examined the normal birth rate in a number of trials of continuity of midwifery care, '... variation in normal birth rates between services ... seems to be greater than outcome differences between "high continuity" and "traditional care" groups at the same unit' (Johanson et al 2002:894). I was forced reluctantly to agree with these authors that the environment within which midwives work is now so medicalised that it appears to over-ride the potential benefits of continuity of care.

This is also evident in New Zealand, where midwifery autonomy has been legislated and over 70% of women choose a midwife as the Lead Maternity Carer. The majority of women therefore receive one-to-one care throughout pregnancy, labour and birth; however, intervention rates are the same as in countries without such advantages (New Zealand Ministry of Health 2003). In the New Zealand unit in which I work, 42.3% of all women in 2002 started labour spontaneously, at term, and gave birth unaided but this figure does not reveal the numbers who also had interventions during labour such as continuous electronic fetal monitoring, artificial rupture of the membranes, oxytocic augmentation of labour and epidural analgesia. For primiparous women the rate of spontaneous onset of labour and vaginal birth at term was only 32.2% (Fisher et al 2003). Holding to the belief that birth is normal, in a medicalised childbirth monopoly where few women give birth without intervention, is almost impossible. However, to '... continuously challenge the culture and constraints of the organisations within which we work' (Downe 2001:11) is just what we need to do if we are to fulfil our primary public health role, which is to keep birth normal.

Continuity, team, case-load midwifery or one-to-one care, whatever the model is called, clearly addresses the public health agenda by preventing many of the potential long-term health consequences of intervention in childbirth for some women. Yet it is still impossible to 'get it happening' throughout the UK and in many other countries (Walsh 2002). Walsh proposes a number of reasons why this is so. He argues that we can hardly claim midwifery as primary care when it is located within acute care settings. Such settings testify to the power of the medical view of childbirth with its secondary prevention approach to reducing infant deaths, dominated by biomedical technologies which say that pathology can be explained in terms of physical and biochemical processes within the individual (Fowler 2000). This approach has been powerful enough to move women from home to hospital for birth and from the care of the midwife to the doctor. This approach remains the dominant model of maternity care in most countries. It results in many midwives defining their role in the narrow terms of antenatal or postnatal care and delivering babies. Locating care within acute settings has undermined midwives' confidence in their ability to provide safe care for women experiencing normal birth, and contributes to the systematic medicalisation of childbirth by all maternity care providers.

What is required is a paradigm shift to see healthy pregnancy outcomes in terms of the public health model (Fowler 2000). The new focus on social determinants of health, rather than solely on individual behaviour and biology, may provide midwives with exactly the kind of support that is needed to improve maternity care in ways that are health-promoting. In this kind of an environment a commitment to keeping birth normal and improving long-term health outcomes through the provision of continuity of care may be easier to achieve.

There are positive signs that change is achievable using the public health model. The high rate of home birth (34%) revealed in the audit of outcomes for the first 50 women cared for by case-loading Sure Start Weston midwives suggests that a new confidence in childbirth as a normal life process is developing in their community (Hutchings & Henty 2002). It is encouraging to read that more case-load practices are being implemented which the midwives see as a validation of their commitment to physiological birth, continuity of carer and informed choice.

Reflection on practice

- Why are the benefits revealed in randomised controlled trials of continuity of care not realised in practice?
- What is meant by the statement 'Continuity of care is a means to an end, not an end in itself'?
- In what ways can continuity of care be enhanced?

REDEFINING THE ROLE OF THE MIDWIFE

While not all midwives will want to work in case-loading models that require midwives to be on call for individual women, there is evidence that many midwives acknowledge the potential health benefits of the model and believe that there are numerous ways of improving continuity (Lavender et al 2002a). A study conducted in seven hospitals in the north west of England revealed that midwives believed that greater continuity could be achieved by extending the duration of contact that midwives have with women from preconception input to additional postnatal visiting (Bennett et al 2001). Whether this would meet women's expressed desire for 'continuity' would need to be evaluated, should such a model be implemented.

The primary aim of the study by Lavender and colleagues was to explore midwives' views of their future in expanded public health roles (Lavender et al 2001, 2002a, 2002b). Midwives were invited to complete a questionnaire which asked their views on participating in opportunistic health promotion, public health and continuity of care, and were invited to describe any barriers they perceived to expanding their role. Midwives who responded believed they have a role in child protection; promoting effective parenting skills; informing young people about healthy lifestyle choices; providing well women clinics; targeting vulnerable groups; and promoting sexual health. There were many and varied responses to the question of involvement in health promotion, with several midwives reporting they had not previously considered issues such as advice on breast examination as part of their role. However, the study also revealed that midwives felt they were inadequately prepared for such role expansion and required further education.

The midwives identified several barriers to expanding their current role. These included a belief that the core role of the midwife was being eroded, either by over-expansion into new territories that left them feeling exhausted at the very thought, or by the inclusion of health care assistants who might relieve some of the pressure but lower the standard of care. Some were concerned that the new roles would require crossing boundaries and stepping on the toes of their colleagues such as the physiotherapist or dietician, as they endeavoured to provide advice and promote exercise and healthy eating.

Some midwives expressed concern that the additional responsibilities being put upon them might deter potential students and cause others to leave midwifery, but others believed the new responsibilities would enhance their job satisfaction. This finding concurs with the ideas expressed by another midwifery leader who considered an enhanced role in public health may be just what some midwives need to keep them in midwifery, while for others it will be the last straw (Warwick 2002).

Reflection on practice

- Are midwives well prepared for a role in public health?
- Is the core role of the midwife being eroded by the public health agenda?
- Will the new public health focus deter potential students and cause others to leave midwifery?

RESOURCING

Many of the surveyed midwives identified that additional resources would be required to extend their role. Financial resources would need to be allocated for updating existing staff, and to employ more midwives, who would expect to be reasonably rewarded for the additional responsibilities they would take on.

Concern was expressed that diverting funds to meet the new requirements might have an effect on the current service provision, which they saw as already under-resourced. This concern is shared by Henderson, who writes '... it is a question of being able to recruit and/or redirect in a way that does not diminish the current quality of services already provided ...' (Henderson 2002a:270).

In an environment where 71% of midwifery leaders in one survey believed their staff establishment was too low to manage the day-to-day delivery of core midwifery services, it seems irresponsible to ask midwives to take on new roles unless there is additional funding provided (Warwick 2002). Midwifery leaders are currently caught in the merry-go-round of having to call in casual staff to make up the shortfall in numbers, which means the budget is overrun and staff have to be cut to balance the budget. As well as placing women and babies at risk of a poor quality service, it is also recognised that having too few midwives to provide core services means that new midwives and return-to-practice midwives may be inadequately supported during their orientation period, '... which is critical to them establishing themselves in their new posts' (Warwick 2002:661). We cannot expect midwives to be able to practise well in environments where they feel unsupported and rushed off their feet, which appears to typify the experiences of many.

Reflection on practice

- What additional resources will be needed to fulfil a public health role?
- Can we afford to provide a broader role in public health?

A further impediment to be considered is the relative powerlessness of most midwives to make independent decisions in the medically dominated maternity care system (Pankhurst & Hart 1999). Given that models of midwifery case loading and continuity place midwives firmly in the front line of decision making which either supports or interrupts normal labour processes, we need to ensure that midwifery autonomy, as well as a view of birth as a normal life process, are upheld (Downe 2001).

MIDWIFERY AUTONOMY AND THE MULTI-DISCIPLINARY TEAM

The public health agenda emphasises working in multi-disciplinary teams in order to address the complexity of inequalities and health outcomes. Ensuring that midwives are properly consulted and involved as autonomous practitioners in such teams is potentially problematic. It has been argued that the position of midwives in the National Health Service in the UK (and I suspect in most countries) mirrors the secondary role of women in society (Bates 1999). In such settings it is unlikely that midwives will easily be able to achieve equal status with doctors and have their autonomy respected. We need to be able to overcome the residue of '... doctor/nurse hierarchies in which predominantly female ... midwives ... diplomatically accommodate the priorities of their predominantly male colleagues (Pankhurst & Hart 1999:632). This can be achieved if midwives believe they are autonomous, are prepared to be accountable and responsible for their practice, and conduct themselves as autonomous practitioners.

My understanding of midwifery autonomy is that midwives use their professional education, clinical skills and judgement to assess, plan and provide care in partnership with individual women and their families, in any setting. A major part of our role is to assist women to make decisions about their maternity care by providing them with information about options. This requires us to keep up to date with new knowledge, be able to appraise evidence critically, to have confidence in our clinical skills, the courage to reflect deeply and to challenge misinformation and poor practice in ourself and others, in order that women are given the best care possible. Midwifery autonomy means there is no need to seek the permission of others before offering women choices and enacting an agreed plan of care.

However, we have all been shaped and our opinions moulded in the process of being born of a particular community and culture and in the process of becoming and being a midwife. Few of us may be aware of the unconscious processes derived from our experiences that influence what information and choices we offer to women (Davies 2001). Experiencing situations of powerlessness in childhood, for instance, may have taught us to avoid conflict and accept domination by others' ideas and opinions. Working within hospitals characterised by hostility and hierarchies may further perpetuate a loss of confidence in our own abilities and opinions (Henderson 2002b). The discovery by Mavis Kirkham and colleagues of the medicalised and limited information provided to women from socio-economically disadvantaged groups during antenatal consultations suggests that many midwives are on 'automatic pilot' and are no longer aware of what unconscious biases are now an integrated part of their midwifery practice (Kirkham et al 2002). Therefore '... the ease with which an individual midwife can make decisions for herself and is able to facilitate this process in others, is now at the heart of the challenge that is woman centred care' (Davies 2001:26). Developing self awareness of how our individual experiences and beliefs shape our behaviour is integral to being an autonomous practitioner and also an essential component of keeping birth normal. Such reflection will enable midwives to assume a role in the multi-disciplinary team that is based on knowledge of their true worth and the contribution they can make.

The hospital-centred, specialist approach to medicine that focuses on the individual rather than society has been challenged by the call for a focus on social inequalities and health outcomes. Here the contribution of midwives will be just as important as that of the many other clinicians and non-clinicians who will be part of the team grappling with the complexities of a holistic approach to health. We need to be constantly aware that the current design of the maternity services is largely accidental, and midwives' roles within it have been systematically medicalised by trying to keep up with and accommodate obstetric interventions as fashions wax and wane (Page 2003). 'Consequently the boundaries of midwifery practice and concepts of normality have become blurred' (Bates 1999: 607). Midwives of the future will need to be clear about the contribution we make to public health priorities by our commitment to keeping birth normal as our core function, in addition to addressing health inequalities. This will require that midwives renegotiate partnerships with obstetric colleagues and develop new alliances with other health professionals and agencies, and with women and communities.

Reflection on practice

- Will multi-disciplinary teams recognise the autonomy of the midwife?
- How autonomous and powerful are individual midwives?
- What experiences have shaped our opinions of ourselves?

EDUCATION FOR A NEW PUBLIC HEALTH PERSPECTIVE IN MIDWIFERY

That women (and midwives) are '… bombarded with information about a range of medical and technological aspects of their pregnancies when many are short on information and support concerning issues such as diet and smoking is one of many paradoxes in maternity care' (Crafter 2002:S9). Paradoxical messages received by vulnerable pregnant women may be such things as 'eat nutritious food' (but we all know it is expensive and you probably can't afford it); 'breastfeed your baby' (but don't do it in public places or you will receive strange looks and comments). Such mixed messages can undermine the confidence of women, especially when midwives unknowingly perpetuate the paradox. A public health perspective in education will enable midwives to consider the inherent paradoxes presented to women, particularly women from disadvantaged groups, and modify their messages accordingly. Hopefully such a perspective will also motivate midwives to lobby governments to make appropriate changes to policy that will remove the paradoxes. A recent publication exploring poverty and diet in pregnancy revealed damaging inconsistencies in UK government policy, where a study which clearly demonstrated that it was impossible for an unemployed, single pregnant woman to eat well enough to have a healthy baby, based on the benefits provided, was ignored by those setting the benefit (McLeish 2002).

Midwives are also subjected to many paradoxical messages. They include such things as a belief in pregnancy, birth and motherhood as normal physiological events in women's lives, but find they work in a medically dominated environment that aims to control and manipulate the events (Crafter 2002). Midwives are told they are an autonomous practitioner but must obey the rules and policies of the organisation in which they work.

Another paradox of relevance to health promotion is that midwives are expected to provide women with information on which to make choices, but will not have the time to make the information relevant and personal to each woman. Such inconsistencies undermine the confidence of midwives and confuse the way we view the world. It is not surprising therefore that Lavender's study highlighted that many midwives feel inadequately prepared to undertake health promotion and many other aspects of an expanded public health role (Lavender et al 2001). Reframing education to emphasise the role midwives have as public health practitioners may be the key to a radical reframing of maternity care away from a medicalised process conducted in acute care settings.

Reflection on practice

- What are the paradoxes that women and midwives experience?
- How can we contribute to social policy?

The educational preparation of midwives to work with disadvantaged groups of women will require greater involvement of local communities in both curriculum design and delivery (Kaufmann 2000, Hart & Hall 2001). This is already evident (at least in the delivery of programmes) in numbers of pre- and post-registration courses reviewed by Hart and Hall. However, they argue for even more involvement of users and recommend that curriculum planning teams should include an identified champion on inequality issues as well as sourcing clinical placements which provide access to women experiencing inequalities.

They caution that including users in the team is often not easy as they may not necessarily be familiar with education jargon and may not be confident in the education setting. They also caution that although including users is a powerful teaching and learning strategy, both students and users must be prepared for the teaching session. Insensitive or prejudicial comments need to be challenged during the session and the opportunity for debriefing afterwards needs to be provided, as students (or teachers) may become defensive when users share negative experiences of service delivery.

Reflection on practice

- Are women from disadvantaged groups involved in curriculum design?
- Are students supported in clinical placements in disadvantaged communities?

PROVIDING EVIDENCE OF EFFECTIVENESS

Providing a new public health perspective in midwifery education is a challenge that our leaders and educators have the skills and abilities to address. Widening the scope of practice of midwives to incorporate new ways to address health inequalities is also achievable. Affirming midwives' autonomy and contribution to multi-disciplinary health care teams will also provide opportunities to renew our primary focus on keeping birth normal. However, the challenge that remains is to provide strong evidence that such an array of educational, policy and practice interventions actually improves health outcomes for mothers and babies from disadvantaged populations.

Social interventions are complex processes requiring careful and rigorous evaluation. As Ann Oakley observed some time ago when discussing the need for randomised controlled studies of health care interventions,

> ... it may seem self-evident that additional feeding of pregnant women will benefit their infants, that hormonal supplementation will increase the chances of successful pregnancy, that new educational curricula will improve children's learning, that additional stimulation in infancy will have long-term cognitive effects, that social work services to socially disadvantaged children will help prevent delinquency; yet in all these cases, comparison of how 'treated' groups fare[d] with those untreated contrast[ed] common sense with the findings of systematic evaluation
>
> (Oakley 1992:74)

Studies without controls may overestimate, or in some cases underestimate, treatment effects, thereby disguising potentially useless or even harmful interventions.

Gaining ethical approval for experimental research in evaluating the effects of social interventions may be difficult since such studies are predicated on the existence of equipoise, that is, that there exists true uncertainty as to the effects of the treatment (Thompson et al 2004). Where government policy has set the public health agenda, inspired by a belief that additional services will improve health outcomes, it will be impossible to gain ethical approval to undertake the necessary controlled studies. Therefore evaluations will require skilled research expertise and careful attention to design in order to discover whether encouraging more public health activities by midwives is a waste of time or whether '... this enhanced activity [will lead] to real breakthroughs' (Hillier & Caan 2002:545).

Reflection on practice

- What kind of evidence will be needed to determine the effectiveness of the midwife in public health?
- What is the 'ecological fallacy'?

CONCLUSION

Working in new ways and with a broader perspective of health will challenge us all. We may need to overcome what Garrod (2002) has identified as territorialism, traditionalism, tribalism, terrorism and timidity that can interfere with effective care. For example, we need to be able to see the peer breastfeeding counsellor as an extra pair of hands and put aside protecting our territory. This may include embracing the health care assistant in maternity care as a valued member of the team. We need to discard 'traditional' views of midwifery to understand that sitting in an inhospitable antenatal or postnatal clinic for many hours for a brief and unfulfilling visit is not appealing to anyone but may be particularly so for women who are dealing with many other stresses in their lives. This will allow us to be innovative in designing new forms of service delivery. We need to see that form filling, negotiating with housing services, encouraging women to read books with their toddlers, etc., are all part of a woman-centred public health service where there are no boundaries, only opportunities, so that tribalism has no place in midwifery. We need to acknowledge that this will be a difficult transition for the timid midwife and provide many opportunities for the saboteur who needs to be managed (Garrod 2002). Tara Kaufmann has also provided a comprehensive vision for the future of midwives in public health (Kaufmann 2000). As a pre-requisite she urges that public health must be well integrated into the core role of the midwife and is not simply a series of extra tasks.

Many challenges exist for our current leaders, both in practice and in education. If midwifery is to take its rightful place as a key contributor to public health, our leaders will need to be strong and united and able to empower midwives to become confident, autonomous practitioners. For educators the challenge is to provide programmes of education that instil an 'inequalities imagination' in graduates, through educating midwives to care for all groups of women and reorienting education from a focus on the acute care setting to the community (Hillier & Caan 2002). For midwifery researchers the challenge will be to design studies to determine whether the new public health focus in midwifery education and practice is achievable, actually improves health outcomes for women and babies, is cost effective and acceptable to the communities we serve.

My vision for the future of the maternity services is one shared with Lesley Page (Page 2002, 2003). My experiences as an independent midwife, in conducting research into continuity of care in Australia and in working in an acute hospital in New Zealand, have led me to see many opportunities for midwives in the call for a public health focus in maternity care. Midwives will be enabled to provide most effective care when they are attached to women and are then located in their local community to provide primary health care, moving in and out of the places in which women give birth. Networks of community-based midwives will then be able to contribute to addressing health inequalities through improving access for all women and maintaining the normal focus which is so easily lost in the acute care setting.

Government calls to refocus health services on public health and away from the acute care setting acknowledge the limited (albeit valuable) contribution that medical science and technology can make to the health of populations. New knowledge is emerging of the influence of prenatal, perinatal and early childhood experiences on the long-term health and well-being of future generations. This includes a growing awareness of the role of socio-economic factors and geographic location in both deprivation and discrimination for certain population groups. Women need midwives who understand how this influences their lives and their health, and that of their unborn children. All midwives are ideally placed to make a considerable contribution to public health, wherever they are located and whatever their role. We simply need to take up the challenge.

References

Barker D 1998 Mothers, Babies and Health in Later Life, 2nd edn. Churchill Livingstone, London

Barker D 2003 The midwife, the coincidence, and the hypothesis. British Medical Journal 327(7429):1428–1430

Bates C 1999 Multidisciplinary care – continuing the debate. British Journal of Midwifery 7(10):607

Bennett N, Blundell J, Malpass L, Lavender T 2001 Midwives' views on redefining midwifery 2: Public health. British Journal of Midwifery 9(12):743–745

Biro M 2003 The Collaborative Pregnancy Care/Team Midwifery Study: A Randomised Controlled Trial. Unpublished PhD, La Trobe University, Melbourne

Crafter H 2002 The practical aspects of health promotion in pregnancy. MIDIRS Midwifery Digest 12(Supplement 1): S8–S11

Davies H 2001 Client-centred midwifery – no easy option. The Practising Midwife 4(6):26–28

Dorling D, Mitchell R, Shaw M, Orford S, Davey Smith G 2000 The Ghost of Christmas Past: health effects of poverty in London in 1896 and 1991. British Medical Journal 321(7276):1547–1551

Downe S 2001 Is there a future for normal birth? The Practising Midwife 4(6):10–15

Fisher K, Foureur M, Hawley J 2003 Maternity Report 1997–2002. Capital and Coast District Health Board, Wellington, NZ

Fowler W 2000 Focusing upstream to analyse perinatal mortality rates. British Journal of Midwifery 8(7):415–420

Garrod D 2002 Sure Start: the role of the public health midwife. MIDIRS Midwifery Digest 12(Supplement 1): S32–S35

Hart A, Hall V 2001 Addressing health inequalities. Implications for curriculum planning and educational delivery. The Practising Midwife 4(9):42–43

Henderson C 2002a The public health role of the midwife. British Journal of Midwifery 10(5):268–270

Henderson C 2002b Terms and conditions: midwives hold the key. British Journal of Midwifery 10(6):344

Hillier D, Caan W 2002 Researching the public health role of the midwife. British Journal of Midwifery 10(9):545–547

Homer C, Davis G, Brodie P et al 2001 Collaboration in maternity care: a randomised controlled trial comparing community-based continuity of care with standard care. British Journal of Obstetrics and Gynaecology 108:16–22

Howden-Chapman P, Cram F 1998 Social, Economic and Cultural Determinants of Health. National Health Committee, Wellington, NZ

Huffman S, Zehner E, Victora C 2001 Can improvements in breast-feeding practices reduce neonatal mortality in developing countries? Midwifery 17(2):80–92

Hutchings J, Henty D 2002 Caseload midwifery practice in partnership with Sure Start: changing the culture of birth. MIDIRS Midwifery Digest 12(Supplement 1):S38–S40

Hypponen E, Davey Smith G, Power C 2003 Effects of grandmothers' smoking in pregnancy on birth weight: intergenerational cohort study. British Medical Journal 327:898

Jacobson B, Bygdeman M 1998 Obsteric care and proneness of offspring to suicide as adults: case-control study. British Medical Journal 317:1346–1349

Jacobson B, Eklund G, Hamberger L, Linnarsson D, Sedvall G, Valverius M 1987 Perinatal origin of adult self-destructive behaviour. Acta Psychiatrica Scandinavica 76:364–371

Jacobson B, Nyberg K, Gronbladh L, Eklund G, Bygdeman M, Rydberg U 1990 Opiate addiction in adult offspring through possible imprinting after obstetric treatment. British Medical Journal 301:1067–1070

Johanson R, Newburn M, Macfarlane A 2002 Has the medicalisation of childbirth gone too far? British Medical Journal 324(7342):892–895

Kaufmann T 2000 Public health: the next step in woman-centred care. RCM Midwives Journal 3(1):26–28

Kirkham M, Stapleton H, Curtis P, Thomas G 2002 The inverse care law in antenatal midwifery care. British Journal of Midwifery 10(8):509–513

Lavender T, Bennett N, Blundell J, Malpass L 2001 Midwives' views on redefining midwifery 1: health promotion. British Journal of Midwifery 9(11):666–670

Lavender T, Bennett N, Blundell J, Malpass L 2002a Midwives' views on redefining midwifery 3: continuity of care. British Journal of Midwifery 10(1):18–22

Lavender T, Bennett N, Blundell J, Malpass L 2002b Midwives' views on redefining midwifery 4: general views. British Journal of Midwifery 10(2):72–77

McLeish J 2002 'All I ate was toast' – poverty and diet in pregnancy. MIDIRS Midwifery Digest 12(Supplement 1): S6–S8

Naagteboren C 1989 The biology of childbirth. In: Chalmers I, Enkin M, Keirse M (eds) Effective Care in Pregnancy and Childbirth Vol. 2:796. Oxford University Press, Oxford

Newton N 1990 Newton on Birth and Women. Birth & Life Bookstore, Seattle, WA
Newton N, Foshee D, Newton M 1966 Parturient mice: effects of environment on labor. Science 151:1560–1561
Newton N, Peeler D, Newton M 1968 The effects of disturbance on labor: an experiment using one hundred mice with dated pregnancies. American Journal of Obstetrics and Gynecology 101:1096–1102
New Zealand Ministry of Health 2003 Report on Maternity 2000 & 2001. Ministry of Health, Wellington
Nyberg K, Allebeck P, Eklund G, Jacobson B 1992 Socio-economic versus obstetric risk factors for drug addiction in offspring. British Journal of Addiction 87:1669–1676
Oakley A 1992 Social Support and Motherhood. The Natural History of a Research Project. Blackwell, Oxford
Page L 2002 Putting the humanity back into maternity. British Journal of Midwifery 10(6):346
Page L 2003 Shaping the future of the maternity services. British Journal of Midwifery 11(3):134
Pankhurst F, Hart A 1999 The impact of team midwifery on GPs. British Journal of Midwifery 7(10):632–636
Ransjo-Arvidson A, Matthiesen A, Lija G, Nissen E, Widstrom A, Uvnas-Moberg K 2001 Maternal analgesia during labor disturbs newborn behaviour. Effects on breastfeeding, temperature, and crying. Birth 28:5–12
Righard L 2001 Making childbirth a normal process. Birth 28(1):1–4
Robinson R 2001 The fetal origins of adult disease. British Medical Journal 322:375–376
Rowley M, Hensley M, Brinsmead M, Wlodarczyk J 1995 Continuity of care by a midwife team versus routine care during pregnancy and birth: a randomised trial. Medical Journal of Australia 163:289–293
Stafford S 2002 Epidurals: a concern for public health? British Journal of Midwifery 10(6):364–367
Thompson H, Hoskins R, Pettigrew M, Ogilvie D, Craig N, Quinn T, Lindsay G 2004 Evaluating the effects of social interventions. British Medical Journal 328:282–285
Torrance E, Thomas J, Grindey J 2003 Outcomes after pethidine or diamorphine administration. British Journal of Midwifery 11(4):243–247
UNICEF UK 2003 Baby Friendly Hospital Initiative. Health Benefits of Breastfeeding. Online. Retrieved December 2004, from http://www.babyfriendly.org.uk/health.asp
Uvnas-Moberg K 1997 Physiological and endocrine effects of social contact. Annals of the New York Academy of Sciences 807(1):146–163
Uvnas-Moberg K 1998 Oxytocin may mediate the benefits of positive social interaction and emotions. Psychoneuroendocrinology 23(8):819–835
Walsh D 2002 Fear of labour and birth. British Journal of Midwifery 10(2):78
Warwick C 2002 How do we prevent midwives from leaving? British Journal of Midwifery 10(11):660–661

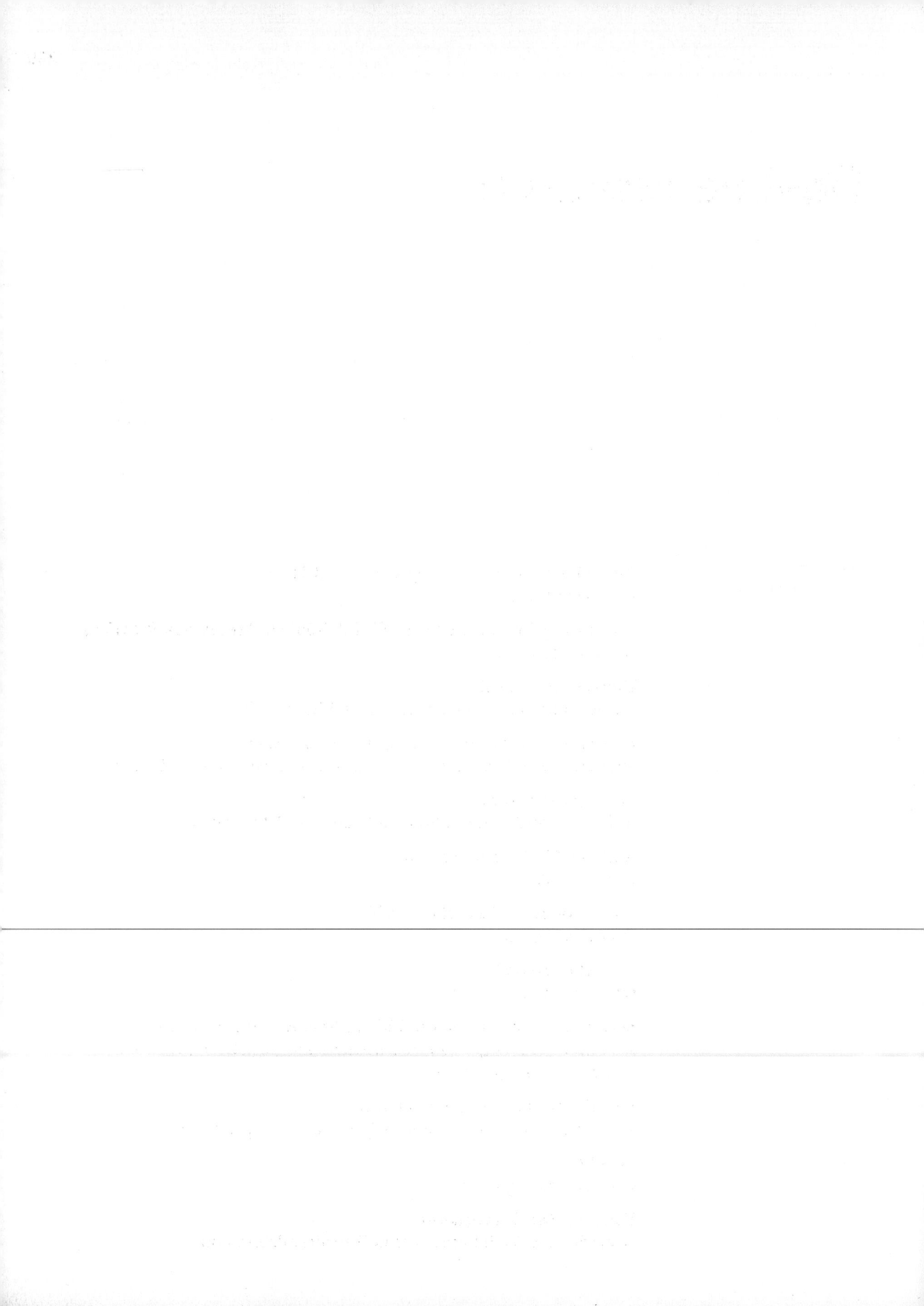

On-line resources

UK ORGANISATIONS

Commission for Health Improvement (CHI)
www.chi.nhs.uk

Community Practitioners' and Health Visitors' Association (CPHVA)
www.msfcphva.org

Delivering the best
www.publications.doh.gov.uk/cno/midwives.pdf

Independent Inquiry into Inequalities in Health
www.archive.official-documents.co.uk/document/doh/ih/ih.htm

Making a difference
www.dh.gov.uk/PublicationsAndStatistics/Publications

National Health Service – UK
www.nhs.uk

Royal College of Midwives – UK
www.rcm.org.uk

Safe Motherhood
www.safemotherhood.org

Securing our future health: Taking a long term view – Wanless review
www.hm-treasury.gov.uk/consultations_and_legislation/wanless/consult_wanless_index.cfm

SEU Report on Teenage Pregnancy
www.socialexclusionunit.gov.uk/publications.asp?did=69

Sure Start
www.surestart.gov.uk

Tackling Health Inequalities
www.dh.gov.uk/PublicationsAndStatistics/Publications

Teenage Pregnancy Strategy
www.teenagepregnancyunit.gov.uk

www.upmystreet.com

INTERNATIONAL ORGANISATIONS

Australian College of Midwives
www.acmi.org.au

European Public Health Alliance
www.epha.org

Public Health Association of Australia
www.phaa.net.au

New Zealand College of Midwives
www.midwife.org.nz

New Zealand Primary Health Care Strategy
www.moh.govt.nz/primaryhealthcare

New Zealand Public Health Advisory Committee
www.nhc.govt.nz/phac.html

The Institute of Public Health in Ireland
www.publichealth.ie

CENSUS INFORMATION

UK – www.statistics.gov.uk/census2001/default.asp
Australia – www.abs.gov.au/
New Zealand – www.stats.govt.nz/census.htm
Ireland – www.cso.ie/census/about.htm
Canada – www.statcan.ca/start.html

COMMUNITY HEALTH NEEDS ASSESSMENT

www.hda-online.org.uk/hdt/1202/skills.html
www.healthaction.nhs.uk/cat.asp?cat=113
www.emh.org/health_needs_assessment.asp
www.ichs.uaa.alaska.edu/acrh/projects/archives/chna.html
www.sph.uth.tmc.edu/admaps/champs/chna/chna.html

Index

Notes: Page numbers in *italics* indicate boxed material, figures and tables.

D

E

F

G

H

T

U

V

W

Y

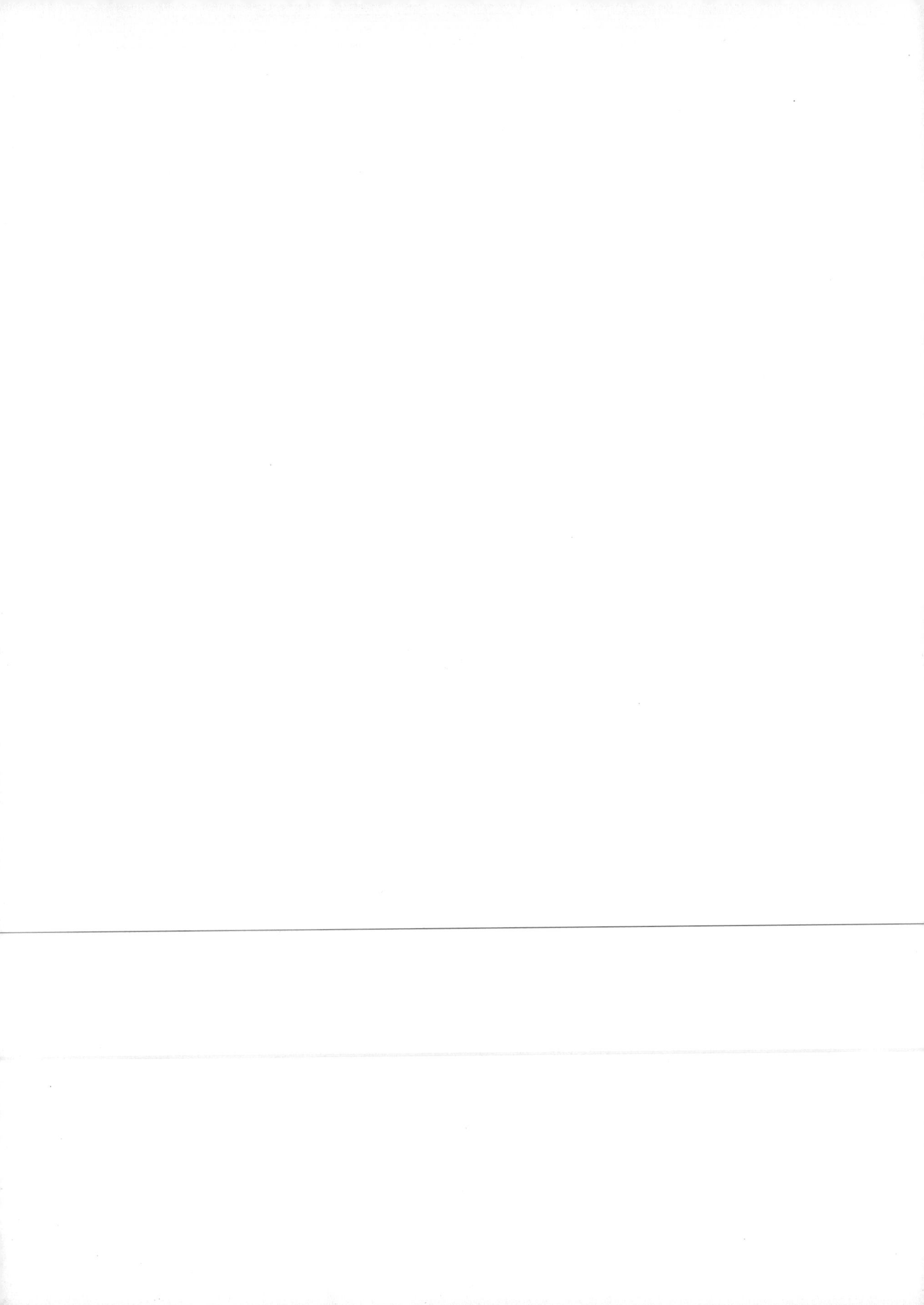

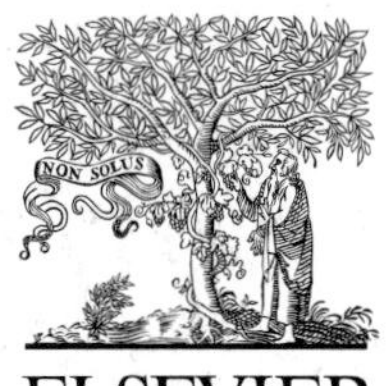

ELSEVIER

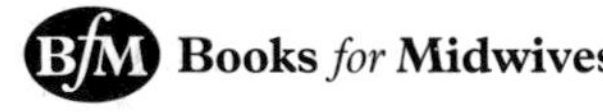

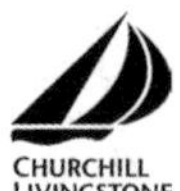

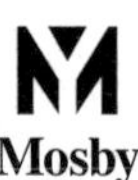

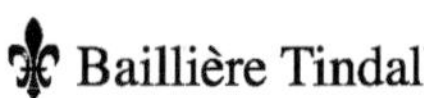

Baillière Tindall

MIDWIFERY PUBLISHERS OF CHOICE FOR GENERATIONS

For many years and through several identities we have catered for professional needs in midwifery education and practice. Leading publishers of major textbooks such as *Myles Textbook for Midwives* and *Mayes' Midwifery: a Textbook for Midwives*, our expertise spreads across both books and journals to offer a comprehensive resource for midwives at all stages of their careers.

Find out how we can provide you with the right book at the right time by exploring our website, **www.elsevierhealth.com/midwifery** or requesting a midwifery catalogue from Health Professions Marketing, Elsevier, 32 Jamestown Road, Camden, London, NW1 7BY, UK Tel: 020 7424 4200; Fax: 020 7424 4420.

We are always keen to expand our midwifery list so if you have an idea for a new book please contact Mary Seager, Senior Commissioning Editor at Elsevier, The Boulevard, Langford Lane, Kidlington, Oxford, OX5 1GB, UK (m.seager@elsevier.com).

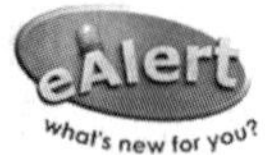

Have you joined yet?
Sign up for e-Alert to get the latest news and information.

Register for eAlert at www.elsevierhealth.com/eAlert Information direct to your Inbox

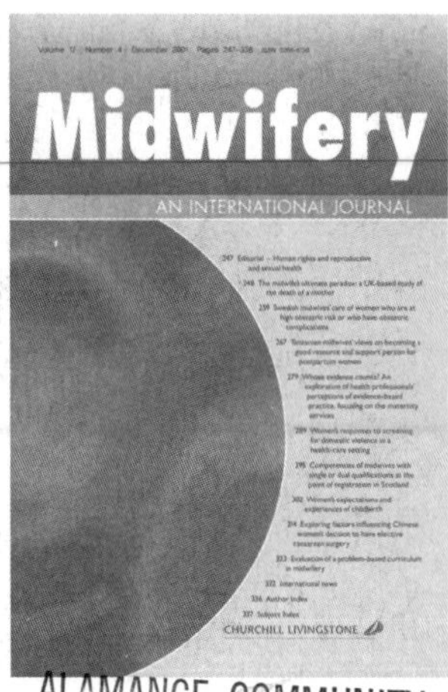

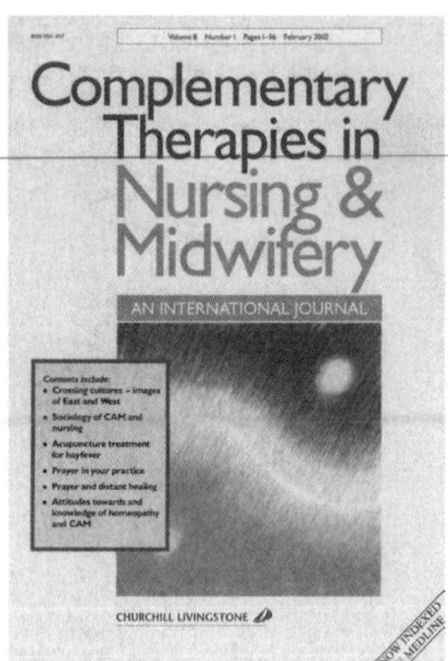